Biostatistics

Without question, biostatistical analysis has contributed to a slew of amazing medical breakthroughs. Yet it also distorts and deforms the holistic and contingent nature of health and medicine. How is it that biostatistics can both sharpen and weaken our understanding of health and medicine? What is unique about the content of health and medicine that so plainly reveals such distortions and deformities? Exploring these questions entails, first, a full survey of the tools and techniques of biostatistical analysis aiding medical breakthroughs. This survey must then be paired with a probe into the conceptual premises of these tools and techniques and how they refashion and reconstitute the inherently qualitative content of health and medicine in preparation for its quantification. We must grasp the statistical machinations at play, both technical and conceptual, that contrive to fit objects to tools rather than fitting tools to objects. This textbook introduces both the procedural methods and the hidden premises of biostatistical analysis.

David Baronov is Professor of Sociology at St. John Fisher University, Rochester, New York, where his current research interests include the ontology of social science methods and the quantitative/qualitative divide. Previous publications include *Conceptual Foundations of Social Science Methods* (2012) and *The Dialectics of Inquiry across the Historical Social Sciences* (2014).

Biostatistics

An Introduction and Conceptual Critique

David Baronov

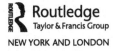

Routledge
Taylor & Francis Group

NEW YORK AND LONDON

Cover image: Classic Image / Alamy Stock Photo

First published 2023
by Routledge
605 Third Avenue, New York, NY 10158

and by Routledge
2 Park Square, Milton Park, Abingdon, Oxon, OX14 4RN

Routledge is an imprint of the Taylor & Francis Group, an informa business

Library of Congress Cataloging-in-Publication Data
Names: Baronov, David, author.
Title: Biostatistics : an introduction and conceptual critique / David Baronov.
Description: New York, NY : Routledge, 2022. |
Includes bibliographical references and index.
Identifiers: LCCN 2022022379 | ISBN 9781032328393 (hbk) |
ISBN 9781032328386 (pbk) | ISBN 9781003316985 (ebk)
Subjects: LCSH: Biometry.
Classification: LCC QH323.5 .B3595 2022 |
DDC 570.1/5195—dc23/eng/20220611
LC record available at https://lccn.loc.gov/2022022379

ISBN: 978-1-032-32839-3 (hbk)
ISBN: 978-1-032-32838-6 (pbk)
ISBN: 978-1-003-31698-5 (ebk)

DOI: 10.4324/9781003316985

Typeset in Adobe Garamond
by Newgen Publishing UK

Contents

Acknowledgments

The unconventional treatment of conventional material presents a good number of hazards and risks. Having the right people to help navigate such obstacles has proven essential. For this project, the rare combination of an appreciation for contradiction, irony, and technical detail was required. Consequently, I am very grateful to a spirited collection of colleagues and scholars whose words of warning, trepidation, encouragement, and bewilderment served me well throughout the writing of this book. In particular, I very much wish to thank Harry Murray, Anand Sridhar, Paul Fuller, Timothy Madigan, Robert Ruehl, Bob Brimlow, Kevin Clarke, Daniel R. Shafer, Richard Crouse, and André Antonio Baronov Torres for all their valuable assistance. In addition, providing tremendous assistance was Dean Birkenkamp, a senior editor at Routledge possessing a rare combination of talent and vision.

Lastly, I wish to acknowledge the essential contribution of Mrs. Druian, without whom this book would never have been possible.

Chapter 1

Just What Is an Introduction *and* Conceptual Critique?

The overriding ambition and conceit of all statistical analysis is to grant authority to certain claims. Within the health and social sciences, there are two sources of this authority. The first source, abstract mathematical rationale, is explicitly acknowledged and transparent. The second source, the conceptual premises of quantified social forms, is ominously unspoken and opaque. With regard to the first source, the technical content presented here resembles that in most introductory biostatistics textbooks. This includes, for instance, all those mathematical tools and techniques fundamental for understanding and conducting biostatistical analysis.

With regard to the second source, the content of this book radically departs from essentially all other introductory biostatistics textbooks. This follows, in part, from a fundamental difference between the application of statistical analysis within the health and social sciences and its application within the natural sciences. Herein lies the uniqueness of our conceptual and critical approach.

This approach requires an inquest into the conceptual premises of biostatistical analysis and a critique of the consequences of these for understanding health and medicine. Importantly, this critique is not a lament of what biostatistical analysis does not do, or cannot do, or what it should do. Rather, this critique engages only with what biostatistical analysis actually does do and the consequences of this—good, bad, and otherwise—for understanding health and medicine.

That said, the findings from this conceptual and critical approach for biostatistical analysis apply equally to statistical analysis in general as applied to other social science fields. In this sense, this introduction to biostatistical analysis serves as a particular case within a larger ambit of investigation—the conceptual premises of statistical analysis and their consequences for various subject matter across the health and social sciences. It just happens that the nature of those phenomena comprising health and medicine make biostatistical analysis an especially apt window into such matters.

We begin then by contrasting our conceptual approach with a conventional, rules-based introduction to biostatistical analysis. By near universal consensus, biostatistical analysis is presented to students as a formal set of rules applied to various subject matter. This is done by choice. Even if it is rarely an informed choice. Here, we introduce biostatistical analysis not via its rules alone, but in combination with its underlying concepts. The rules are essential. However, the rules guiding biostatistical analysis are grounded in the concepts from which they arise. Hence, both the rules and the concepts behind these rules are presented in parallel fashion.

Rules are sequential operations that are necessary to obtain some outcome. These operations follow from certain defined *a priori*, syllogistic rationale. This deductive procedural rationale thus guides how we approach different subject matter for investigation and

DOI: 10.4324/9781003316985-1

analysis. Moreover, rules are abstract and universal. They apply to all phenomena in the same manner. And so it is with the mathematical tools and techniques that comprise biostatistical analysis. Concepts reveal premises about the nature of things in our world that—in this case—permit the application of certain *a priori*, syllogistic rationale.

These conceptual premises are discovered inductively via the observation and analysis of how researchers (such as biostatisticians) approach their subject matter for investigation. Thus, whereas rules are abstract and universal, concepts are grounded and contingent. They result from concrete practices—such as biostatistical analysis—that are products of historical and cultural epochs.

Consider, for example, the standard deviation both as a set of rules and as a concept. In accord with certain mathematical rationales, the rules determine (a) how to calculate the standard deviation and (b) how to interpret the meaning of the result. The rules for calculation prescribe a sequence of operations that include addition, subtraction, division, exponents, and a square root. The meaning ascribed to the result of these operations is the degree of variability among certain quantitative values attached to things in a sample.

As a set of rules, the standard deviation is an abstract tool indifferent to content. As a concept, the standard deviation brings our attention to the interpretive consequences of applying this abstract tool to social phenomena, such as those comprising health and medicine. Thus, the quantitative values originally attached to abstract "things" via general rules are now attached to concrete individuals within a sample.

The mathematical rationale behind the standard deviation further presumes that these operations can be performed on "fragments" of human beings. Indeed, the properties of human beings (such as a resting heart rate) are treated as if they were discrete and alienable and, in fact, can continue to exist even after separated from a human being. The consequences of this concept of a human being as an abstract "thing" comprised of divisible parts—versus a "person," or an indivisible whole—are fundamental to understanding biostatistical analysis.

Given the predominance of a rules-based approach in biostatistics textbooks, it is the ordinary experience of most students to end their introductory course knowing a good deal more about certain mathematical tools and techniques and comparatively less about health and medicine—the actual subject matter of investigation. The reasons for this are simple. The mathematical tools and techniques were not designed to conform to health and medicine. Rather, these were designed to facilitate a particular (positivist) interpretation of this subject matter. This requires reframing health and medicine as subjects of study in a manner that removes it from its original holistic and social contexts.

Consequently, the application of biostatistical analysis requires a certain "willful suspension of disbelief" on the part of a student. This phrase is lifted from Samuel Coleridge, a 19th-century English poet, to suggest a person's momentary tolerance of an implausible premise for the telling of a tale. For the poet, this might open one's mind to human flight to explore humankind's limitless aspirations. For the student of biostatistical analysis, this implies a provisional suppression of the holistic nature and sociocultural context of health and medicine for the purpose of applying a set of abstract mathematical tools and techniques to this subject matter.

Our aim here then is to present these mathematical tools and techniques (without abridgement!), while retaining the conceptual complexity of those phenomena comprising health and medicine. Accordingly, we hope that readers will end this book knowing much more about these tools and techniques—and their conceptual premises—*as well as* much more about the conceptual "DNA" of health and medicine as subjects of investigation.

Throughout this text, particular emphasis is given to the conceptual premises that are required for a certain approach to the investigation of some subject matter. These premises reflect the nature of what a thing is thought to be. For example, a premise for the qualitative analysis of childbirth might emphasize subjective criteria, such as a woman's personal experience. A premise for the quantitative analysis of childbirth might emphasize observable criteria, such as the heart rate of a fetus or the duration of a woman's contractions. These are simply two ways to understand the same phenomenon that operate from different conceptual premises about the nature of childbirth.

To begin, it is essential to recognize that significant qualitative and subjective judgment precedes all quantitative and objective biostatistical analysis. Consider an ordinary circumstance. Ayesha works at the local health department tracking and cataloguing injuries and accidents for Gottaouchie County. Her oldest child is in high school and participates on the track team as a long-distance runner. Through casual conversations with colleagues about their children, the health and safety of students engaging in extracurricular sports activities became an interest of Ayesha.

Everyone shared stories and examples about their children's experiences (qualitative description), good and bad (subjective judgments). This led Ayesha to wonder how highschool long-distance running might impact a student's health and safety. Many health concerns came to mind, including obesity, cardiovascular fitness, substance abuse, physical injuries, or mental health.

Given limited time and resources, Ayesha relied on her subjective judgment to choose among the possible health conditions. Which aspects of health did she wish to explore? Which might she ignore? Personal preference was the main driver to this point and she chose cardiovascular fitness. Next, she had to choose how best to understand and measure cardiovascular health. For largely practical reasons, she chose the resting heart rate as her measure of cardiovascular health.

Notice three things to this point. First, we began with anecdotal observations and descriptions that followed from chance conversations among a small group of random people. Second, the questions shaping Ayesha's thinking are entirely qualitative and subjective. What is health? What aspect of health should we focus on? If we investigate this aspect, how should we try to capture it?

Third, resolving each of these questions results in a narrowing and a winnowing. "Health" begins as a general category of well-being before it is narrowed to an arbitrary list of medical concerns. Each item on the list is judged for its practicality, to account for Ayesha's finite time and resources. The specific item that she chooses (cardiovascular health) is then further narrowed, for convenience, to a quantitative measure (the resting heart rate). The resting heart rate is thus a proxy for cardiovascular health.

On the one hand, we move from the general (health) to the specific (resting heart rate) via this process. On the other hand, we move from qualitative and subjective conversations among colleagues to quantitative and objective measurements. We gain specificity. We lose generality. But we lose something else. We lose the originating, subjective rationale. In fact, Ayesha built layer upon layer of abstraction. Cardiovascular fitness entered as a proxy for general health and safety and a resting heart rate entered as a proxy for cardiovascular fitness. When the study is complete we will—*by intentional design*—know a great deal about resting heart rates and very little about health in general.

Ayesha may personally think of health in general as holistic and integrative, akin to an orchestra. However, when framing it as a subject for (biostatistical) investigation, she has been trained to view it as discrete and reductive, like a jigsaw puzzle. It is thus from early in the research process that we find ourselves relying upon our willful suspension of disbelief for the telling of a tale.

Indeed, a major reason for treating holistic subjects—such as health and medicine—as discrete and reductive is to facilitate the use of biostatistical tools and techniques. As a *temporary* willful suspension of disbelief, this makes sense. For instance, it would be difficult to enjoy a television medical drama if one chose not to look past the rather rare (or even impossible) medical events somehow encountered on a weekly basis. In the same manner, to gain some limited insights from a particular measure of health (such as a resting heart rate) we too must temporarily suspend our disbelief and offer a wink-and-a-nod to the discrete and reductive conceptual premises of biostatistical analysis.

To confront head-on the supreme challenge of holding this mix of contradictory ideas in our head, we purposely begin our introduction to biostatistical analysis with two of its more challenging mathematical tools. These are linear and logistic regression. (To simplify, unless speaking of one or the other specifically, we refer to both as "regression analysis.") We open with regression analysis for two reasons. First, introductory textbooks generally present these as tools that allow one to account for the context and interrelationships of variables in a quasi-holistic fashion. Thus, dissecting regression analysis provides unique insights into the conceptual premises of health and medicine that underlie biostatistical analysis.

Second, the general form and logical structure of regression analysis provides some of the most fully developed expressions of the biostatistical principles and rationale that students typically encounter in an introductory textbook. This points to a fairly counterintuitive notion that shapes the design of our approach. It is by grappling first with its more advanced forms that we are better able to understand the implications of "simpler" biostatistical tools and techniques that lie ahead for us, such as the standard error or confidence interval estimation.

It is certainly true that the standard error is necessary for regression analysis. However, it is regression analysis that provides the grounds for bringing in the standard error, not the other way around. Hence, we begin with the broader grounds, not with a collection of otherwise abstract and isolated operations. Indeed, it is the grounds that provide the logical form and predicate for each operation. Put simply, one does not grasp the purpose of the house by studying a doorknob. One grasps the purpose of the doorknob by studying a house.

Beginning with regression analysis also reinforces a further theme shaping our approach to biostatistical analysis. By their manner of presentation, most introductory textbooks infer that regression analysis is *more complex* than other tools and techniques, such as univariate or bivariate analysis. Insofar as the former requires a higher level of technical operations than the latter, this may be true. However, regression analysis is not more complex merely because it incorporates and builds upon these "simpler" tools.

Obviously, there are common elements across all biostatistical tools and techniques, such as probability theory. But regression analysis is not some Frankenstein-like amalgamation of simpler forms. From the simple to the complex, each is merely one particular tool to address one particular type of research problem.

Thus, adhering to some *pro forma* procession of tools and techniques from univariate analysis to regression analysis is not an orderly and cumulative progression from the simple to the complex. From our angle, it is an arbitrary parade of different tools and techniques, each of which is germane to particular research circumstances. The notion of complexity thus pertains not to any tool or technique, but to the full research project which draws upon these tools and techniques. Indeed, many research projects that rely only on rudimentary bivariate analysis address far more complex research circumstances than other projects deploying more complicated tools, such as regression analysis.

That said, our approach is deceptively simple. We begin, in Chapter 2, at the highest level of procedural sophistication, where the underlying conceptual premises that we discuss are often obscured by the dizzying and frenetic technical steps and language. We then proceed in subsequent chapters to bring in all those further tools and operations that make regression analysis possible, such as the standard normal distribution and least squares estimates. In this way, we introduce readers to both (a) the mathematical and technical scaffolding that is a basic feature of any introductory biostatistics course, as well as, (b) the conceptual premises and logic that shape how biostatistical analysis conceives of health and medicine.

Along the way, we introduce two further innovations to more clearly lay out the technical aspects of biostatistical analysis. Biostatistics textbooks typically draw from an array of health-related scenarios for this purpose. It is common to introduce each new tool or technique with an example from a completely new scenario. Here, we limit ourselves to the same hypothetical scenario throughout the entire textbook. By returning to the same scenario, the reader's focus can remain fixed on the various tools and techniques without continuously shifting between stories about teachers or nurses or animal husbandry.

Admittedly, the topic of our common scenario—high-school long-distance runners—may not be the most riveting. But this will allow us to illustrate all manner of mathematical tools and techniques via a single, unchanging reference point.

We then introduce a second innovation. A principal aim of biostatistical analysis is to analyze different types of problems (or circumstances). In fact, at an introductory level, we can distinguish between nine types of problems (or circumstances), based on different combinations of four basic elements. These elements are the outcome (or dependent) variable, the number of groups, the dependent or independent relationship between groups, and the number of causal (or independent) variables. We refer to each of the nine unique combinations of elements as a configuration.

These nine configurations then help us to organize our presentation of various biostatistical tools, techniques, and tests via the distinct types of problems (or circumstances) associated with each. The conceptual rationale for these configurations—along with examples lifted from high-school long-distance running—are presented in Chapter 4. The technical application of biostatistical tools, techniques, and tests to these examples for each configuration is then taken up in Chapters 5, 6, and 7.

The reader will benefit by keeping in mind the following organizing principles for the material in this textbook.

- Biostatistical tools and techniques are best presented alongside their implicit conceptual premises.
- All quantitative and objective data originate from qualitative and subjective observations.
- A full understanding of biostatistical analysis requires a person's willful suspension of disbelief.
- A single, common scenario—high-school long-distance running—can facilitate moving between different biostatistical tools and techniques.
- Applications of biostatistical tools, techniques, and tests can be demonstrated with nine configurations that capture the common types of problems (or circumstances) encountered in an introductory biostatistics course.

The first three principles follow from a single calamity. This is the common practice to present biostatistical analysis as the unexceptional application of a set of rote mathematical tools and techniques, grounded in probability theory, to a particular subject matter—health and medicine. Hence, biostatistical analysis and *general* statistical analysis are considered interchangeable. This is profoundly mistaken. It is not that the mathematical tools and techniques of each differ. Rather, it is precisely because these are the same that biostatistical and general statistical analysis differ.

If the tools and techniques of each differed, this would indicate some attempt to adapt these to the unique subject matter of biostatistical analysis. Instead, it is the subject matter of biostatistical analysis that must be adapted to fit the tools and techniques of general statistical analysis. It is the *manner of this adaptation* that distinguishes biostatistical analysis from general statistical analysis.

For example, much of the subject matter comprising health and medicine that we encounter is inherently holistic and contingent, such as the nature of illness or palliative care. However, the tools and techniques of biostatistical analysis that we apply to this subject matter operate from premises that are reductive and universal. Thus, it is true that biostatistical analysis does not generally advance beyond the rudimentary mathematical tools and techniques that it borrows. However, it is also true that, as a specific application of general statistical analysis, biostatistical analysis introduces novel complications for how we navigate between the holistic and reductive premises that emerge from the nature of the subject matter of health and medicine itself.

In this way, biostatistical analysis represents a unique and compelling contribution to science and a course in biostatistical analysis differs fundamentally from a course in general statistical analysis. This is because the former course must present the tools and techniques of general statistical analysis (in full!) and it must *simultaneously* account for the conceptual consequences of adapting this subject matter to the reductive and universal mathematical premises of general statistical analysis.

It is, in part, due to this ideological notion of biostatistical analysis and general statistical analysis as interchangeable, that no introduction to biostatistical analysis would be complete—save for most all hitherto published works—without brief attention to the political circumstances surrounding the origins of biostatistical analysis and its eventual supremacy as a mode of explanation across health and medicine. By general consensus, the origins of biostatistical analysis—and statistical analysis more generally within the social sciences—mark a triumphant moment in positivist interpretation that its champions modestly christened the "scientific method."

Credit for this great leap forward can be traced to the work of an assortment of philosophers with training in physics, mathematics, and other natural sciences, beginning in the 1940s. Among others, this included the efforts—both intellectual and evangelical—of Karl Popper, Hans Reichenbach, Otto Neurath, Ernest Nagel, Carl Hempel, and Imre Lakatos.

The principal contribution of these individuals was to translate the language of the natural sciences into a kind of creole dialect for the social sciences. The modified scientific method that resulted was believed to offer a sensible set of ontological principles and epistemological guidelines that could safeguard truth claims and, thereby, also the integrity of any social scientific investigation or discovery. Truth claims could be assessed by a number of practices that upheld deductive-nomological principles, such as falsifiability (contra historicism), fallibilism (contra apodictic truth), and probability (contra radical empiricism). Investigation of the social world, by and large, has thus been guided ever since by certain formal techniques that comprise the scientific method, including biostatistical analysis.

The design of nearly all introductory biostatistics textbooks today provides a showcase for this positivist project within the social sciences. The unstated goal of such textbooks is to introduce and reinforce an ideological viewpoint which is smuggled part-and-parcel into the training of each generation of scientists and scholars across the fields of health and medicine. One of the aims of this textbook, therefore, is to better allow readers to make an informed choice regarding this ideological commitment. Many readers will find the conventional, positivist viewpoint quite sufficient after reading this textbook. That is fine. Our goal is merely to present this conventional viewpoint alongside concepts and ideas critical of this viewpoint and allow readers to judge such matters on their own.

Three final notes

We close with three further preparatory remarks for the task ahead. First, among researchers across health and medicine there is increasing recognition of gender non-conforming identities that undo the orthodox binary categories of male and female. This complicates the practice of treating "sex" as a biological category and "gender" as a social construct. Our imperfect remedy is to limit ourselves to the categories of "cis female," "cis male," and "gender non-conforming." Cis female and cis male refer to persons who are comfortable with the gender identity that they were assigned at birth. Those who identify as gender non-conforming are not comfortable with aspects of the gender identity that they were assigned at birth.

Nearly all studies within health and medicine collect and report the sex or gender of participants. However, almost no studies conduct biological tests to determine the sex or gender of participants. Thus, by default what they actually collect is a person's self-identity. Consequently, the distinction between "sex" as a biological category and "gender" as a social construct is largely meaningless within these studies. Moreover, studies within health and medicine increasingly ask participants to select among some options resembling cis female, cis male, and gender non-conforming. These we refer to as a person's gender identity.

Secondly, we offer a word about repetition. Repetition is not redundancy. Beethoven's Fifth Symphony opens with four poignant notes. These notes then recur throughout the entire symphony. Far from senseless redundancy, with each recurrence, Beethoven builds upon and further develops an increasingly complex theme contained within those four original notes. Granted, the majesty of the present work falls well short of Beethoven. However, it is this notion of repetition as an instrument for ongoing development that is intended here.

Certain ideas and concepts, such as holism or odds ratio, are presented first in plain form and then repeated in subsequent applications throughout the text. The hope is that, similar to Beethoven's opening notes, the first mention of an idea or concept may plant a seed and that each ensuing return to that same idea or concept will deepen the reader's understanding and broaden her or his grasp of its applications and consequences. Alas, no symphony will result. Rather, our goal here is simply to foster a greater appreciation for the key ideas and concepts that allow a reader to better assess the role and value of biostatistical analysis tools and techniques for exploring phenomena across health and medicine.

Lastly—and echoing elements of repetition—we add a note regarding a most unsexy topic, the index. Few people give much thought to an index and here we will spend only two sparse paragraphs on the matter. The index is a listing of general topics (concepts, schools of thought, or political ideologies) and concrete things (people, places, events). For concrete things, this is unremarkable. For general topics, however, this presents certain complications.

Our approach is to introduce a concept initially and to then revisit, embellish, and often contradict our initial description. This is not because the earlier account was mistaken. Rather, this is to emphasize that a concept has manifold meanings and that what is true in one context may prove untrue in another. Therefore, when the index indicates that a concept (such as the standard deviation) appears on several occasions throughout the book this signals that different aspects of that concept's meanings are developed with each appearance. Thus, should a concept appear ill-conceived or incomplete it is always advisable to turn to the index to help piece together each of the multiple renditions for the fullest representation of that concept.

Chapter 2

Regression Analysis
Concepts and Groundwork

Textbooks generally present biostatistical analysis as a rich array of sophisticated tools and techniques that only a software engineer could love. Within this array, regression analysis is considered one of the more complex tools. Its introduction is thus ordinarily reserved for later in the procession of tools and techniques. However, it just so happens that along with greater complexity, regression analysis also presents one of the more complete (and ambitious) expressions of the rationale and conceptual premises upholding biostatistical analysis.

Insofar as these rationales and premises are a principal concern for this introduction to biostatistical analysis, we prefer to begin with that which best expresses it. That said, the mathematical rules and technical operations that propel regression analysis need not deter us at this early stage. Instead, these enter in Chapter 7. However, to understand the fantastic potential, the severe limitations, and the most intimate hopes and dreams that researchers attach to biostatistical analysis more broadly, there is no better place to begin than regression analysis.

There are four forms of regression analysis to consider:

- simple linear regression;
- multiple linear regression;
- simple logistic regression; and
- multiple logistic regression.

These four forms introduce two basic differences. These are a difference between simple and multiple regression and a difference between linear and logistic regression. The principal difference between simple and multiple regression is that the former analyzes situations with one independent (or causal) variable and one dependent (or outcome) variable, while the latter analyzes situations with multiple independent (or causal) variables and one dependent (or outcome) variable.

The principal difference between linear and logistic regression is that:

- Linear regression ALWAYS, ALWAYS, ALWAYS requires a *continuous* dependent (or outcome) variable.
- Logistic regression ALWAYS, ALWAYS, ALWAYS requires a *dichotomous* dependent (or outcome) variable.

Put aside for a moment the distinction between a continuous and dichotomous variable. We address this soon enough. For now, all that matters is that *the type of dependent (or outcome) variable* leads to all manner of differences between linear and logistic regression. In fact, as

DOI: 10.4324/9781003316985-2

soon will be apparent, the type of dependent (or outcome) variable is one of the most conse-quential factors for a great many aspects of biostatistical analysis!

One further concern is terminology. An "independent" variable is a causal factor, such as smoking. A "dependent" variable is an outcome variable, such as lung cancer. On the one hand, it is critical that the reader become familiar with these terms. On the other hand, referring to a "causal factor" and an "outcome variable" tends to be more intuitive for those first learning biostatistics. These more intuitive terms are thus generally adopted here.

Some not-so-concise preliminaries

Standard introductory biostatistics courses will introduce regression analysis as tools of seduction after subjecting students to a steady diet of univariate and bivariate analysis. Univariate analysis describes the distribution of a single aspect of health, such as asthma, within some group. Thus, if we discovered that 30% of the students in a high school had been diagnosed with asthma, this would be an example of univariate analysis. Bivariate analysis examines the link between a single causal factor and a single outcome. Thus, if we discovered a link between smoking and cardiovascular disease, this would be an example of bivariate analysis.

The moment of seduction occurs around the ninth or tenth week when the instructor suddenly stumbles across the dilemma of "confounding" variables. Perhaps—after weeks of bivariate analysis—she suggests that cardiovascular disease may not actually be associated with smoking alone. Indeed, she asks, what if there are a slew of factors (exercise, age, diet) that further complicate the (bivariate) relationship between smoking and cardiovascular dis-ease? Then promises are made.

To set this up, the instructor first insists that she is shocked ... shocked to learn that univariate and bivariate analysis alone may be inadequate for this problem. But the damage is done. The first eight weeks have already laid the conceptual groundwork for a reductive, discrete, and decontextualized approach to health and medicine. (Fear not, we will address these notions in short order.) So what of those promises offered up by our frazzled instructor who appears to be reading the textbook for the first time along with her students?

There are two aspects of these promises. First, a vow is made that regression analysis will allow us to contextualize health and medicine. Investigating the role of confounding variables (and of effect modification) is an example of this. Second, regression analysis will allow us to assess the relationships between the causal variables (both individually and in combination) and the outcome variable.

To begin, however, one of the purposes of the material from the previous eight weeks had been to introduce certain notions which students are expected to treat as simply emerging organically from the nature of the world as we find it. One example of this is the idea that our world can be organized around four types of variables. There are three considerations in this regard:

- A variable's functional role within the analysis.
- The type of thing a variable represents (or measures).
- The mathematical rules for measuring the type of thing a variable represents.

The first consideration juxtaposes dependent and independent variables. Regression analysis proceeds based on an independent variable (smoking) affecting a dependent variable (car-diovascular disease). This is determined by the researcher when she or he hypothesizes that *some* independent variable will have *some* impact on *some* dependent variable. This presumes a one-way relationship between an independent and dependent variable and presents few problems, given the transparency of the researcher via her hypothesis. In other words, the premise behind the functional roles of dependent and independent variables within regression analysis is explicit and, therefore, lies open to debate.

The second and third considerations, the type of thing a variable purports to represent and its measurement, introduce different challenges. With regard to the type of thing a variable represents, the matter is not terribly onerous. All phenomena across health and medicine are believed to fit one of four types of variables. These types are labeled continuous, dichotomous, ordinal, and categorical variables.

- Continuous variables pertain to things (or phenomena) whose values can (theoretically) be infinitely large or small and include whole numbers or the tiniest fractions. Values can run from zero to infinity. Examples include a person's height or weight. Note that discrete variables are a subtype of continuous variable. These pertain to things (or phenomena) that are only enumerated in (non-divisible) whole number units that also (theoretically) run from zero to infinity. Examples of discrete variables include a patient's number of white blood cells or the number of patients in a hospital.
- Dichotomous variables pertain to things (or phenomena) that are binary and thus provide only two options. Examples include a positive/negative biopsy or the presence/absence of asthma.
- Ordinal variables pertain to things (or phenomena) that present a rank order of items. This rank order indicates the relative position of items, such as "greater than" or "less than." But the degree of difference (or distance) between items is unknown. Examples include the rank order in which runners complete a race or the rank order in which patients recover from back surgery.
- Categorical variables pertain to things (or phenomena) that belong to nominal groups or classes. Examples include a person's religion or a person's ethnic identity.

Having said that ... there is a complication. It turns out that there is a second set of measures associated with a different collection of variables. Our first set contains four types of variables—continuous, dichotomous, ordinal, and categorical—based on the type of thing they represent. This second set introduces four scales of measurement. These are labeled nominal, ordinal, interval, and ratio.

These scales are distinguished by the different mathematical rules that apply to the four types of variables in the first set (see Table 2.1). For instance, the mathematical rules of a nominal scale apply to categorical variables. However, dichotomous variables are also subject to the nominal scale and are thus treated as a subtype of categorical variable. (We will return to the consequences of treating dichotomous variables as a type of categorical variable.) Not surprisingly, the mathematical rules of an ordinal scale apply to ordinal variables. Lastly, both the interval scale and the ratio scale apply to continuous variables. By extension, the rules of interval and ratio scales also apply to discrete variables.

Those are the basics. Let us now bring in some examples to illustrate how the four types of variables can be reconciled with the mathematical rules introduced by the four scales of measurement. We begin with categorical variables and nominal scales.

At Archduke Franz Ferdinand Carl Ludwig Joseph Maria of Austria High School in Tipping Point, Illinois, there are 25 long-distance runners. Each runner competes in only one type of race. Eight compete in 3k races, five compete in 5k races, eight compete in 10k races, and four compete in 15k races (see Table 2.2). In this case, the "type of race" is a categorical variable with a nominal scale.

Table 2.1 Type of variable matched with its type of scale

	Nominal scale	Ordinal scale	Interval scale	Ratio scale
Categorical variable	X			
Dichotomous variable	X			
Ordinal variable		X		
Continuous variable (with no zero point)			X	
Continuous variable (with zero point)				X

Table 2.2 Number of runners competing in each type of race at Archduke Franz Ferdinand Carl Ludwig Joseph Maria of Austria High School, n = 25

Type of race	Number of runners
3-kilometer races	8
5-kilometer races	5
10-kilometer races	8
15-kilometer races	4
Total	25

The data in Table 2.1 are (discrete) whole numbers that produce counts and sums of runners in each category, such as the eight runners who compete in 10k races. Thus, the mathematical rules for a nominal scale allow only a few operations for purposes of comparing the number of runners in each category. We are generally limited to measures of more or less of this kind or that. For instance, there are four more runners who compete in 3k races than compete in 15k races.

Fortunately, we further learn that four types of data are collected for these 25 runners. First, coach Dragutin Demitrijević records if a runner suffers an ankle injury. Whether or not a runner injures her or his ankle (yes/no) is a dichotomous variable on a nominal scale. Notice that, whereas we have four (nominal) categories of races, here we find two (nominal) "categories" pertaining to an ankle injury—yes or no. Nonetheless the same mathematical rules of nominal scales apply.

This allows us to compare the number of runners injuring an ankle with the number not injuring an ankle. We can then report our findings as the proportion of those who suffer an ankle injury. Notice that a proportion is a "quantitative" measure of a qualitative property, the presence/absence of some quality. This is true even when that quality is presented in explicitly quantitative terms, such as a white blood cell count above 11,000 cells per microliter.

A second measure of interest to coach Demitrijević is the rank order that each runner finishes a race, from first place to last place. Here we have an ordinal variable. Because we record the actual placement—first, twelfth, fifteenth—but not the distance between these placements, we use an ordinal scale. This tells us the order of finish, but little more. Thus, for purposes of comparison this is quite limited.

For our third source of data we administer the Demitrijević Self-Esteem Inventory, a creation of coach Demitrijević. This is a set of 41 questions that measures a runner's self-confidence. All runners complete the Demitrijević Self-Esteem Inventory at the beginning of each track season and their scores are recorded. The possible scores are 0–41. A score of 41 indicates the highest self-confidence and zero indicates the lowest self-confidence. This is a continuous variable with an interval scale. This measure is continuous (or discrete) because the gradients between 0 and 41 are equally spaced.

This requires an interval scale, insofar as a score of zero does not indicate an absolute absence of self-confidence and a score of 41 does not indicate a cosmic state of pure self-confidence. All runners have *at least* very low self-confidence and no runner's self-confidence can reach a possible maximum. Furthermore, we cannot say that a runner with a score of 30 is twice as self-confident as a runner with a score of 15. This is because there is no theoretical (or absolute) zero point. However, we can say that a runner whose score increases from 12 to 22 is equivalent to an increase for another runner from 22 to 32. This is because the value of the increments between scores are uniform.

We can thus compare a runner with her/himself and determine if her or his self-confidence increased or decreased over time, as increments along the scale. For instance, we can say that this particular runner increased her level of self-confidence by eight points on the Demitrijevíc Self-Esteem Inventory over the track season. In addition, we can compare the increase or decrease among several runners and say that for these runners there was, on average, an increase of 13.4 points on the Demitrijevíc Self-Esteem Inventory over the track season.

The fourth measure that coach Demitrijevíc records is each runner's completion time for a race. The time it takes to complete a race is a continuous variable with a ratio scale. The time to complete a race for each runner is measured by the same units of time with a theoretical (absolute) zero point. Therefore, we can make direct comparisons between racers based on the mathematical rules of a ratio scale.

Note that the theoretical zero point applies to mathematical principles and *not* to the theoretical possibility of completing a race in 0:00. (Again, no such zero point—even theoretically—exists in the Demitrijevíc Self-Esteem Inventory.) Thus, if one runner completes a 5k race in 13 minutes and 14 seconds and a second runner completes the same race in 26 minutes and 28 seconds, we know that the first runner completed the race in one-half the time of the second runner. She ran twice as fast as the second runner.

Curiously, these four scales of measurement—nominal, ordinal, interval, and ratio—were only first stumbled upon relatively recently (in the 1940s) and were not broadly put to use by social scientists until the 1950s. This timing is hardly accidental. As noted in Chapter 1, the 1950s was a transitional period, ushering in the wholesale adoption of quantitative statistical analysis as the gold standard for true scientific knowledge across the social sciences. Social phenomena were re-imagined in that period to better fit the new tools of statistical analysis.

Far from discovering some universal—and hitherto hidden—properties of social phenomena, these four scales of measurement were a historical contrivance to reconfigure our understanding of the social world and promote an emerging consensus about this. Again, detailing the consequences of this mostly veiled consensus is central to this book.

Let us continue with our weary instructor's two promises. Again, these are, first, that regression analysis will allow us to better contextualize the subject matter of health and medicine and, second, that these tools will allow us to better account for the relationships between independent (or causal) variables and dependent (or outcome) variables. The ostensive purpose of regression analysis is to account for any differential impact of one or more independent (or causal) variables on a single dependent (or outcome) variable.

While these causal variables can be categorical, dichotomous, ordinal, or continuous, the outcome variable must always be *continuous* in the case of linear regression and *dichotomous* for logistic regression. As detailed below, this distinction—between continuous and dichotomous variables—is fundamental within biostatistical analysis for reasons related more to the nature of inquiry than the nature of the subject matter within health and medicine. For now, we focus on the implications of those elements that are shared by linear and logistic regression.

We turn to a further example to illustrate these two promises. Jordan Sotirov is the track coach at Manol Vassev High School in Vlassovden County. Coach Sotirov wants to know what factors determine who are the best long-distance runners. He suspects that diet, experience on the track team, and hours of training are the key factors. But coach Sotirov is not certain which of these has the biggest impact. First, he examines data for all 5k races over the past five seasons and determines the mean completion times for all runners. After combining this with data for each runner pertaining to diet, experience, and training hours, coach Sotirov discovers—via multiple linear regression—that, with regard to completion time, diet explains 12%, years of experience 20%, and hours of training 22%.

Notice, however, that the supposed starting point—examining data for 5k races over five seasons—is not the *actual* starting point. Prior to that, coach Sotirov identified what he believed to be the key factors. But prior even to this, he stated his originating desire to discover who are his best long-distance runners. For this, he chose the criterion of finishing 5k races in the shortest time and this became his dependent (or outcome) variable. Certainly, there were other possible criteria for assessing the "best" long-distance runners.

Who is the most reliable and supportive teammate? Who made the greatest improvement over the past year? Who most effectively maximizes her or his abilities? It happens that the coach chose a measure that uniquely fits the premises of biostatistical analysis. Indeed, this happy coincidence will recur throughout different examples in this book. It is good to remember that, in each case, the path chosen was not the only path available.

The goal of a race is to complete it in the shortest possible time. So this choice of criterion makes sound intuitive sense. However, the fact that it is *a choice* means that it necessarily precludes other choices. It is a narrowing of the concept of "best" runner. The question is not whether or not there are better measures of a runner. The question is, if there were other tools—besides statistical analysis—that were equally accessible (and culturally acceptable), might coach Sotirov have chosen a different measure of the best runner? Absent such options, the choice of "fastest" runner is no mere arbitrary narrowing. It is simply the configuration of a concept (best runner) to fit a tool (statistical analysis) that is culturally acceptable and easily accessible.

Now consider the three independent variables. Again, with respect to explaining a runner's time, coach Sotirov found that diet contributes 12%, experience 20%, and training 22%. We will address the mechanics of how he derived these numbers in Chapter 7. For now, let us take up the conceptual premises behind the mechanics—and that which makes necessary our willful suspension of disbelief in this case. The variables represent the factors (or conditions) determining the length of time a runner needs to complete a race. Several implications follow.

First, we observe that both diet and training are vestiges of local culture and a given stage of historical-material development. The findings of coach Sotirov are thus limited to a very small population. Indeed, so small is this population that it might better represent an ethnographic snapshot—that is, a more qualitative than quantitative study. After all, replicating this same study with long-distance runners from a high school in the Watts neighborhood in southern Los Angeles and runners from a high school in Beverly Hills would no doubt reveal significant differences in diet and training that reflect local cultural practices.

Or imagine comparing long-distance runners from a Boston high school in the 1940s with runners attending that same high school in the 1990s. In the Boston example, we would find equally sharp differences in historical-material development—such as the quality of the track and equipment or the depth of nutritional knowledge—in addition to differences in local cultural practices.

Second, in coach Sotirov's study at Manol Vassev High School each independent (or causal) variable is treated as a discrete factor that can be isolated from the others. As discrete factors, they can be combined and aggregated. Coach Sotirov considers the three independent (or causal) variables that he chose to be especially important. However, in theory, there exists some larger, finite collection of discrete factors that, when aggregated, would constitute the most complete constellation of factors possible for determining a runner's speed.

Moreover, as noted, the variables here are treated as discrete parts that can be combined to form the larger context. In this sense, the context (or the whole) is treated as some sterile and vacuous arena. Its organizing characteristics (or constituting logic) plays no role in our analysis. For example, the poor nutritional content of the diet within a particular community is framed as a collection of food items occupying the "arena" of food choices in that community. Consequently, the origins of this arena and precisely how it shapes and determines food choices are masked within regression analysis.

Alternatively, coach Sotirov could treat the whole as constituted—not as an aggregation of discrete parts—but by a host of reciprocally conditioning relationships between dynamic parts. We explore this alternative below via the metaphor of a farm.

Third, in selecting diet, experience, and training for our independent (or causal) variables, it is hoped that we have isolated (and highlighted) the most salient factors determining who are the best runners. Based on the findings of coach Sotirov, these three variables theoretically account for 54% of all factors explaining the speed of a long-distance runner. (This is the R square value that, again, we detail in Chapter 7.) This points to a core principle of biostatistical analysis—its thirst for parsimony. This drives a researcher to feverishly reduce the number of variables to the fewest possible that will still have a meaningful impact on a certain outcome.

A major motive for this is the desire for practical and efficient solutions. For example, had coach Sotirov found that training time alone explains 60% of a runner's speed, we would want runners to focus more narrowly on this factor. Complexity and nuance are thus the natural enemies of parsimony. And to a large extent these must be sacrificed for regression analysis. A holistic and contingent analysis would severely hamper the search for explanations that rely upon the fewest possible factors.

For example, based upon biostatistical analysis, poor health outcomes for African Americans are commonly attributed to certain discrete factors, such as hypertension, obesity, and glucose levels. Attributing these outcomes to structural conditions—such as the social reproduction of racialized poverty—is not an option within such an analysis. This is *NOT* because regression enthusiasts are somehow ignorant of (or unsympathetic toward) such an interpretation! It simply follows from the operating logic of regression analysis. This (parsimonious) operating logic requires that any systemic origins of poverty be stripped of their (holistic) operating logic. The "origins of poverty" can then be reframed as discrete parts (or proxies), such as unemployment figures, high-school completion rates, or incarceration rates.

A two-step process is envisioned in this regard. First, one set of social scientists deploys regression analysis to complete the preliminary work of *exposing* certain discrete parts via its findings. Then, it is left to another set of social scientists to explain the origins of these parts. From this perspective, regression analysis can be understood as playing an integral, yet circumscribed role, within social analysis. Whereas, for coach Sotirov and many others it is an endpoint.

On the one hand, treating these three independent (or causal) variables as "discrete" entities that can be "aggregated" obscures a complex and holistic reality that might better explain why some runners are faster than others. On the other hand—and equally importantly—this parsimonious treatment of independent variables allows us to isolate and analyze certain elements of the larger reality, such as diet. This isolation then suggests strategies for manipulating different features of that larger reality to achieve certain concrete ends, such as improving a runner's time.

In this way, we gain specificity and efficiency. Thus, the error is not the willful suspension of disbelief that in this case treats a given context as an aggregation of discrete parts. The only error would be to treat that aggregation of discrete parts as an unmediated reflection of true reality.

In other words, once we discover that training time explains 22% of a runner's time, we must return our analysis from the level of the parts (our three independent variables) to the level of the neighborhood or context (the whole) from which those variables were temporarily separated. We can then use these data (such as training time) to better understand the context—allowing the part to inform the whole—before again returning to certain isolated elements of the whole (perhaps the type of running shoe) for further study. Ideally, we thus enter an ongoing analytical movement forward-and-back between part and whole.

Again, it is understood that any introduction to biostatistical analysis must remain largely fixated on analysis at the level of isolated parts. That is the nature of the immediate task. Therefore, it can be a considerable challenge for students to maintain this understanding of biostatistical analysis as a deliberate and strategic set of tools within a much larger analytical process. Problems only arise when the findings from biostatistical tools and techniques are treated as the endpoint and are thus allowed to upend a broader and deeper analysis.

Thus, properly applied, the intricacies of biostatistical analysis detailed throughout this book are an indisputable good. The problem occurs only if, after applying our biostatistical tools and techniques, we fail to return to our original holistic level of analysis that generated our research question. This is the only way to properly understand and make use of the lessons learned from biostatistical analysis.

The difference between a tool (such as regression analysis) and an analysis (such as investigating the impact of track team participation on student health) is like the difference between a fork and preparing a meal. Certain aspects of preparing a meal require a fork, but no one holds up the fork as somehow equal in importance to the meal preparation itself. This is the perspective that we must maintain throughout this book, while still plumbing the depths of the many amazing techniques for using a fork.

With this in mind, let us then explore how one deploys regression analysis as a strategic tool. Recall that the present chapter is limited to the conceptual premises and implications behind these tools. The fun times are postponed for reviewing the mathematical rules and techniques of regression analysis in Chapter 7. In fact, accounting for the weighted impact of multiple independent variables on a single dependent variable is something that most of us do on a daily basis without giving it much thought. Examples include discussions with friends about anything from which is the best movie from the *Big Momma's House* trilogy to who is the better badminton player, Lin Dan or Taufik Hidayat, or when is the best time of year to plant a garden.

You and your friends each line up your criteria (or independent variables)—perhaps the plot, characters, and dialogue in the case of the *Big Momma's House* trilogy. You then weight these independent variables. For example, Lin Dan had the better serve and Taufik Hidayat was the master of the hairpin net shot and you think that serving is more important than overall skills because of this or that reason, or vice versa. Then you put these together to better define your dependent variable—what it means to be a great *Big Momma's House* movie, a superb badminton player, or an outstanding gardener. The point is that the basic idea underlying regression analysis is not at all foreign for any of us.

To illustrate just one of hundreds of ordinary, everyday encounters with regression analysis, we recount a story ripped straight from the headlines of the local periodical in Any Town, USA.

Two people watch a movie together on a Tuesday and catch a comedy show on a Thursday. Friday morning, one of the two is found dead in a pool of blood and the other is arrested for murder. Tragedies like this can be read about every day. As in this case, they follow inevitably from neither person knowing the basics of regression analysis. Let's examine the facts.

After leaving the movie house Tuesday evening, witnesses describe a friendly discussion that suddenly turned heated when the two could not agree on the basic criteria to judge the picture show. The first person emphasized the plot, casting, and acting. The second person emphasized the scenery, dialogue, and ending. Eventually, they came to agree on the same four criteria (or independent variables)—the plot, acting, dialogue, and ending. Then things turned ugly.

There was agreement that the acting was subpar and the plot was wonderful. But sharp differences remained over the integrity of the ending and the authenticity of the dialogue. The conversation eventually broke down when neither person knew how to weight the criteria to better form the argument. Two days later, after the pair attended a comedy show, violence erupted. The two initially agreed on three crucial independent variables for gauging the performance—material, delivery, and originality. But again, a failure to properly weight these variables led eventually to further conflict and then … murder.

We hear about such situations most every day. Had either of the two possessed even a rudimentary grasp of regression analysis the gruesome outcome surely would have been averted. Their first step would have been to settle on either a proper continuous or dichotomous dependent variable. The easiest option would arguably have been a dichotomous variable (good movie/not good movie). This would have led them safely to multiple logistic regression.

All too commonly, however, in the heat of passion, combatants reach for a continuous outcome variable instead, such as, how many stars to give a movie. This can work. But often the need for agreement over a specific interval scale or ratio scale can prove too much. Their second step would have then been to agree to a common set of independent variables and to specify ways to weight each of these based on their relative importance. Notice, however, that assessing a single movie (or case) in this manner is not illustrative of multiple regression, *per se*. Let us turn to common examples that compare a number of cases.

Again, there are many everyday examples of this. For instance, we might argue with a friend about why *Big Momma's House I* was the highest earning movie in the *Big Momma's House* trilogy ($117 million US box office). Or we might explain why Taufik Hidayat defeated Lin Dan at the 2005 Badminton World Championship. In these cases, we implicitly summon key principles of regression analysis. To argue, we must (a) specify the dependent variable—the highest earning movie in the *Big Momma's House* trilogy or the winner of the 2005 Badminton World Championship, (b) identify the criteria (or independent variables) explaining this outcome (or dependent variable), and (c) detail the role and relative importance of each of the independent variables in our explanation.

In the course of research within health and medicine, there are certain common research problems for which these regression tools are thought to be uniquely well-suited. Two such problems concern confounding variables and effect modification. A third (related) concern is the need to *simultaneously* assess the relative importance of certain attributes or exposures (risk factors) *vis-à-vis* a given dependent (or outcome) variable. Note that these attributes or exposures are both types of independent variables.

Importantly, to address the twin problems of confounding and effect modification, we must steel ourselves to enter this realm of analysis in which variables are treated as discrete and aggregated. Thus, a (temporary) willful suspension of disbelief will be necessary for the reader to continue beyond this point. That is, for now, the holistic and contextualized nature of health and medicine must be put aside.

The nature of the problem—confounding, effect modification, and the differential impact of attributes and exposures

Confounding occurs when the effect of some exposure (such as long-distance running) on an outcome variable (such as a resting heart rate) is impacted by the presence of a third variable (such as daily meditation). *Importantly, to be confounding, this third variable must directly interact with both the exposure and the outcome variable.* In this scenario we want to know if long-distance running (the independent variable, or exposure) reduces a high-school student's resting heart rate, the dependent (or outcome) variable.

In the course of our study, we learn that daily meditation is required of all high-school long-distance runners as part of their training and we grow concerned that daily meditation may act as a confounding variable. After all, perhaps daily meditation itself is sufficient to explain a lower resting heart rate, regardless of participation in long-distance running.

Our difficulty stems from the fact that there is a direct interaction between daily meditation and long-distance running (the exposure) because meditation is required for all runners. There is also a strongly suspected direct interaction between daily meditation and a resting heart rate (the outcome). Therefore, we must distinguish between three types of possible impact. These are:

- The impact of long-distance running *alone* on a resting heart rate.
- The impact of daily meditation *alone* on a resting heart rate.
- The impact of long-distance running and daily meditation, *in combination*, on a resting heart rate.

The technical steps for assessing this are detailed in Chapter 7. The general idea is the following. For purposes of comparing the resting heart rates for each of these situations, we must draw samples from three groups of high-school students.

- Group 1: high-school students who are long-distance runners AND who meditate daily.
- Group 2: high-school students who are NOT long-distance runners AND who meditate daily.
- Group 3: high-school students who are NOT long-distance runners AND who do NOT meditate daily.

After comparing these three groups, we found that both group 1 and group 2 had mean resting heart rates that were considerably lower than that for group 3. However, the mean resting heart rate for the members of group 1 was also notably lower than that for group 2.

On the one hand, given that the mean resting heart rate for group 2 was considerably lower than that for group 3, it certainly appears that meditation is acting as a confounding variable.

On the other hand, given that the mean resting heart rate for group 1 was below that of group 2, there is also reason to suspect that long-distance running *alone* might affect a resting heart rate. However, without performing a full analysis, it remains uncertain if the size of this difference between groups 1 and 2 is large enough to be definitive. Hence, the statistical significance of this example aside, this represents the nature of the question that is being addressed in the case of confounding.

Two further terms are in order before leaving confounding variables. This concerns an important distinction between "crude" and "adjusted" rates (or measures), which emerges from the idea of confounding. A crude rate refers to the rate for some condition within the general population. An adjusted rate refers to the impact of other factors on that same rate. Let us examine this difference between a crude rate and an adjusted rate.

Imagine we wish to calculate the US death rate due to cancer. If we simply divide the total number of deaths due to cancer for a given year by the total number of people in the US population we produce the crude death rate. However, we recognize that cancer deaths are not evenly spread across the population. Far more older people die of cancer than younger people, for example. Age acts as a confounding variable. To account for this, we produce an adjusted US death rate due to cancer that incorporates these age differences. This produces an age-adjusted death rate for cancer in the US.

There is a related distinction between crude measures and adjusted measures. Imagine there are four independent (or causal) variables explaining a resting heart rate (a continuous outcome variable). If we were to correlate each variable with the resting heart rate *independently* we would have four crude measures of correlation. Alternatively, if we were to apply multiple linear regression, this would allow us to simultaneously account for the impact of the other variables and produce an adjusted measure of correlation for each independent variable. This is a stupendously important application of regression analysis, as demonstrated below.

Effect modification occurs when the *magnitude of the effect* of some exposure (such as long-distance running) on an outcome (such as a resting heart rate) differs based on the level of exposure to a third variable (such as caffeine). In this example, we again want to know if long-distance running—the exposure—reduces a high-school student's resting heart rate. For this, we start by comparing the mean resting heart rates of two groups.

- Group 1: high-school students who are long-distance runners.
- Group 2: high-school students who are NOT long-distance runners.

Our initial results suggest that it may be that the mean resting heart rate of high-school long-distance runners is lower than that of students who are not long-distance runners. But our results are not conclusive. We suspect caffeine consumption may be distorting (or masking) our results. Therefore, we next gather all high-school students who are "low" consumers of caffeine and create two groups.

- Group 1: low consumers of caffeine who are high-school long-distance runners.
- Group 2: low consumers of caffeine who are NOT high-school long-distance runners.

Our results indicate that the members of group 2 have a higher mean resting heart rate than the members of group 1.

Thus, we find a clear association between competitive long-distance running and a lower mean resting heart rate among all persons who are low consumers of caffeine. Based on this, we conduct a further comparison. This time, we gather all long-distance runners and create two groups of low and high consumers of caffeine.

- Group 1: high-school long-distance runners who are low consumers of caffeine.
- Group 2: high-school long-distance runners who are high consumers of caffeine.

This time we find an elevated mean resting heart rate for group 2 compared to group 1. This suggests that caffeine consumption may be modifying our results based on the level of caffeine consumption. Hence, it is true that long-distance runners have lower resting heart rates than those who are not long-distance runners. However, the *magnitude of this difference* in heart rates is impacted by a person's level of caffeine consumption.

You will be familiar with the phrase commonly attached to this situation. Researchers might report: "Long-distance runners have lower resting heart rates than those who are not long-distance runners, *all things considered.*" "All things considered" is simply "CYA" language for researchers, indicating the assumption that there are no other significant differences between a long-distance runner and a person who is not a long-distance runner. This can include any number of factors, such as caffeine consumption, gender identity, or age.

Notice that, unlike the prior scenario for confounding, in this case there is no direct interaction between the third variable (levels of caffeine consumption) and the exposure (long-distance running). *This is a fundamental test for distinguishing between confounding and effect modification.*

In the case of effect modification, there is no interaction between caffeine consumption and long-distance running because the distribution of low, moderate, and high levels of caffeine consumption is the same among all students, regardless of whether or not she or he competes in long-distance running. Thus, there is no benefit to creating a set of three groups in the same manner as we did in the case of confounding. Instead, we create three subgroups only among our long-distance runners.

- Group 1: high-school long-distance runners who are low consumers of caffeine.
- Group 2: high-school long-distance runners who are moderate consumers of caffeine.
- Group 3: high-school long-distance runners who are high consumers of caffeine.

After comparing the mean resting heart rate of these three subgroups our suspicions are confirmed! We find that the positive effect of long-distance running on a student's resting heart rate is *modified* by her or his level of caffeine consumption.

Thus, it is true that a long-distance runner is at less risk for an elevated resting heart rate than a student who does not compete in long-distance running, all things considered. However, it is also true that a long-distance runner who is a low consumer of caffeine is at less risk for an elevated resting heart rate than a long-distance runner who is a high consumer of caffeine. In other words, the *magnitude* of the effect of the exposure (long-distance running) on the outcome (a resting heart rate) is modified by *the level* of a third variable (caffeine consumption).

We turn now to a third purpose of regression analysis. This is to better understand the differential impact of multiple independent variables on a dependent variable. To illustrate, we turn to a recent concern for coach Bimala Maji. She has noticed a growing number of ankle injuries among her long-distance runners at Tebhaga High School in Jalpaiguri County. Our dependent variable (or outcome) is thus ankle injuries.

Note that the dependent variable (resting heart rates) in our previous example was a continuous variable. Here, our dependent variable (ankle injuries) is dichotomous (yes/no). As (very loudly) mentioned above, continuous outcome variables require *linear* regression and dichotomous outcome variables require *logistic* regression. Continuing with our spate of ankle injuries, coach Maji suspects a few different causal factors (or independent variables).

Her first thought is that a runner's years of experience may be associated with ankle injuries. Second, she wonders about the new running shoes adopted by about one-third of her long-distance runners earlier this season. She surmises that the new shoe may be linked to the increase in ankle injuries. Third, coach Maji is curious if a runner's gender identity might somehow explain these ankle injuries. Our three independent variables are thus years of experience, new shoes, and gender identity.

After running her multiple logistic regression analysis, coach Maji concludes that years of experience increase the odds of ankle injury by about 10%, new shoes increase these odds by about 30%, and the gender identity of a runner has no effect. In this way, she identifies the differential impact of the three independent variables on the dependent variable (ankle injuries). Little more can be detailed here, without turning to the technical side of things. To set this up, we turn to the "secret sauce."

The secret sauce—key elements distinguishing linear and logistic regression

As mentioned, there are a number of far-reaching consequences based on the differences between the continuous outcome variables of linear regression and the dichotomous outcome variables of logistic regression. One such consequence follows from a contrast between the internal logic of each. The internal logic of linear regression flows from two impressive operations, correlation and the least squares estimates. The internal logic of logistic regression, meanwhile, relies on two very different operations, the odds ratio and the logit.

We begin with linear regression and the roles of correlation and least squares estimates. Indeed, linear regression cannot proceed without either one. The technical details of both require only basic mathematics and can be mastered with relatively brief practice. These are presented in Chapter 7. At the same time, it is essential to grasp the underlying concepts for each operation to understand the more fundamental rationale behind linear regression.

Correlation allows us to estimate the strength and direction of a relationship between two variables. A correlation coefficient is an estimate of the strength and direction of the relationship between two continuous variables. In fact, there are many types of correlation coefficients. For purposes of illustration, however, we draw upon the ever-popular Pearson Product Moment correlation coefficient—or Pearson's r. (Note that r is the Greek letter *rho* and this is pronounced "row.")

The direction of a correlation between variables can be "positive" or "negative." Given a positive correlation, the value of one variable rises (or falls), as the value of another variable rises (or falls). A simple example of a positive correlation is an increase in caffeine consumption that leads to an increase in a resting heart rate. In the case of a negative correlation, the value of one variable rises as the value of another variable falls, and vice versa. A simple example of a negative correlation is an increase in weekly hours of meditation that leads to a decrease in a resting heart rate. (Arguably, a more intuitive term for this is an "inverse" correlation.)

The purpose of correlation within linear regression is thus to quantify the strength and determine the direction (positive or negative) of an association between two continuous variables. For instance, a correlation can provide a measure of the degree to which caffeine consumption may alter a person's resting heart rate and, if so, in what direction (an increase or a decrease).

The purpose of **least squares estimates** within linear regression is two-fold. First, it details the linear relationship between a continuous outcome variable (such as a resting heart rate) and one or more attributes (such as gender identity) and/or exposures (such as caffeine consumption). Second, it estimates the value of other unknown variables based on the details of that linear relationship. For instance, after specifying the linear relationship between caffeine consumption and a resting heart rate, we can estimate a random person's resting heart rate based on her or his level of daily caffeine consumption.

Now we turn to logistic regression and the roles of the odds ratio and the logit. Again, logistic regression cannot proceed without either one and—as with linear regression—the underlying technical details of both require only high-school mathematics. (See Chapter 7 for details.) Once more, it is essential to grasp the underlying concepts for each operation to understand the rationale behind logistic regression.

An **odds ratio** tells us the odds that the members of group 1 will experience a certain outcome (such as an elevated resting heart rate) compared to the odds for the members of group 2. For instance, if an odds ratio is 2:1, this indicates that for every two members of group 1 who experience a certain outcome, one member of group 2 will experience that outcome. The secret to understanding the odds ratio is to unravel the relationships between it and the concepts of probability and odds. For this, we bring in a quick example in which we produce a probability, odds, and an odds ratio.

Coach Sliman Kiouane directs the track program at Sail Mohamed Ameriane ben Amerzaine High School in Kabylie County. He is concerned that high caffeine consumption is harming the performance of his 30 long-distance runners. He creates two groups of 15 runners in each. He instructs those in group 1 to eliminate all caffeine consumption for three weeks. He instructs those in group 2 to increase their caffeine consumption to at least six cups of coffee per day over the same three weeks.

After this, he determines how many persons in each group had a resting heart rate above 80 bpm. For those in group 1, three of 15 (or 20%) had a resting heart above 80 bpm. For those in group 2, this was 12 of 15 (or 80%).

Thus, he observed a 20% probability that a runner who eliminated all caffeine would have a resting heart rate above 80 bpm and an 80% probability that a runner who drank six cups of coffee per day would have a resting heart rate above 80 bpm. Probability, therefore, is an (uncomplicated) empirical description of the situation. This probability, however, does not indicate the "risk" that actual runners in each group face. This is because probability is a measure for the group *as a whole* and is not directly applicable to the individual members of a group. Risk applies to individuals.

The risk for an individual is determined by the odds. The odds thus apply to the members of a group, not to the group as a whole. The odds introduce a slightly confusing formula in which p = probability:

$$\frac{p}{1.0 - p}$$

To interpret the odds, remember that these are the odds for an individual either (a) to experience a certain outcome or (b) NOT to experience that outcome. Thus, for odds, two possible outcomes are considered. For probability, only one outcome is considered—to experience a certain outcome.

For the current example, we have:

$$\text{group 1}: \frac{p}{1.0 - p} \rightarrow \frac{0.2}{1.0 - 0.2} = 0.25$$

The odds are thus 0.25:1. For greater clarity, this can be rewritten as a ratio of 1:4. (We divide each side of the ratio by 0.25 to derive 1:4.) This can then be read as: For every one person in group 1 who has a resting heart rate above 80 bpm, there are four persons who do not have a resting heart rate above 80 bpm. It is four times more likely that an individual in group 1 will NOT have a resting heart rate above 80 bpm than it is that she or he will have a resting heart rate above 80 bpm.

Notice in this example that the odds are originally reported as 0.25. This is always the case. We then reformat this as 0.25:1 to frame it as actual odds. The reason, again, that we convert this to 1:4 is merely for ease of interpretation. Generally speaking, it is easier to understand a ratio if the left side of the ratio—representing persons in group 1 who have a resting heart rate above 80 bpm—is written as a whole number. When the left side of a ratio is a decimal less than 1.0, we make this a whole number by dividing both sides of the ratio by the decimal value on the left side.

$$\text{For example: } 0.44:3 = \frac{0.44}{0.44}:\frac{3}{0.44} = 1:6.82$$

Moving to group 2, we find:

$$\text{group 2: } \frac{p}{1.0-p} \rightarrow \frac{0.8}{1.0-0.8} = 4.0$$

The odds are 4:1. For every four persons in group 2 who have a resting heart rate above 80 bpm there is one person who does not have a resting heart rate above 80 bpm. Thus, it is four times more likely that an individual in group 2 will have a resting heart rate above 80 bpm than it is that she or he will NOT have a resting heart rate above 80 bpm.

Probability and the odds are, therefore, two different ways to express our findings for each group. Probability is a measure for the group as a whole. The odds is a measure of risk for the individuals in a group.

However, our actual interest is how group 1 compares to group 2. For this, we have the odds ratio. The odds ratio is a ratio between the odds for the members of group 1 and the odds for the members of group 2. In this case, we have:

$$\frac{0.25}{4.0} = 0.062$$

This is an odds ratio of 0.062:1. Again, we divide each side of the ratio by "0.062" and we find a ratio of 1:16.13. For every one member of group 1 who has a heart rate above 80 bpm, there are 16.13 members of group 2 who have a heart rate above 80 bpm. Thus, it is 16.13 times more likely that a member of group 2 will have a resting heart rate above 80 bpm than it is that a member of group 1 will have a resting heart rate above 80 bpm.

The value of the odds ratio, therefore, is that it allows us to compare the odds of some outcome for the individual members of two different groups. Moreover, its importance for logistic regression is that the outcome for an odds ratio is always dichotomous—such as, outcome A or NOT outcome A.

The **logit** works in tandem with the odds ratio and, however brief, some initial remarks regarding the logit can further help set the table. Among other things, full consideration of the logit will require a quick excursion into natural logarithms, exponentiation, and antilogs. For now, the seed we wish to plant regarding the logit is that it provides a tool for calculating the probability of an outcome that favorably aligns these probability values with the mathematical rules of the standard normal distribution. In short, it allows dichotomous outcomes to mimic the characteristics of continuous outcomes. The details of this, however, mathematical and otherwise, will need to wait for Chapter 7.

A return to those two promises

Let us now step back a moment to take in the big picture and return to those two promises of regression analysis. You will recall, first, that there was an assertion that regression analysis would allow us to better contextualize health and medicine. Investigating the role of confounding variables (or effect modification) is a purported example of this. Second, there was the claim that regression analysis would allow us to assess the relationships between the independent variables and the dependent variable, both individually and in combination. We have seen how regression analysis attempts to fulfill both these promises. Let us now consider the conceptual implications of regression analysis and how it depicts health and medicine in this regard.

For this, we consider two competing frames for contextualizing the subject matter of health and medicine and for understanding the relationships between variables. To anticipate, our contention is that each frame is appropriate depending upon one's stage of research. The frame that we associate with regression analysis—and with biostatistical analysis more generally as a specific stage of research—we label reductive. The second frame admittedly is not precisely a "stage." Rather it is better thought of as how we frame a research project in its entirety. This we label holism. Holism accommodates the reductive frame as a temporary strategy—that is, a willful suspension of disbelief—before returning one's analysis to a holistic frame.

So what are these two frames and why does this matter? The reductive frame and the holistic frame offer four contrasts (Table 2.3 summarizes these). First, the reductive frame views the subject matter of health and medicine as conforming to—and as explicable through—universal rules (or laws). This premise is lifted directly from the natural sciences and can work very well for certain subjects, such as disease diagnosis. Biostatistical analysis thus provides findings with a degree of certainty that abstract from particular conditions in a manner that is consistent with the application of universal rules.

The holistic frame replaces universal rules (or laws) with contingent and provisional explanations. On the one hand, this frame acknowledges the "truth" of biostatistical findings—at least, within the self-limiting conditions of the reductive frame. On the other hand, it views these findings as conditional, not universal. There is an assumption that all findings are determined by the conditions under which they were produced and that ultimately they are likely destined to be surpassed. Hence, the occasional need for the willful suspension of one's disbelief.

The second contrast compares the conceptual models associated with each frame. The reductive frame views a collection of interacting phenomena—such as a slate of independent and dependent variables—as forming an aggregation of discrete parts. This supposition is essential for regression analysis and axiomatic for biostatistical analysis more generally. We can analyze the relationship between two variables precisely because they are discrete and independent of each other. Were the two variables somehow connected this would "contaminate" the dynamic between them. This is the entire rationale for why we must account for confounding variables.

The holistic frame rejects this premise and treats a collection of interacting phenomena as a whole with inter-related parts. It is this interaction of parts that creates the whole and

Table 2.3 Comparison of reductive and holistic frames

Research concern	Reductive frame	Holistic frame
Goal of investigation	Discover or apply universal rules (or laws)	Develop contingent and provisional explanations
Conceptual models	Aggregates with discrete parts	Wholes with inter-related parts
Research imperatives	Parsimonious variables	Context-based variables
Ideal research design	Experimental design	Ecological design
Metaphor	Machine	Farm

it is the whole that then reconstitutes the parts. If this is so, the notion of two independent variables is not logically possible. This is because (a) it is only through these relationships that the whole is formed and (b) once formed, the whole further develops the relationships between these parts (or variables).

While this distinction between the two frames—as aggregates versus wholes—can be admittedly less than self-evident, it is hoped that two metaphors (a machine and a farm), described below, will better illustrate these differences. In addition, the conceptual implications behind claims that two variables are dependent or independent of each other are further developed in Chapter 10.

A third contrast between these two frames is the research imperative of each that juxtaposes parsimonious and context-based variables. For the purposes of fine-tuning its universal laws and better defining the discrete variables to test these laws, the reductive frame emphasizes parsimony when selecting variables. The goal is to draw upon the fewest necessary variables for any explanation. This is a hallmark of regression analysis. The holistic frame counters that the criteria for the number of variables is always context-based and cannot be held to any generic, a priori criteria, such as parsimony. This difference between frames follows logically from the first two differences.

A fourth contrast, with ties to parsimony, concerns the ideal research design. Those adopting a reductive frame favor an experimental research design that maximizes (and magnifies) the linkages between certain causal factors and an outcome. The two principal types of causal factors within biostatistical analysis of health and medicine are attributes and exposures.

When we compare two groups that differ based on personal characteristics—such as age, religion, or gender identity—these are attributes. When we compare two groups that differ based on certain experiences—such as a low-fat diet, radiation treatment, or a new medication—these are exposures. The aim of an experimental design is to isolate these as causal factors and to minimize the impact of conditions external to these on the outcome.

By contrast, the ideal research design for those working with a holistic frame tends to be an ecological model. An ecological model stands opposed to the experimental model, insofar as the former views causal factors as embedded within dynamic social contexts. It is argued, therefore, that any ascribed linkages between certain causal factors and outcomes are conditioned (and qualified) by social conditions and historical developments.

To better illustrate these differences between the two frames, we offer two metaphors. These are a machine and a farm, representing a reductive and holistic frame, respectively. A machine operates in the same way and via the same mechanisms always and every time. When it breaks, its repair requires restoring the machine's original mechanisms of operation. In this way, it follows universal principles (or laws) that apply to every other machine like it, no matter if it is five years old or brand new. No matter if it is in Japan or Moldova.

In addition, a machine is comprised of an aggregation of discrete, interacting parts. When one part breaks it is replaced by an identical part and the machine continues to operate no differently. Each part is thus independent of the machine itself, insofar each is easily replaced. It is the unique combination of parts and not the relationships between parts—except as required by the functional design—that matters. The functional design further determines the precise number of necessary parts. The aspiration of this design is efficiency. This means keeping the number of necessary parts as low as possible. A machine thus oozes parsimony.

Many machines operate on farms and are designed to replace (or supplement) human labor. This is the social context for its creation. The farm itself is a hive of productive activities that must account for a great many inter-related factors, such as soil quality, the climate, the seasons, the types of crops and livestock, and local land prices. A farmer must constantly adapt herself or himself to this volatile set of contingent factors that make universal rules (or laws) highly unstable and dependent on local conditions. All work plans are thus contingent and must be constantly re-thought. The specific intricacies of farm life are inherently uncertain and unstable week-to-week and month-to-month, requiring constant adjustment to a mix of vacillating conditions.

Furthermore, it is the incessant interaction of these factors—such as climate, crops, and soil quality—that matters, not merely each factor's individual characteristics. No one of these factors can be evaluated independently of the others. Rather, a farmer must observe and assess how these interact and how each impacts the web of productive activities comprising the farm as a whole. Lastly, the number of factors (or variables) to consider is determined by ever-shifting conditions, the time of year, the current weather forecast, the latest market values, etc. The number and types of factors are thus always context-based.

The point in emphasizing the distinctions between these two frames is to avoid the trap of a one-side or partial understanding of health and medicine, and of biostatistical analysis. One danger is that some researchers will treat the reductive frame—or biostatistical analysis in general—as the default or primary frame for understanding health and medicine. The holistic nature of health and medicine is, thereby, ignored or denied. An equal danger is that researchers will remain stuck at the level of holism and fail to appreciate the benefits of a reductive frame to analyze fundamental aspects of health and medicine. As such, a holistic frame is mistakenly treated as primary—to the *exclusion* of a reductive frame—rather than understanding a reductive frame as a further lens *available to* holism.

Lastly, there is one further frame that merits mention. The so-called "multiple methods" frame within the social sciences has been a popular (pragmatic) research strategy for several decades. Unlike the reductive or holistic frame, multiple methods purposely eschews rigid, conceptual commitments. Selecting a particular method (or tool) is situational and based on some current need. This can be mistaken for holism at times, which also moves between different methods at times.

The principal difference between holism and multiple methods is the conscious and deliberate use of the willful suspension of disbelief. This is crucial because there are fundamental conceptual differences between certain methods—biostatistical analysis and ethnography, for instance. On the one hand, biostatistical tools and techniques appear to be reductive and quantitative. Its subject matter has thus been rendered discrete and "measurable." On the other hand, ethnographic tools and techniques are holistic and qualitative. Its subject matter—by all appearances—presents itself unrendered, as it truly is, and directly observable and contextual.

The pragmatic and *ad hoc* movement between contradictory modes of understanding can then create challenges for the interpretation and presentation of findings. Indeed, it is common for "reductive" researchers to occasionally masquerade under the banner of "multiple methods," thereby, treating this eclectic approach as a work-around to aid in addressing qualitative matters that lie beyond the scope of biostatistical analysis. In this way, too often, a multiple methods frame is simply reductive research supplemented with holistic insights. Without the *intentional* movement between frames, the guiding principles of the research project as a whole—a holism that makes room for a reductive frame, for example—dissolve in the final product of the research. In that case, there is a default to a conventional reductive frame.

Again, biostatistical analysis in general—and regression analysis in particular—fit the conceptual premises of the reductive frame. Importantly, we argue that where regression analysis falls short regarding its two promises is NOT its reliance on reductive methods.

Rather, it is the failure to take lessons learned from these reductive methods and reintegrate these insights into a holistic whole, such as our farm.

Instead, regression analysis (via its reductive frame) too often is simply substituted for the full research project and its holistic principles. For example, many research articles are little more than a recitation of the results from a person's regression analysis that either confirm or refute a certain proposition. In this way, a (temporary) willful suspension of disbelief becomes a (permanent) delusional state.

Our purpose in this chapter has thus been two-fold. On the one hand, we have reviewed the conceptual foundations of regression analysis so that the reader can better understand and engage with these tools when appropriately deployed in research. On the other hand, we worked consciously and *explicitly* within the conceptual premises of regression analysis so that the reader does not misread or misuse these otherwise helpful tools. We reserve for a later chapter, in the context of conducting biostatistical analysis, the technical steps and mathematical premises necessary to carry out regression analysis.

There remains, however, the question of how it is that regression analysis—or any other biostatistical tool or technique—is initially taken up and absorbed within one's analysis. One of the early moments in this process is the selection of a study design. Too often, this is represented by a plainly fictitious sequence of events. For example, as we shall see, ultimately it is our biostatistical tools and techniques that determine our choice of study design and not our study design that determines our choice of biostatistical tools and techniques. The reason behind this confusion—and what it reveals about certain premises of biostatistical analysis—is one of the principal reasons for turning now to study designs, as an integral stage of biostatistical investigation.

Chapter 3

Study Designs and Sampling

A Beginning ... or the End?

We have been introduced to linear and logistic regression as important tools of biostatistical analysis. However, as applications of general mathematical principles, these tools require no prior knowledge of health and medicine—or of *any* specific subject matter. Thus, regression analysis is a necessary feature of biostatistical analysis, but this necessity does not arise from the unique content, or subject matter, of health and medicine. Rather, this subject matter— its presentation and depiction—appear to arise from the nature of regression analysis. The tool seems less a window into the reality of health and medicine and more an abstraction from that reality.

To make sense of this, we must retreat to that moment *prior* to the application of biostatistical analysis to the subject matter of health and medicine that brings about the need for regression analysis (or other such tools) to try and jerk our analysis forward. This prior moment involves the general schema and plans for the collection and analysis of material pertaining to health and medicine (in the form of data) that provides the pretense for the use of certain biostatistical tools, such as regression analysis.

Our attention thus moves backward in the sequence of events from the deployment of biostatistical tools to the deliberate reconfiguration of health and medicine for the purpose of generating specific forms of data. This reconfiguration begins with study designs and then, as detailed in Chapter 4, results in nine unique research configurations. Each configuration reflects a specific set of research circumstances. Based on these, a configuration provides a mode of investigation to generate specific forms of data suitable for certain biostatistical tools and tests.

At a surface level, study designs may thus seem to be an early step in research. But this impression is deceiving and we will see how the most consequential decisions are, in fact, taken long before a researcher chooses between a randomized controlled trial, a cohort study, or a case-control study.

That said, selecting a study design is a critical step in a deliberate strategy to frame and manipulate those conditions and factors that a researcher believes help to explain certain health outcomes. Moreover, this step is critical for assuring the compatibility between the data from our study and the tools and techniques of biostatistical analysis. Thus, while the choice of study design follows, in part, from the nature of the subject matter under study, this choice also follows from the technical imperatives imposed on that subject matter by the mathematical premises and rationale of biostatistical analysis.

Given the centrality of these mathematical premises, it is helpful to begin our overview with that study design considered purest in technical form and thus best suited for biostatistical analysis. That would be the randomized controlled trial. This is the mode of investigation that sits most high in the hierarchy of study designs within the world of health and medicine. Moving from the apex of this hierarchy to the cellar, we then hope to demonstrate

DOI: 10.4324/9781003316985-3

both the pragmatic and conceptual consequences of these choices for any study in-and-of-itself, as well as, for the subject matter at hand.

The hierarchy of study designs determines not only the outlines of one's investigation, but which questions are permissible and which are not. The twin tenets upholding this hierarchy are parsimony and control. It is by these criteria that a study design will rise or fall in stature. Parsimony ensures that we reduce the explanation of any outcome to the absolute fewest possible variables (or factors). Control ensures that the conditions under which certain causal factors—specific attributes or exposures—are isolated, observed, and measured are identical for all research participants.

To reiterate, attributes are the personal characteristics of research participants, such as age, religion, or gender identity. Exposures are the personal experiences of research participants, such as a low-fat diet, radiation treatment, or a new medication.

Note, however, that this clean distinction between attribute and exposure has certain peculiarities. Attributes are properties attached to an individual. Exposures pertain to environmental conditions or certain phenomena external to an individual. The implicit assumption is that an attribute holds some physiological significance that may interfere (or interact) with an exposure. This is the basis for confounding. For example, when studying diet as an exposure linked to heart disease, a person's age may make a person more susceptible to disease. In the case of certain attributes—such as age, gender identity, body mass index—this is uncomplicated. The "physiological" implications of other attributes are less clear.

For example, race, zip code, marital status, or occupation are common attributes whose principal impact seems more *experiential* than physiological. In this sense, they are more akin to exposures than attributes. For instance, longevity studies that compare married persons and single persons appear to assess two life experiences (or lifestyles), rather than a property (such as marital status) that is attached to a person as an attribute.

Consider a further example, variations of which we see reported all the time in medical journals. Imagine a scenario in which researchers test a new hypertension drug. For this, they create an experimental group and a control group and put protocols in place to assure that the only difference between groups is exposure to the new medication. Imagine then a second scenario in which researchers want to study differences in the mean systolic blood pressure between African American persons and white persons to understand the impact of race (an attribute) on hypertension.

That which accounts for any difference in the first study—between the experimental group and the control group—is clearly an exposure (the new medication). That which accounts for any difference in the second study—between African American people and white people—is ostensibly an attribute (race). This attribute, however, is inseparable from an exposure, such as the life experiences of an African American person in the US.

In fact, within studies that rely on biostatistical analysis, there is a persistent (and peculiar) desire to isolate attributes (such as a person's race, gender identity, or age) from a person's life experiences—something that is obviously inseparable from that attribute. An attribute is assumed to distinguish one group (with the attribute) from another group (without the attribute). But the basis of this distinction goes unstated. Thus, framing the differences between both the experimental group (with new medication) and the control group (with placebo) *as well as* between the African American subjects and the white subjects as differences *of exposures* seems quite sensible.

There is, of course, a difference between exploring the correlation between an attribute and some outcome and declaring the attribute to be the cause of that outcome—as in an experimental design. However, biostatistical analysis maneuvers with shark-like focus to pinpoint those factors that account for some outcome. And it is quite common to find certain attributes well represented among these factors. The inference is clear. For instance, to be African American in the US causes hypertension. Attribute and exposure are one, insofar as the experiences attached to the attribute constitute an exposure. For now we must put aside this dubious categorical partition of attribute and exposure and continue on with things.

With respect to our criteria of parsimony and control, the randomized controlled trial remains the gold standard by which all other research designs are judged. So what exactly is a randomized controlled trial? And how do its elements adhere so well to these criteria? Furthermore, what are the practical and conceptual consequences of this adherence for health and medicine? Likewise, what, if anything, is omitted or distorted by this study design?

Within health and medicine, the randomized controlled trial comes as close as is practically possible to the design of experimental research in the natural sciences. Most other study designs only exist because they probe areas of health and medicine that are not conducive to the strict protocols of randomized controlled trials. Thus, in the case of researchers adopting these *lesser than* study designs, it is the subject matter—and not the researcher's professional aspirations or ideological commitments—that distinguishes their work from the *greater than* work of their peers. This indeed is our reason for beginning with randomized controlled trials.

Given this rationale, it is good to recall that the history of any science is a history of two simultaneous processes—retooling and reconceptualizing. All present-day biostatistical tools and techniques were created to solve some unique problem(s) that existing tools and techniques could not adequately address at some time in the past. Those past problems led to a surprisingly small pool of basic (or boilerplate) study designs, which have themselves evolved and developed in response to further unique problems arising from their application to different subject matter.

The goal with each new iteration has been a set of tools and a collection of study designs believed more adequate for its subject matter. In turn, the subject matter itself—in dialectical fashion—came to be reconceptualized to better fit the emerging tools for its investigation. Of course, one of the major themes for us is the extent to which the subject matter of health and medicine has been forced to conform to the conceptual premises of biostatistical tools and techniques, rather than conforming these tools and techniques to the subject matter.

Randomized controlled trials—the back story

It is essential to recognize, and to keep ever front of mind, that the principal purpose of a randomized controlled trial is to generate data. Moreover, these data must satisfy the operational precepts of certain biostatistical tools and techniques. (This is, of course, no less true for all research designs.) In this sense, biostatistical analysis *precedes* the selection of a study design and determines the protocols for each study design—notwithstanding the order by which research appears to be carried out.

Indeed, there is a broadly held and mistaken notion of how scientific research proceeds. This follows from certain myths propagated by introductory research methods textbooks—and many advanced textbooks—suggesting that research unfolds as a series of sober choices governed by the objective judgments of researchers seeking only pearls of hidden truths.

The mythical story is this. Research follows sequential, lock-step stages that emerge largely from the mind of a researcher. The process begins when researcher X is inexplicably possessed by an interest in some random subject Y. Researcher X then formulates a research question for subject Y and develops a falsifiable hypothesis based on this. *After this,* researcher X selects a study design to confirm or refute this hypothesis.

Researcher X then follows a set of protocols dictated by the study design that she or he chose and generates data. After this, researcher X consults with a statistician and determines which tools and techniques will be best to analyze the data. Researcher X carries out this biostatistical analysis and discovers whether she or he has confirmed or refuted the hypothesis. If confirmed, researcher X goes on to publish the study. If refuted, researcher X humbly absorbs lessons learned from failing to generate significant findings and moves on to another research question.

This, of course, is a fantasy world—though not an especially interesting or magical one. In reality, the process is far murkier than this. First, researcher X develops an expertise in subject Y over an extended period of study and research. Given this, researcher X selects a (micro) subtopic within subject Y. This selection is based both on her or his expertise along with hours of scouring over which current research subtopics are (a) getting published, (b) attracting grants, and (c) leading to tenure. Second, researcher X formulates a research question. The research question must mimic those questions guiding recently published studies. This is because the research question must fit within current debates to increase its odds of publication. Novelty or originality is highly discouraged.

Third, researcher X selects a study design. This is a rote exercise that varies, if at all, only slightly from previously published hypotheses. At the same time, researcher X will consult with a statistician and select a falsifiable hypothesis consistent with the generation of data (and related biostatistical analysis) found in recently published studies. Fourth, researcher X then follows a set of protocols for the study design that she or he chose and generates the same panel of data—with different actual values—as that from recently published studies. Incidentally, in many other professions this practice of blatantly replicating the work of other colleagues (or plagiarism) would not be well-received.

Incidentally, notice a glaring oddity in both of these portrayals of research protocols. This concerns the refusal to publish results that refute a hypothesis. The idea that negation is not as relevant a finding as an affirmation seems counter to our ordinary life experiences. It would be akin to sending in teams of detectives, one-by-one, to solve a crime and yet refusing to tell each new team what theories of the crime had been ruled out by previous teams of detectives. This would then continue until, by dumb luck, one team of detectives stumbled upon the solution.

Fifth, researcher X carries out the biostatistical analysis and discovers whether she or he has confirmed or refuted the hypothesis. If confirmed, researcher X goes on to publish the study and—statistically speaking—will most probably go on to conduct further research on the same (micro) subtopic within subject Y, with only the slightest amendments to the research question, hypothesis, study design (based on generating the same data), and biostatistical analysis. If her or his hypothesis is refuted, researcher X dejectedly absorbs lessons learned from failing to find publishable results and recommits herself or himself to move on and this time hew more closely to the hypotheses, study designs, etc. of recently published studies.

Few researchers are more attentive to the realities of the research process—and its inverted sequential logic—than those conducting randomized controlled trials. The protocols for these trials provide strict guidance and any deviation from the script is roundly punished. These protocols demand four cardinal steps:

- Simple random sampling from the population of interest (with adequate size and power).
- Random assignment to experimental and placebo groups.
- Double-blind design.
- Placebo-controlled design.

Let us review each of these steps. The first step, sampling, is more fully detailed later in this chapter. Here we lay bare its conceptual premises. Sampling techniques are borrowed from the natural sciences and mathematics and their adoption requires some explanation. Indeed, a great deal hinges on this otherwise routine activity. This is because sampling makes visible a number of critical research concerns, including the classification schemas across health and medicine, the notion of inclusion or "representativeness," the determination of statistical significance, and the concept of "power."

We begin with classification and the natural sciences. Given the massive number of fish, fauna, fossils, frogs, flies, fjords, etc., it is only possible to study the tiniest fraction of the natural phenomena all around us. The natural sciences thus developed convenient typologies for distinguishing and organizing all of the stuff we find crammed onto our planet. The criteria distinguishing the contents of each typology then determine what items are included or excluded from this or that type of thing and thus define the boundaries for each area of research. For example, within the biological sciences there are seven nested classifications for all living organisms—kingdom (all living organisms), phylum, class, order, family, genus, and species.

Simultaneously, mathematicians handed us—via set theory—a souped-up rationale for selecting individual items from each typology to generate "representative" samples of these. The rationale is labeled "random." This indicates that each element within a typology (or each person within a population) has an equal likelihood of selection for the sample and that the methods for assuring this are carried out in a consistent manner. (The techniques for this are detailed below.)

Mathematical principles thus determine (a) how many items from a particular typology are needed for a sample and (b) how it is decided which of the many available items are chosen to be in a sample and which are chosen not to be.

Note how this entails initial subjective judgments followed by the application of objective rules. That is, we must determine the (subjective) criteria by which we will constitute a typology and the (objective) rules by which we will decide upon the necessary number of items from a given typology to include in a sample and how to select these.

Researchers across health and medicine soon set out to emulate these sampling practices from the natural sciences.

The classification schemas had already been largely built up over many decades. Indeed, given the high level of intersubjective agreement among researchers regarding these formal categories, most sampling concerns fell on the shoulders of biostatisticians. They proceeded with two preoccupations—how many items to choose and how to choose these items. How many, is a matter of statistical significance and the concept of power. How to choose, engages with representativeness. Let us address these in reverse order.

We begin with the general notion—adopted from the natural sciences and mathematics—that a proper sample can only be derived from a category of things that can be represented. This follows, in part, from a presumption of sufficient homogeneity among those items comprising the category. The consistency of sameness among this type of tree, or that kind of beetle, must be so invariant and render it so distinguishable from all other types of trees or beetles that we could select any 10 trees (of this type) and the defining properties of any one of those trees would make it utterly indistinguishable from the others.

On the one hand, this is obviously a contrived homogeneity that follows from the criteria that we chose and applied to trees—its leaf structure, bark, climate adaptation, etc. On the other hand, this is an empirical homogeneity that follows from the botanical properties of trees that we can objectively observe and document. This presumption of homogeneity among the items comprising a category within the natural sciences thus follows, first, from the subjective criteria of the natural scientists and, second, from the inherently homogeneous nature of items across the natural world.

Our concern thus turns on how well the homogeneity among maple trees can mirror the homogeneity among homeless African American youth in Biloxi, Mississippi, or among women diagnosed with breast cancer in Denver, Colorado, in March 2026. After all, if the cost of representation is either to denude our research participants of all meaningful substance or to distort the presentation of our research participants beyond recognition then what is the value of representation? Indeed, this trade-off between what is necessary to generate a representative sample and the reduction of research participants to vapid, one-dimensional forms is a very real concern for research within health and medicine that we will return to in Chapter 10.

Compare this treatment of representativeness with two further notions borrowed from mathematics—statistical significance and "power." Statistical significance and power are derived from mathematical rules that determine how many items should be chosen for a sample. Subjective judgment is limited here to a researcher's preferred degree of precision—ordinarily, 95% or 99%. Statistical significance indicates whether or not a finding meets a threshold of "certainty" and, therefore, can be reported as "significant."

A common threshold for statistical significance is a p-value of less than 5%. (This is written $p < 0.5$. Note that "p" stands for probability.) A p-value of less than 5% indicates a 95% probability that our findings represent the way things truly are. As detailed in Chapter 8, one of the key determinants of the p-value—and thus statistical significance—is sample size.

"Power" introduces a defensive tactical maneuver for avoiding a certain type of error when assessing statistical significance. A type one error occurs when we celebrate a significant finding that, in fact, is not significant. A type two error occurs when we torment ourselves over a finding not deemed to be significant when, in fact, it is. Much of this hangs on the sample size. Thus, we desperately strive to avoid a sample that is too small, leading ordinarily to a type one error, or a sample that is too large, costing us time and resources.

But power also plays a central role in avoiding type two errors. Hence, there is a sweet spot that avoids a sample size that is too small or too large and it is our determination of the level of power that, in part, allows us to find this. (Statistical significance and power are addressed in greater detail in Chapters 8 and 9.)

The final three elements of randomized controlled trials are random assignment, a double-blind design, and a placebo-controlled design. The distinction between random sampling and random assignment is essential to keep in mind. Random sampling refers to how we create a sample. Random assignment refers to how we create an experimental group and a control group. These are separate procedures that occur at separate stages of research. The random assignment of participants to the experimental and control groups minimizes any differences between the two groups. All participants have an equal likelihood of assignment to either group.

The prior stage of random sampling is designed to assure a pool of participants who represent the population of interest. Hence, each person is identical to that degree. Any additional criteria for assigning persons to the experimental and control groups would create a distinction between the two groups beyond simply being representative of the population. *Importantly, the most common reason for choosing a research design other than a randomized controlled trial within health and medicine is the inability to conduct random assignment.* For example, in a study comparing persons with cancer and persons without cancer, we cannot randomly determine who goes into each group. This limitation only enhances the importance of biostatistical tools and techniques in health and medicine. Measures of statistical significance become tools (and proxies) to compensate for the lack of a proper experimental research design.

The double-blind design is a further contrivance to minimize bias. This is, in part, related to the need for a placebo-controlled design. The placebo effect is one of the few explicitly metaphysical concepts that shapes human subject research. It has been long recognized that a portion of persons who believe that they are receiving treatment for some condition will experience improvement, regardless of whether they receive the true medication or the placebo. This subverts the most basic precepts of Western medical science. Consequently, lacking any acceptable scientific explanation, researchers snatched a Latin term for "to be pleasing" (placebo) and slyly added a placebo group into experimental research.

For example, in testing a new drug it is assumed that there will be some measurable improvement for most participants by virtue of everyone knowing that they are involved in medical research. The success of a new drug, therefore, is not merely some improvement but some improvement in the experimental group above that for the control (or placebo) group. Naturally, for many health and medical studies including a placebo group is less feasible. Examples include special diets or health interventions, such as peer-based programs.

The double-blind design conceals from both participants and researchers who belongs to the experimental group and who is in the control (or placebo) group. With regard to participants, this minimizes the placebo effect. With regard to researchers, this minimizes the risk of unintentional bias by a researcher toward a participant based on the researcher's knowledge of her or his role in either the experimental or control group. The severe limitations for double-blind research with human subjects are further reasons why randomized controlled trials within health and medicine face significant challenges.

Notice that these four steps—simple random sampling, random assignment, double-blind design, and placebo-control design—are all innovations and strategies for bridging research from the natural sciences with research in the social sciences. The first two are standard procedures for the natural sciences that have been significantly overhauled to accommodate the more complex settings and random idiosyncrasies of social science research. The last two are new creations made necessary to meet the strictures of human subject research in randomized controlled trials.

Health and medicine, whose subject matter straddles the natural and social sciences, seeks both the status and legitimacy of the natural sciences as well as the agile flexibility of the social sciences. Upholding randomized controlled trials as the lodestar for true scientific research, while furiously working to develop cheap study design knock-offs—underwritten by flashy biostatistical tools and techniques—is a reflection of this.

Randomized controlled trials—an example

For the details of our randomized clinical trial we travel to Elizavetgrad County—a county known for its fast talkers, all night diners, and spot-on, impromptu moon walkers. This might just be the perfect place to study the association between caffeine consumption and the risk of elevated resting heart rates among high-school long-distance runners. This, of late, has been a growing concern for coach Olga Taratuta at Black Cross High School. Coach Taratuta has been tasked to run a county-wide study to get to the bottom of this matter.

She begins by enrolling 100 high-school long-distance runners recruited from across Elizavetgrad County for an eight-week study. Runners are taken to a mountain retreat set up for the study. Upon arriving, researchers assess the general life stressors for each runner and score each of these on a 10-point scale. Stressors include personal relationships, family life, schoolwork, etc. Researchers then send each runner to her or his room and begin to tightly control each person's diet, sleep pattern, medications, and physical activities. For example, participants are permitted two hours of light physical activity per day and all potential stressors—such as cell phones or access to international news—are forbidden.

The first two weeks provide a wash-out phase with zero caffeine consumption for everyone. After this, the resting heart rate is recorded for all participants prior to the random assignment of each participant to one of four groups. These are three experimental groups and one control group. Group 1 will consume 100 micrograms of caffeine per day, group 2 will consume 250 micrograms, and group 3 will consume 450 micrograms. Group 4 is a control group and will consume zero micrograms of caffeine per day. (For reference, there are approximately 95 micrograms of caffeine in an eight-ounce cup of coffee.)

The study is double-blind. No participant is told which group she or he belongs to and no on-site researcher knows any participant's group. Caffeine is administered to participants three times per day via a beverage that is identical in color, temperature, viscosity, odor, and taste. Each beverage is prepared at an off-site lab and delivered to the mountain retreat in a cup marked with a participant's unique identifier code. On-site researchers then distribute the beverages to the participants.

After six weeks, each participant's resting heart rate is again recorded. We then compare each participant's resting heart rate before and after her or his participation in one of the four groups. This allows us to assess the impact of different levels of caffeine consumption on a participant's resting heart, after controlling for diet, sleep pattern, medications, physical activities, and other potential stressors. (The biostatistical tools and techniques for assessing this are detailed in Chapters 6 and 7.)

For now, it is crucial to recognize that these protocols are not *in addition to* biostatistical analysis. These are dictated by the operative premises of biostatistical analysis. Hence, biostatistical analysis is not adjunctive to the randomized controlled trial. Rather, our randomized control trial is an extension of biostatistical analysis.

Beyond randomized controlled trials

When either random assignment to the experimental or control group, a double-blind design, and/or placebo-controlled design are not practical options, there are four principal research designs we turn to. These are cohort studies, case-control studies, ecological studies, and case reports or case series.

Cohort study

A cohort study recruits a large number of participants from a defined population and follows them over an extended period. A "large number" of participants is typically anywhere from 50 to 50,000. The "extended" period can be six months to six decades. The number of participants and the length of time depend on resources and the nature of the study. The defined population can be as broadly or narrowly drawn as the researcher wishes. Again, this is based on resources and the nature of the study.

Importantly, the original participants in a cohort study generally do not have the condition that researchers are investigating at the time of enrollment into the study. Rather, the purpose of the study is to monitor all participants for the emergence of some condition. For this reason, the extended period of a cohort study is ideal for late-onset, long-term, and chronic conditions that require study over long periods of time, such as cardiovascular disease or cancer.

In our case, coach Taratuta recruits 100, ninth-grade high-school long-distance runners from across Elizavetgrad County. She chooses ninth-graders so that we can follow participants over four years of high school to better understand any association between caffeine consumption and an elevated resting heart rate. She records the resting heart rate of all participants in the first week of the school year when they enter the ninth grade.

Over the next four years coach Taratuta continues to record each participant's resting heart rate on a monthly basis. Participants maintain a weekly log of their caffeine consumption and they submit this at each monthly check-in. In addition, participants complete a "consequential" events report form at the monthly check-in to identify any anomalous developments that might account for a change in a participant's resting heart rate.

Consequential events include notable changes regarding behaviors (such as diet, exercise, or sleep patterns) or life stressors (such as personal relationships, family life, or school work). Coach Taratuta is thereby able to identify patterns across the study participants that associate changes in the resting heart rate with variations in caffeine consumption, while controlling for behaviors and stressors. (Biostatistical tools and techniques relevant for this are discussed in Chapter 5.) A cohort study thus allows us to pinpoint aspects of linkages between caffeine and elevated resting heart rates in relation to other possible factors. These factors can then be more precisely investigated later in a randomized controlled trial.

Case-control study

A case-control study begins with a group of participants who are chosen because they all share some condition that researchers are investigating. Ordinarily, these are relatively rare conditions, such as Legionnaires' disease. Thus, a run-of-the-mill, random sample from the general population would not likely capture many persons with that condition. (A cohort study, by contrast, is better suited for investigating more common conditions, such as asthma.)

Case-control studies are also common designs for investigating a sudden outbreak of an infectious ailment with an unknown origin, such as food poisoning, among a small set of people. After recruiting a group of persons with some rare condition—commonly 20 to 40 persons—researchers catalogue an array of pertinent attributes (such as age, gender identity, and body mass index) and exposures (such as medications, diet, and exercise) for each person. Based on this, researchers develop a detailed profile for each person with the condition.

Researchers then seek out persons in the general population who match the profile of a participant but do NOT have the condition. The goal is to create matched pairs of people with very, very similar profiles, one of whom has the condition and one of whom does not.

The next step is to compare those attributes and exposures of persons who have the condition with the attributes and exposures of those without the condition. It is hoped that a pattern will emerge from this comparison that indicates which attributes and exposures are most unique to those persons with the condition.

The good people of Durruti County, for example, are very concerned about possible links between caffeine consumption and elevated resting heart rates among high-school long-distance runners who may be trying to get an edge on the competition. Because the level of interest for an elevated resting heart rate (above 95 bpm) is relatively rare, researchers develop a case-control study. George Sossenko, the track coach at Sébastien Faure Century High School, first identifies 30 high-school long-distance runners from across Durruti County who have a resting heart rate above 95 bpm.

Researchers then develop a detailed profile for each of these runners. The profile includes four attributes (age, gender identity, BMI, and zip code) and four exposures (years of running experience, diet, medications, and stressors). Based on these attributes and exposures, each runner with a resting heart rate above 95 bpm is matched with a runner with a similar profile and a resting heart rate below 80 bpm. Lastly, the exposure level of daily caffeine consumption is also collected for all participants.

Researchers then compare the daily caffeine consumption level for each matched pair to determine if variations in caffeine consumption between those with elevated heart rates and those with heart rates below 80 bpm are associated with an elevated heart rate. Ideally, the matched pairs design will eliminate all other attributes and exposures as factors and the only remaining factor explaining the elevated heart rates will be the daily caffeine consumption. As we will see, an odds ratio is an ideal tool for assessing case-control studies and other circumstances when the outcome of interest is very rare within the general population.

Ecological study

It is not generally the primary purpose of an ecological study to generate data for biostatistical analysis. The primary purpose is to explore features of the social and environmental conditions that contribute to certain health conditions. A typical research question might ask: How do impoverished living conditions contribute to lead poisoning or childhood asthma? Or: How do working conditions on industrial farms contribute to physical injuries among migrant farmworkers? In such cases, it is a complex web of social and environmental factors that contribute to these conditions.

Given this vexing combination of factors, it is not a simple matter to isolate specific variables that can be linked to this or that health condition. Thus, ecological studies are often viewed as *preliminary* investigations that are akin to a case report or case series—discussed below—that can lead to later studies that identify specific causal factors associated with a particular health outcome.

For Durruti County there are several social and environmental factors that coach Sossenko might investigate. Notice however, that he faces an initial dilemma, insofar as he is working with different operational assumptions that do not allow us to think in terms of links between *a specific causal* factor (such as caffeine) and *a particular* outcome (such as a resting heart rate above 95 bpm). Rather, coach Sossenko might simply identify a condition that he wishes to better understand. For example, this could be elevated resting heart rates among the high-school long-distance runners of Durruti County.

To get a handle on this he might begin by sketching out the general social conditions, economic opportunities, and any major environmental concerns within the county. This could lead us to better understand what factors—including caffeine—might account for elevated resting heart rates among these runners. This, however, would not necessarily result in findings relevant for biostatistical analysis. Thus, coach Sossenko's ecological study of Durruti County would remain a preliminary study. The follow-up might be a case-control study that isolates a specific suspected causal factor.

Case reports and case series

Case reports and case series are in-depth, qualitative descriptions of certain health conditions with uncertain origins. A case report concerns a single patient, or a small number of patients over a relatively small geographic area. A case series contains a larger number of patients across a broader geographic expanse. A detailed description is necessary because either the condition itself, or its origins and transmission, represent a novel encounter for health practitioners. Consequently, the objective of a case report or case series is to provide a detailed account of the condition and its circumstances. This includes the condition's biological markers, the patients' symptoms and personal backgrounds, and the social and environmental factors that may be relevant to its origins and transmission.

The details of a case report or case series then allow researchers to place this condition within the taxonomy of known medical conditions. An example of this would be early cases of COVID-19 *vis-à-vis* severe acute respiratory syndrome (or SARS). In addition, these details allow researchers to link a small number of isolated cases with similar cases emerging in other areas. An example of this was the early isolated cases of what later came to be known as HIV/AIDS. Thus, like ecological studies, case reports and case series are generally treated as very early stages of investigation prior to the development of protocols for the generation of data appropriate for biostatistical analysis.

Sampling

As noted above, study designs begin with one crucial task. This is sampling. Here we present the fundamental elements of sampling. These elements emerge from a general desire to bring order to an unruly world. The world we initially encounter appears arbitrary and chaotic. This is true for both the natural world and the social world. Over and against this untidiness we impose structure and order. We do this, in part, through sampling, which helps us to sort and classify all manner of social phenomena.

In the social world, sampling begins at the broadest level by identifying some population. Simply put, a population is any collection of interrelated things. How these things interrelate is determined by specific qualities that identify them as members of the same population.

For example, "all (200) high-school long-distance runners in Nasser County" might be our population. We could then draw a sample from this population of 200 high-school long-distance runners. Alternatively, our population might be "all (80) cis-female high-school long-distance runners in Nasser County." Again, we could then draw a sample from this more specific population of 80 long-distance runners. Or we may want to narrow our population even further and consider "all (40) senior cis-female high-school long-distance runners in Nasser County."

In each of these instances, all members of each population are interrelated because they share a set of attributes (and/or exposures) that no person outside that population shares. This links them with one another and excludes all others. This, in fact, is one of three premises with which sampling begins its work. These three premises are:

- All populations are distinguishable by the attributes and/or exposures of its members.
- All populations are scalable.
- All populations are divisible.

Working with these premises, researchers thus choose (or create) the population with which they work. In addition, insofar as the combination of attributes and/or exposures is concerned, each member of the population is indistinguishable from one another and so each is a potential unit of observation. For this reason, our data pertaining to this population can be based on measures for any combination of these individual members.

Thus, in choosing the attributes and/or exposures that define a population, we determine our unit of observation. In turn, the population is our unit of analysis. The unit of observation refers to a group from whom we collect data. The unit of analysis is a group about whom we wish to draw conclusions.

The second premise is that all populations are scalable. This allows researchers to expand or contract a population by adding or removing certain attributes or exposures. Our previous example began with the population of "all (200) high-school long-distance runners in Nasser County." We then scaled this down to "all (80) cis-female high-school long-distance runners in Nasser County." Alternatively, this can be scaled up to "all (2,000) high-school long-distance runners in Louisiana." From there, we could continue to "all (10,000) high-school long-distance runners in the Southeastern United States," and so on.

Notice that when scaling up from "all runners in Nasser County" to "all runners in Louisiana," the original population of 200 runners at the county level now become the members of a new population at the state level. Hence, an individual is ordinarily a member of multiple (potential) populations simultaneously. This highlights how the choices that researchers make in defining a population directly impact the results of any study. That which is true of one population at one scale (Nasser County) may not be true of another population at another scale (the state of Louisiana).

Imagine that we believe long-distance running has a negative impact on the resting heart rate for high-school students. We then run a study that includes high-school long-distance runners from 12 Louisiana counties and our results are inconclusive. However, we discover along the way that if we remove the data for three of the 12 counties then *voila!*—magically, we find results more to our liking. It is true that such a maneuver would be hard to conceal and there are professional sanctions for such misdeeds. The take-away for us more fundamentally, however, is that in choosing the scale of one's population a researcher determines her or his unit of analysis.

The third premise of sampling is that all populations are divisible. If populations were not divisible, there would be no reason to draw a sample. For example, no meaningful sample can be retrieved from a jar of 3,000 identical marbles. That which is true for one marble is true for all marbles. A divisible population thus permits comparisons between (and among) a collection of interrelated—but distinguishable—things. This allows us to discover things that are true for the population as a whole and things that may only be true for certain subgroups with distinct attributes and/or exposures. The importance of this premise for bio-statistical analysis cannot be exaggerated and is illustrated in Chapters 4 through 7.

Imagine our population is "all (200) high-school long-distance runners in Nasser County." We thus have 200 persons who are (a) interrelated via certain common attributes and exposures (for example, long-distance running) and (b) divisible into numerous subgroups. Above, we began with the population of "all (200) runners" and derived a population of "all (80) cis-female runners" and then a population of "all (40) senior cis-female runners." We treated each of these as a different population.

Alternatively, we could have retained the original population of "all (200) runners" and broken these populations into subgroups, such as "cis-female runners" and "cis-male runners" or "senior cis-female runners" and "junior cis-female runners." (Note that the term "subgroup" always presumes that the members of the different subgroups all share a common membership in some larger population.) This allows comparisons among the members of the *same population* based on certain attributes and/or exposures that distinguish certain members of the population. This is the entire rationale, for example, for randomized controlled trials.

Examples of divisibility (and subgroups) to be found in Chapters 5 and 6 are distinctions based on gender identity (cis female/cis male), caffeine consumption level (low, moderate, high), and blood type (A, B, and O). It is this divisibility that allows us to compare the resting heart rates of persons who all share one common exposure (long-distance running) yet differ based on certain attributes and/or exposures. By creating subgroups, a researcher thus further fine-tunes her or his choice of unit of observation and unit of analysis.

Let us step back for one moment. Our ability to freely scale a population up or down, combined with its divisibility into subgroups of varying kinds, would appear to seriously compromise the conceptual integrity of a population. What kind of thing is it that can be so easily turned inside out and remade into so many other things? One thing made clear is the importance of the criteria determining a population's unique membership—such as, "all (200) high-school long-distance runners in Zabalaza County."

On the one hand, the purpose of sampling is to better understand our population. On the other hand, the purpose of better understanding our population is to bring further structure and order to the larger world. But does this structure and order follow from certain inherent properties of populations that we discover via different objective tools, such as sampling? Or do these "inherent" properties simply follow from how we subjectively impose structure and order on a chaotic and unpredictable world? Moreover, is this an empirical question? A rational deduction? Or perhaps an ideological preference?

However one answers such questions, sampling clearly offers a powerful tool to bring structure and order to our world. Each act of sampling is a reification of some population (presumably, as an actually existing thing) and a gesture toward order out of chaos. In this sense, we operate at an empirical level. At the same time, each vanishing of a population into a larger population—the move from all high-school long-distance runners in a county to all high-school long-distance runners in a state—confirms the relative, contingent, and provisional nature of a population, and thus the enduring chaos just beneath the order we impose. This we discover by rational deduction.

Then again, the specific details of any particular order seem less important than simply curbing chaos. This is presumably, in part, an ideological choice. In fact, curbing chaos and imposing order are purposes behind all biostatistical tools and techniques. Therefore, it is only right that this artifice should be present (and prominent) at one of the earliest procedural moments (sampling) within biostatistical analysis. Let us now see what this looks like for sampling *vis-à-vis* the subject matter comprising health and medicine.

Sampling techniques are framed as either probability or non-probability. That said, the role of so-called non-probability sampling is extremely limited. Generally speaking, things that are identified by that which they are not—such as non-probability—are not especially well-defined things. We do not refer to a car as a non-bike. We call it what it is, a car. We do not adopt non-dogs. We adopt cats. Only a thing lacking in any unique quality is referred to by qualities that it does not possess. Hence, we have non-probability sampling.

The chief distinguishing quality of probability sampling concerns the likelihood of including members of the population in a sample. Commonly, probability sampling provides an equal likelihood that each member of the population will be selected. That said, there are also probability sampling techniques in which researchers select units (such as clusters) rather than individuals to create their sample. In such cases, it is not that each unit has an equal likelihood of selection. Rather, each unit has a predictable (and calculable) likelihood of selection. An example of this discussed below is cluster sampling.

Not surprisingly, the chief distinguishing quality of non-probability sampling is that each member of the population does *not* have an equal likelihood of selection. You can achieve this goal by any number of "techniques." Three exemplary approaches are wading into a crowd, snowball sampling, and quota sampling. These are common tools for journalists, for instance, seeking varying perspectives for background on a story.

Wading into the crowd is essentially the person-in-the-street interview. This we call convenience sampling. There may be some topic of interest to the general public, such as a new zoning restriction, and local journalists can gather quick reactions from members of the public with this approach. For example, a journalist might attend a county fair and ask 30 people for their opinions about the new zoning restriction. Snowball sampling is a method whereby the people you initially meet at the county fair refer you to certain friends, relatives, or colleagues who share a certain attribute or experience of interest to your study.

The sample that results is thus not only non-representative of any population but, in addition, it is biased toward persons within common social circles.

Lastly, quota sampling is a variation on wading into the crowd that includes attempting to speak with a certain number of persons based on some attribute or experience, such as men *and* women, children *and* adults, Puritans *and* heretics. For example, a new zoning restriction may impact homeowners and renters differently. So a quota sample would ensure that one spoke with an equal number of homeowners and renters. However, these people would not be *representative* of homeowners and renters.

In each of these cases, the population is, at best, poorly defined, and there is no effort (or intent) to create a representative sample. Therefore, each of these approaches has limited value for biostatistical analysis.

The closest we come to so-called non-probability sampling within biostatistical analysis may be case reports and case series. Not surprisingly, such studies are treated as anecdotal and are not considered generalizable. Their use is limited to exploring some newly encountered health phenomenon presenting certain novel features. The purpose of such studies, therefore, is to document these phenomena in scrupulous detail and to frame this *vis-à-vis* our current knowledge of health and medicine. Hence, a case study or case series is a quintessential example of bringing order to chaos.

It is notable that there are no inferential biostatistical tools associated with case reports or case series. These tend to be narrowly empirical studies that make abundant use of descriptive statistics and qualitative accounts. Case studies and case series are thus outliers of a sort. They do not apply inferential statistics. Yet, as hybrid studies that combine qualitative and quantitative elements, they do not fit cleanly within the rubric of descriptive statistics. They are treated as narrative-driven exercises that are primarily qualitative.

This points to a cardinal distinction conventionally drawn between descriptive and inferential statistics within biostatistical analysis (and statistical analysis in general). Here we outline only the basics of this distinction, while exploring the rationale for this division more fully in Chapter 10.

Not surprisingly, descriptive statistics help *describe* a sample or population. This allows us to look for patterns within the data to guide us in how we approach and set up our research. Thus, descriptive statistics use data to summarize the characteristics of a population or sample. Such data might include the mean or median age of a population to gauge the predominance of younger or older persons or the range or standard deviation to estimate the variability of the ages within the population.

Note incidentally that the term "statistic" refers narrowly to data pertaining to a sample and the term "parameter" refers to data for a population. For instance, the mean can be either a sample statistic or a population parameter.

Inferential statistics provide data that assist us with two basic tasks. First, these data allow us to generalize from a sample to a population. For example, if the median weight of our sample of high-school students were 71.4 kilos, we might be able to infer that the mean weight for the population of all high-school students is 71.4 kilos. Second, inferential statistics reveal degrees of probability with regard to a difference (or similarity) between two or more groups that differ based on some attribute or exposure. Such groups include samples and populations or experimental and control groups. In this sense, a "sample" technically differs from a "group." The members of a sample stand in relation to the members of some population. The members of a group stand in relation to the members of another group (or other groups).

Let us then turn to probability sampling. By convention, probability sampling refers to four types of sampling. These are:

- Simple or systematic random sampling.
- Simple or systematic random sampling with clusters (or cluster sampling).
- Simple or systematic random sampling with subgroups (or stratified sampling).
- Simple or systematic random sampling with clusters and subgroups (or stratified cluster sampling).

All four variations are random samples that rely on either simple or systematic techniques for selecting the members of the sample. Two have subgroups, two do not. Two have clusters, two do not. One has both subgroups and clusters. Let us consider each of these, in turn, and see how each demonstrates aspects of the three premises of sampling and populations.

Simple random sampling and systematic random sampling differ by their manner of selecting the members of a sample. In each case, we begin with a defined population and a list of all persons in that population. For simple random sampling, we might assign a random number to each person in the population. Numbers are then drawn by some random technique in which all numbers have an equal likelihood of selection. The persons associated with each number then become members of the simple random sample.

At times, the number of persons in a population may be very large. For example, our population may be all 20,000 workers in a major hospital system. Systematic random sampling may be more feasible in such cases. Here we obtain a list of all 20,000 workers and, depending on the sample size we desire, we select every 20th, every 50th, or every 75th person. Given the broad availability today of such lists in electronic form, along with ordinary computing capacity, the simple random sampling technique is increasingly the default option. For this reason, we will focus here on simple random sampling.

Again, simple random sampling is always preceded by defining one's population. However, discussions of this sampling technique too often simply assume that the often complex process of defining a population has taken place—and it has. This complex process thus merits one's attention. Our simple random sampling technique is the first explicit recognition of the first premise of sampling, that a population is defined by certain attributes and/or exposures that distinguish its members from persons outside that population. Thus, the formation of a sample is the actual method by which this premise transitions from an idea to become a concrete feature of a study.

Consequently, sampling is not just a set of procedural steps. It is the way in which a certain population is constituted and represented. Of course, depending upon the historical treatment and experiences of that population, this may carry certain moral or political considerations beyond clinical precision. For example, if working with populations of Lakota or Seminole peoples, it is essential to work within the framework of how these peoples themselves understand the criteria for inclusion in their population.

There is one further initial concern. This is the technique of sampling with replacement. This technique is in order when we are drawing multiple samples from the same population and we want all members to have an equal likelihood of selection for any of these samples. We, therefore, return all members of each sample back into the population before selecting the next sample. The common purpose of this is to estimate some parameter for a population based on a great many samples. (This is discussed in Chapter 9 and is especially relevant for configurations #1 and #6.) Here we are discussing how a single sample is drawn and so sampling with replacement does not apply.

The second probability sampling technique is simple random sampling with clusters. (This is often shortened to cluster sampling.) Again, in theory, this could be carried out with systematic random sampling. The difference between this technique (with clusters) and the previous technique (without clusters) is the manner by which the physical (or virtual) location of the members of the population influences how researchers recruit them for the sample.

While conventionally there is an emphasis on spatial or "physical" clusters, it is also the case that online (or virtual) clusters can serve the same purpose. Examples include online affinity groups who follow sports or fashion and are distinguishable by the team or clothing designer who they follow.

This sampling technique presumes the identification of (a) specific population attributes and/or exposures and (b) a technique for random selection. This is the same technique detailed above for simple random sampling.

A "cluster" is any site where members of the population congregate. Common clusters include built environments (such as townships or neighborhoods) and/or physical structures (such as churches or schools). For instance, a statewide study of "all (2,000) high-school long-distance runners in Louisiana" might treat each of the 63 counties in Louisiana as a cluster. Our simple random sampling technique is then applied to these 63 counties. Based on this, we randomly select 23 counties to represent the 63 counties and all 785 runners from these 23 counties form the sample for our statewide study, representing 2,000 runners.

To further clarify, for simple random sampling with clusters, *the process of selecting clusters* is randomized and all the members of a cluster enter the sample. It is each cluster that has an equal likelihood of selection. By contrast, for simple random sampling (without clusters), *the process of selecting individual members of the population* is randomized and each person who is selected enters the sample. It is each individual member of the population that has an equal likelihood of selection.

Naturally, it would be very unusual for a population to be equally distributed across all counties. Some counties may have very large populations and some may have very small populations. However, unless there is something unique about persons in certain counties, it does not matter if we select all small counties or all large counties as long as we meet our optimal sample size requirement. If there is something unique about the residents of different counties, we would want to switch to either a simple random sample with subgroups or a simple random sample with clusters and subgroups.

Importantly, while certain mechanics differ between simple random sampling (with or without clusters), the underlying rationale for each is identical. This is because *a cluster is NOT a subgroup*. The population attributes and/or exposures of interest for the runners in our statewide study are identical in every county—"any high-school long-distance runner." Thus, no matter what combination of counties we select, the members of the population drawn into our sample share the same attributes and/or exposures that define our population of interest.

Reliance on a county—or any other cluster—is largely a matter of convenience. If it simplifies sampling while meeting the requirements of simple random sampling, do it. If not, do not. The unit of observation (the individual runner) and the unit of analysis (all runners in the state of Louisiana) are identical for simple random sampling, *with or without a cluster*. Recall that a unit of analysis is the group about whom we wish to draw conclusions. A unit of observation is the group (or individual) from whom we collect data. Generally speaking, a cluster is *never* a unit of observation or a unit of analysis.

At times, we may want to take advantage of the second premise of a population, its scalability, and shift our study from the state level to the county level. Imagine our population is "all (200) high-school long-distance runners in Zabalaza County." In that case, an obvious choice for clusters would be the 41 high schools in that county with long-distance running teams. We would then apply simple random sampling techniques to select 11 of these high schools. All 62 runners in those 11 high schools would then represent a sample from our county-wide population of "all (200) high-school long-distance runners." Again, with or without clusters, the unit of observation for our study remains the individual runner and the unit of analysis remains all runners in Zabalaza County.

The third probability sampling technique is simple random sampling with subgroups. (This is often shortened to stratified random sampling.) This technique demonstrates the third premise of populations, their divisibility. Simple random sampling with subgroups again presumes the identification of (a) specific population attributes and/or exposures and (b) a technique for random sampling.

The technique in this case requires that we identify certain subgroups (or strata) within the population and draw a random sample from each of these. Importantly, "subgroup" is not the conventional term for this sampling technique. Subgroups are referred to as "strata" and the technique itself is thus "stratified random sampling." However, the term strata is both obscure and, worse, it carries a connotation of hierarchy (or layers) that may or may not fit a given population. Thus, we find "subgroup" more suitable.

Imagine that our population is "all (200) high-school long-distance runners in Zabalaza County." We decide to create one sample of 60 runners that includes two subgroups within the population. The first subgroup is 30 cis-female runners. The second subgroup is 30 cis-male runners. We create the sample—and each subgroup—via simple random sampling. This allows us to compare the resting heart rates of the two subgroups who differ based only on the attribute of gender identity.

Now suppose that our results indicate no significant differences in mean resting heart rates. However, we suspect that age may be a factor. We again create a sample with two subgroups of 30 cis-female and 30 cis-male runners. But this time we assure that each of these subgroups is further subdivided into 15 freshmen and sophomores and 15 juniors and seniors.

To do this, we reset the scale by now creating two subgroups of "all (80) cis-female" and "all (120) cis-male runners." In this manner, each of these subgroups is then treated as a population. The first is defined as "all (80) cis-female long-distance runners in Zabalaza County." The second is defined as "all (120) cis-male high-school runners in Zabalaza County."

From the first population we create two subgroups of 15 cis-female runners who are freshmen and sophomores and 15 cis-female runners who are juniors and seniors. From the second population we do likewise and create two subgroups of 15 cis-male runners who are freshmen and sophomores and 15 cis-male runners who are juniors and seniors.

Our results now indicate that there are differences among these four subgroups regarding their mean resting heart rates. Cis-female runners who are freshmen and sophomores have a mean resting heart rate that is significantly above the means for the other three subgroups. This example of simple random sampling with subgroups thus demonstrates how both the divisibility and scalability of populations are essential for sampling.

Obviously, these choices of subgroup are arbitrary. We can choose any subgroup we wish, as long as it is available within the population. This follows from the premise that a population is divisible. However, because the population is also scalable some intriguing juxtapositions emerge. In relation to the world outside the population of high-school long-distance runners in Zabalaza County, each of the two original subgroups (cis-female and cis-male runners) is a population unto its own. In relation to the population of all high-school long-distance runners in Zabalaza County, each is a subgroup. In relation to one another—absent any reference to Zabalaza County—each is again a population.

Oddly, it is only in relation to itself that each subgroup is a "sample." For instance, the subgroup of (30) cis-female runners is a sample that is representative of "all (80) cis-female high-school long-distance runners in Zabalaza County." Hence, it is only in relation to itself—our 30 cis-female runners in relation to the 80 cis-female runners from which they were selected—that a subgroup is a sample.

This is because a subgroup is itself not *representative* of anything. It is simply a collection of persons within a defined population who share some attribute and/or exposure that distinguishes them from all other members of the population. This, of course, tracks pretty closely with the definition of a population—a collection of persons who share some attribute and/or exposure that distinguishes them from all others outside the population.

The fourth sampling technique, simple random sampling with clusters *and with* subgroups, follows from what has already been discussed with the first three techniques. This sampling technique mirrors simple random sampling with subgroups (and *without* clusters) except that (a) we select clusters for our sample, not the individual members of a population, and (b) we select clusters that are divisible into subgroups. Hence, this combines what is commonly referred to as cluster sampling and stratified random sampling.

For example, imagine that our population is "all (2,000) high-school long-distance runners in the state of Louisiana." We choose all (63) counties in Louisiana as our clusters. We first select 23 counties via our simple random sampling technique. We then identify two subgroups in each cluster—again, such as cis-female runners and cis-male runners. We now gather data for all members of the two subgroups in each of the 23 counties. This generates data that allow us to compare all cis-female and cis-male runners across the 2,000 high-school long-distance runners in the state of Louisiana.

It may be prudent to reiterate two fundamental assumptions of sampling with clusters. First, all members of a cluster are members of some larger population that includes persons outside that cluster. Second, membership in a specific cluster is NOT itself an attribute and/or exposure that distinguishes an individual from other persons in that larger population who are not in that cluster. Thus, if some attribute and/or exposure is an exclusive criterion for membership in a cluster, then this is not a cluster. It is a subgroup.

Where matters now stand

Conventional wisdom holds that research begins with a research question. More accurately, however, it seems that basic research—or at least that undertaken in anticipation of biostatistical analysis—begins less with a research question and more with practical considerations of the research circumstances. These circumstances are evaluated for their proximity to the premises of a randomized controlled trial. Specifically, is it practical to randomly assign participants to an experimental group and a control group? Are we able to hide this assignment from both participants and researchers? Can we exercise effective control over each participant's exposure to different risk factors?

These practical considerations, in fact, have two effects. First, they create a bias toward selecting research topics conducive to circumstances accommodating the conditions for randomized controlled trials. This follows, in part, from the desire to produce a publishable study. Second, when circumstances are not ideal, there is an incentive to force the issue and find half measures that imitate the conditions of randomized controlled trials.

Furthermore, notice that for the sake of our example of a randomized controlled trial above, we created a representative sample from among long-distance runners across Elizavetgrad County. However, the principal purpose of each of these study designs is not a representative sample *per se*. Rather, the purpose is to devise protocols that isolate certain attributes and exposures as a means to prepare data for biostatistical analysis.

Thus, notwithstanding specific differences in protocols, the overriding purpose of each study design is to identify risk factors (or protective factors, such as vaccines) associated with some outcome. These factors include both attributes and exposures. Once these factors have been identified, accounted for, and measured in a manner consistent with the rules and techniques of biostatistical analysis, the level of probability that each is associated with the outcome is determined.

As described above, there are important differences between the ecological research design and the first three research designs (randomized controlled trials, cohort designs, case-control designs). The main purpose of these three research designs is to generate data for biostatistical analysis, while ecological studies are more exploratory and descriptive and less hypothesis-driven. Consequently, certain differences between ecological studies and these three study designs help to further illustrate how the protocols (and assumptions) of randomized controlled trials influence interpretations of these other study designs.

For instance, it is not that ecological factors are absent from these three studies. However, ecological factors are *implicitly* treated as if they are attributes of individuals and not exposures. For instance, Daiyu is identified as the type of person who lives in a neighborhood with or without a bank, with or without a grocery store with fresh produce, or with or without an unemployment rate above 10%. The features of the ecological space are thus transferred to the persons living in that space.

These features become attributes attached to a person to permit comparisons with persons who live in other ecological spaces. These features are treated as the properties of people precisely because the social origins (or context) of such features are omitted from the analysis. Our commonsense language might misplace this attribute, suggesting that, "this is a poor neighborhood." But a proper study, if framed for purposes of biostatistical analysis, would clarify that, "this is a neighborhood where poor people are gathered."

This treatment of ecological features as attributes of the persons living in a particular ecological space points to a further peculiarity. The first three study designs examine associations between a person's exposure (or non-exposure) to certain risk factors and that person having a certain condition, such as diabetes. And, naturally, these studies also consider associations between persons with or without certain (conventional) attributes—such as age or gender identity—and that person having a certain condition. However, in the case of attributes, this introduces almost the reverse situation of that when considering ecological features as risk factors.

For instance, clearly age and BMI are integral biological attributes (or measures) of a human being. Each of us has an age. Each of us has a BMI. Yet, for purposes of biostatistical analysis, we must treat these as attributes *external* to any one human being. Our commonsense language may suggest that, "Daiyu is 44 years old." For research purposes, however, it is more accurate to say that, "Daiyu belongs to that class of persons who have lived 44 years."

Framing Daiyu's age as external to her, allows us to treat it as a peculiar type of exposure. Just as we may want to know the rate of lung cancer among smokers, we may want to know the rate of osteoporosis among persons who fit the category of being 44 years old. In other words, a person's age does not belong to her or him. Rather, a person belongs to a category of people who have lived a certain number of years.

Further mischief ensues when we move from biological attributes to social or cultural attributes, such as gender identity or race. Every conceivable effort is made to construe these as biological categories—or at least as objective categories beyond the reach of subjective judgment. That this is not conceptually possible and, therefore, the entire world of subjective, socially constructed identities appear to lie outside the ken of biostatistical analysis is a story for another day. That said, all this only reinforces the need for a temporary willful suspension of disbelief as a premise for conducting even the most rudimentary biostatistical analysis.

We see then that these study designs reflect and reify the troublesome heterogeneity of the actually existing social world and our best efforts to remap that world to better match the homogeneity and regularity of the natural world—for which the tools and techniques of biostatistical analysis are ideally suited. Put differently, a major goal of these study designs is to bring the collection and production of data into alignment, as closely as possible, with the collection and production of data *vis-à-vis* a randomized controlled trial. This is because this is the study design closest in kinship to the natural sciences. It may be true that only God can make a tree. But only a biostatistical researcher can see that tree and view it as made in her or his own image.

When beginning this chapter we recognized that regression analysis was an essential tool for the biostatistical analysis of health and medicine. But we also understood that this tool did not originate from—and was not unique to—the subject matter of health and medicine. Indeed, regression analysis is a general mathematical tool that can be applied to most any subject of investigation. Reversing our steps, we found that the choice of regression analysis—or any other biostatistical tool—actually *precedes* and is a determinant of one's choice of study design.

Upon further scrutiny of these study designs, it is evident that most of these are mere exercises in isolating attributes and exposures to better link these to a certain outcome. Cohort studies and case-control studies, for example, are efforts to better approximate the rarefied experimental premises of randomized controlled trials. The unspoken role of all these study designs is thus to provide the muscle to force the subject matter to obey the mathematical rules of biostatistical analysis. Hence, our instinct to move backwards in the process was correct. But it seems we may not have gone back far enough.

For this, we must further regress to the actual original research conditions that confront our subject matter as objects of investigation. This is the moment prior to both the introduction of regression analysis and the choice of study design.

Confronting the original research conditions lands us at the broad intersection of those chaotic circumstances to which we must bring order to move forward. In this case, to "bring order" implies reconfiguring the subject matter before us to have it better align with the tools and techniques of biostatistical analysis and other such tools retrieved from the natural sciences. This search for order leads us to nine constructs for the mathematization of health and medicine. We label these constructs "configurations."

Very simply, a configuration results from a contrived reorganization of certain inherently qualitative and contingent subject matter. Each configuration invokes specific tools of investigation appropriate for that configuration. For instance, regression analysis can be reframed—and reintroduced—as a tool that addresses the analytical needs of two particular configurations, configurations #5 and #8.

Thus reborn, regression analysis is no longer an indifferent and generic set of abstract mathematical operations. It is a specialized instrument to interpret material that has been lifted up from its original context and origins and reconfigured as an orderly collection of quantified things, much like happens to objects from the world of natural sciences. A cohort study is no longer understood as a fluid set of protocols that can be adapted to certain research questions. It is a set of rigid protocols to which muddled and haphazard research circumstances must adapt to better isolate particular attributes or exposures *vis-à-vis* some outcome.

Integral to all this, of course, is the miracle of one's willful suspension of disbelief. Without this, we would have pure fetish. Consideration of configurations makes this all the more evident by laying bare the project of biostatistical analysis as a deliberate and strategic distortion. Indeed, the nine configurations introduced in Chapter 4 can be distinguished, in part, by their manner of adapting different subject matter from health and medicine for various reductive protocols originating from the natural sciences. Let us now turn to these configurations to help us better understand the processes and consequences of this mathematization of health and medicine.

Configurations for Biostatistical Analysis
Conceptual Matters

Our aim in this chapter is to provide a clear and complete—yet reasonably succinct—overview of all tools and techniques required of biostatistical analysis at an introductory level. To do so, we introduce (and organize) these tools and techniques as elements of nine "configurations." Each configuration is a unique combination of four basic elements of biostatistical research. Hence, the nine configurations allow us, first, to present the essential tools and techniques for introductory biostatistical analysis and, second, to demonstrate how varying the arrangement of these four elements allows us to consider a range of different research questions. These four elements are:

- The type of outcome (or dependent) variable—continuous, dichotomous, ordinal, or categorical.
- The number of groups.
- The type of relationship between groups (dependent or independent).
- The number of causal (or independent) variables.

Table 4.1 presents the nine configurations and details the unique arrangement of these four elements for each. The type of outcome variable weighs heavily in determining which biostatistical tools, techniques, and tests that we deploy. This is, therefore, the primary element organizing these configurations. We have five configurations with continuous outcome variables, three with dichotomous outcome variables, and one with ordinal or categorical outcome variables.

Importantly, biostatistical research largely hinges on the relationship between one or more causal (or independent) variable(s) and one outcome (or dependent) variable. With the exception of configurations #1 and #6, the nine configurations can be seen most simply as variations on this relationship between causal and outcome variables. This begins with the type of outcome variable that then shapes the types of measures (means versus proportions) and the types of tests (a two-sample t test versus a chi square test of independence) that are available to us.

Second in importance is the number of groups. Each group represents the presence, absence, or level of some causal variable. For example, groups 1, 2, and 3, respectively, may consume zero daily caffeine beverages, two daily caffeine beverages, and four or more daily caffeine beverages. Not surprisingly, with regard to the number of groups, it is mathematical rationale that guides our selection of an appropriate biostatistical tool or technique.

Remarkably, these two features—the type of outcome variable and the number of groups—account for nearly all variation among the nine configurations. The third feature distinguishing configurations is the nature of the relationships between groups (dependent or independent). This is certainly important. However, it is only configuration #3 that

DOI: 10.4324/9781003316985-4

Table 4.1 Elements of the nine configurations

	Outcome variable	Number of groups	Relation of groups	Independent variables	Confidence intervals	Hypothesis testing	Type of analysis
#1	Continuous	1	–	1	Yes	No	Univariate
#2	Continuous	2	Independent	1	Yes	Yes	Bivariate
#3	Continuous	1 or 2	Dependent	1	Yes	Yes	Bivariate
#4	Continuous	3+	Independent	1	No	Yes	ANOVA
#5	Continuous	2+	Independent	3+	No	Yes	Regression
#6	Dichotomous	1	–	1	Yes	No	Univariate
#7	Dichotomous	2	Independent	1	Yes	Yes	Bivariate
#8	Dichotomous	2+	Independent	3+	No	Yes	Regression
#9	Ordinal or categorical	2+	Independent	1	No	Yes	Chi square

operates with dependent relationships between groups. (We explore the consequences of dependent versus independent relationships between groups below.)

The fourth feature is the number of causal (or independent) variables. Again, while quite important, this only pertains to configuration #5 (and multiple linear regression) and configuration #8 (and multiple logistic regression). All other configurations operate with one causal variable, though some have a single causal variable with multi-levels, such as configurations #4 and #9.

There are two further considerations regarding causal variables when working through these nine configurations. First, the causal variable always takes the form of either an attribute or an exposure. Second, the causal variable can be continuous, dichotomous, ordinal, or categorical. Both of these characteristics are present in the nine configurations, however, neither of these help to distinguish between configurations. (Note that, technically, configurations #1 and #6 do not have "causal" variables. They examine the distribution of a certain variable within a population.)

Each configuration will be approached from two angles. The first angle is conceptual. For this, we explore the presuppositions behind each configuration and how a configuration takes up and reconstitutes certain subject matter as a prelude to its absorption into biostatistical analysis. This makes it possible, for example, to frame a causal variable *vis-à-vis* an outcome variable. The second angle is technical. For this, we detail the mathematical tools, techniques, and tests that each configuration adopts in order to apply its subject matter to certain research questions. The purpose of the present chapter is to address the conceptual content. The purpose of Chapters 5, 6, and 7 is to address the technical content.

As promised, each configuration will work with examples that draw from the familiar scenario of our intrepid high-school long-distance runners. Again, our purpose behind this is to better steady the reader's attention on the conceptual differences between configurations by minimizing the shifting details of different scenarios.

There are two final considerations for Table 4.1. The column for "type of analysis" identifies four types—univariate, bivariate, regression, and chi square. The term univariate is slightly misleading. The prefix "uni" implies an interest in one variable. In truth, we often consider a variety of variables for univariate analysis. However, we treat these individually and not in relation to other variables. For example, if we collect the age, height, weight, and hat size of 200 persons this would be univariate analysis, insofar as we record these measures to merely describe a sample of 200 persons and not to relate these to a person's diet, income, or zip code.

When we attempt to link one measure (or variable), such as age, with another, such as weight, this is bivariate analysis. This requires two variables and the goal for bivariate analysis is to determine how one variable covaries with another variable. An example of covariation might be the relation between long-distance running and her or his resting heart rate.

When we increase the number of variables explaining a person's resting heart rate (beyond long-distance running), then it is advantageous to shift from bivariate analysis to regression analysis. This allows us to understand how other factors, such as caffeine consumption, may also influence a person's resting heart rate. Regression analysis can also indicate when one variable (long-distance running) may be impacted by another variable (caffeine consumption). Perhaps, the impact of long-distance running on a person's resting heart rate is severely reduced by high levels of caffeine consumption.

Lastly, we have chi square analysis. This is helpful when we want to compare the distribution of responses across several categories, such as a low, moderate, or high resting heart rate. Over the next few chapters we will see how different circumstances call for different types of analysis.

Importantly, in the course of examining these nine configurations, we introduce two technical frameworks that are essential for biostatistical analysis. These are confidence interval estimation and hypothesis testing. In fact, it is here that we begin.

Confidence interval estimation and hypothesis testing

Confidence interval estimation and hypothesis testing address related, yet distinct, questions. In applying these frameworks it is, therefore, helpful to present each side by side for purposes of comparison. This will allow us to simultaneously expand and build upon certain aspects of a scenario. It remains a question, however, how much this expansion follows from the complexity of the subject matter comprising health and medicine and how much the complexity of the subject matter is brought to heel by the mathematical rationale of these frameworks.

It will surprise no one that confidence interval estimation produces intervals. An interval is a range of values that aims to capture the true value of some measure. This measure could be the true mean weight of a population of high-school students based on the mean weight of a sample of students from that population. Or it might be the true difference in resting heart rates between the members of an experimental group and the members of a control group. The "confidence" of an estimated confidence interval refers to a degree of certainty—a confidence level—that the researcher chooses. Commonly, researchers choose a 95% confidence level. Thus, one might say, "We estimate, at a 95% confidence level, that the true mean weight for all high-school students lies between 68.4 and 74.4 kilos."

Having said that, it is technically the case that this 95% confidence level does *not* refer to the actual interval from our one sample. Rather, this refers to the probability that if we drew 100 samples of high-school students, 95% of those samples would produce an interval that contained the true mean weight of the population of high-school students—and 5% of the samples would not. Thus, we do *not* produce a "probability" for the interval range of any particular sample. To capture this subtle distinction, convention instructs us to adopt a lawyerly turn-of-phrase, substituting "confidence" for "probability."

Whereas confidence interval estimation produces intervals, hypothesis testing gives us "significant differences." The principal measure of a significant difference is the *p*-value. The *p*-value pertains to the likelihood of finding a difference of a certain size. Thus, to grasp the p-value, we must first understand the nature of the hypothesis that is being tested. Hypothesis testing is a lot like professional wrestling. During the pre-match interview, the wrestler uses a lot of overheated rhetoric describing how he will pulverize his opponent. Then he looks into the camera and tearfully pledges that all he really wants is a good, clean fight to prove that he is the better wrestler. But once the match begins it does not seem like he really wanted a good, clean fight after all.

For hypothesis testing, our researcher acts in similar fashion. She begins by boastfully introducing some miracle new drug that will crush its opponent. Then, turning to the imaginary camera, she sheepishly begins by hypothesizing, well in fact there is a good chance that this drug will make no difference. This we call the null hypothesis. Then, half-ashamed, as a token, she offers an alternative hypothesis that maybe her drug will make some small difference, saying, "All I want is a good, clean competition."

The basic idea of hypothesis testing is simple. Imagine our high-school long-distance runners are divided into two groups of 15 runners. Group 1 is the experimental group and its members consume large amounts of caffeine over a six-week period. Group 2 is the control group and its members consume zero caffeine over the same six-week period. If the mean resting heart rate for group 1 is higher than the mean resting heart rate for group 2 after six weeks, this indicates *some* difference between the two groups that differ based on caffeine consumption. If the size of this difference in mean resting heart rates meets a certain threshold, this indicates a *statistically significant* difference.

This threshold indicates the probability of finding a difference of this size. The smaller the probability of finding a difference of this size, the more likely that caffeine consumption is associated with the difference in resting heart rates. By popular acclamation, the appropriate smallness of this probability is a p-value of 0.05 or smaller. A p-value of 0.05 indicates that there is only a 5% probability of finding a difference of that size. Hence, we say that there is a 95% probability that the difference—whatever it is—indicates a true difference between the two groups. Technically, to be statistically significant, the p-value must be *less than* 0.05.

Our nine configurations

To proceed, let us first pause to bring together three essential elements of biostatistical analysis now available to us:

- study designs;
- confidence interval estimation and hypothesis testing; and
- configurations.

Study designs indicate the data that will be generated. The purpose of a study design is to assure that a research question is properly framed and that the subject matter is suitably adapted for research protocols that originated in the natural sciences. The overriding concern of these designs is to provide conceptual techniques for linking attributes or exposures (as causal factors) with an outcome variable that allows us to gauge the impact of the former on the latter. A randomized controlled trial remains the gold standard for study designs in this regard.

Confidence interval estimation and hypothesis testing help us to interpret the meaning of the data that are generated. The purpose of an estimated confidence interval or a hypothesis test is to determine the likelihood that certain attributes or exposures have had an impact on some outcome variable. They provide mathematical techniques for measuring degrees of certainty with regard to any difference between two or more groups whose members differ based on some attribute or exposure. The estimated confidence interval and the p-value are the principal forms of "proof" for any difference for confidence interval estimation and hypothesis testing, respectively.

Configurations identify the conditions for linking the generation of data (study designs) with the interpretation of data (confidence interval estimation and hypothesis testing). The purpose of a configuration is to distinguish between nine types of research projects that differ principally based on the nature of how attributes or exposures are linked to an outcome variable. (Configurations #1 and #6 compare samples and populations technically without an outcome variable.) Configurations identify the specific biostatistical tools, techniques, and tests for analyzing this link when applying either confidence interval estimation or hypothesis testing.

The type of outcome variable and the number of groups are the primary determinants for which biostatistical tools, techniques, and tests to apply. All but two of the nine configurations are compatible with hypothesis testing. Five are compatible with confidence interval estimation. Linear and logistic regression are examples of tools that make use of hypothesis testing, but not confidence interval estimation. These apply to configurations #5 and #8.

What follows is a description of the conceptual content of each of the nine configurations. In particular, we want to know how each configuration contributes to biostatistical analysis and what types of problems it helps us resolve. For this, we first identify a configuration's general goal. This distinguishes it from the other configurations. We also specify the four elements distinguishing each configuration and identify its principal biostatistical tool or test.

For example, when a configuration employs confidence interval estimation, the biostatistical tool will be an estimation equation. When a configuration works with hypothesis testing, there will be a specific biostatistical test, such as a one-sample t-test.

There are important differences between the purposes for the use of confidence interval estimation and hypothesis testing, even when addressing the same configuration. Given this, we encounter competing methods that generate distinct, yet related, findings. Below, we explain these differing purposes and then provide examples that fit a purpose pertaining to either confidence interval estimation or hypothesis testing. This allows us to better illustrate the concepts behind the technical operations that are detailed in Chapters 5, 6, and 7.

In this sense, Chapters 4, 5, 6, and 7 can be understood as parts of a single unit. Their presentation across four chapters is for the better digestion of a great many details. The operational logic and guiding conceptual principles are largely contained here in the present chapter. We begin.

Configuration #1

Goal: To estimate a population mean for some continuous variable based on a sample mean.

(Configurations #1 and #6 are similar in form and differ only regarding the type of outcome variable. The examples for both configurations are, therefore, alike for purposes of comparison.)

outcome variable:	continuous
number and relation of groups:	one group
number of independent variables:	one independent variable
biostatistical tool or test:	estimation equation; one-sample t-test

Confidence interval estimation and configuration #1

PURPOSE

We apply confidence interval estimation to configuration #1 to discover an unknown population mean based on a sample mean. For this, we must estimate—at a certain confidence level—a range of values to capture the true population mean.

EXAMPLE

There are 200 high-school long-distance runners in Lumumba County. We have limited health data for these runners. We want to know the mean resting heart rate for all high-school long-distance runners in Lumumba County. For this, we recruit a random sample of 40 high-school long-distance runners and find a mean resting heart rate of 73 bpm for this sample, with a standard deviation of 8.0.

Given these results, we must estimate—at a certain confidence level—a range of values that aims to capture the true mean resting heart rate for all high-school long-distance runners in Lumumba County.

HYPOTHESIS TESTING AND CONFIGURATION #1

We cannot apply hypothesis testing to this scenario, without more data to construct null and alternative hypotheses.

Importantly, there is another scenario that can be confused with both configurations #1 and #6. Imagine there are 200 high-school long-distance runners in Lumumba County and we have limited health data for these runners. It happens that we have statewide data indicating that four years earlier the mean resting heart rate for all high-school long-distance runners was 70 bpm. We want to know if the current mean resting heart rate for all high-school long-distance runners in Lumumba County differs from the earlier statewide data.

Technically, what we have here is a comparison between a mean resting heart rate for population 1 and a mean resting heart rate for a sample that is taken from population 2. We infer the mean for population 2 based on the sample mean. Given this, we want to know if there is any difference between the mean of population 1 and the mean for population 2.

Therefore, we are comparing the mean of two populations that differ by attribute or exposure. In this case, they differ by the attribute of different "ages" marked by a four-year passage of time. We want to know if the mean for these two populations, four years apart, differs. Thus, this scenario better fits configuration #2 (for a continuous outcome variable) and configuration #7 (for a dichotomous outcome variable).

This is equally true for configuration #9 (for ordinal or categorical outcome variables). Therefore, we include this scenario as example C for configurations #2 and #9 and hypothesis testing to illustrate this application. We also include it as configuration #7, operation 7.0.

Configuration #2

Goal: To compare the means of two independent groups for some continuous outcome variable based on a difference in attribute or exposure.

(Configuration #2 and configuration #7 are similar in form and differ only regarding the type of outcome variable. The examples for both configurations are, therefore, alike for purposes of comparison.)

outcome variable:	continuous
number and relation of groups:	two independent groups
number of independent variables:	one independent variable
biostatistical tool or test:	estimation equation; two-sample t-test

Confidence interval estimation and configuration #2

PURPOSE

a.   One reason we apply confidence interval estimation to configuration #2 is to detect any difference in the means between two independent groups that differ based on some attribute, such as gender identity. For this, we estimate—at a certain confidence level—a range of values that aims to capture any difference in means.

b.   A second reason we apply confidence interval estimation to configuration #2 is to detect any difference in the means between two independent groups that differ based on some exposure, such as caffeine consumption. For this, we estimate—at a certain confidence level—a range of values that aims to capture any difference in means.

EXAMPLE

a.   There are 200 high-school long-distance runners in Mandela County. Of these, 110 identify as cis males and 90 as cis females. We want to know if there is any difference between the mean resting heart rates of our cis-male and cis-female runners. We recruit a random sample of 40 cis-male and 40 cis-female high-school long-distance runners. We find a mean resting heart rate of 70 bpm for cis males, with a standard deviation of 9.0, and 76 bpm for cis females, with a standard deviation of 7.0.

   Given these results, we must estimate—at a certain confidence level—a range of values that aims to capture any difference in means between these two groups.

b.   There are 200 high-school long-distance runners in Mandela County. We are concerned that caffeine consumption may be elevating the resting heart rate of our runners. We recruit a random sample of 80 high-school long-distance runners and randomly assign 40 to group 1 and 40 to group 2.

   Over six weeks, group 1 consumes three caffeine beverages per day and group 2 consumes no caffeine beverages. We record the resting heart rate for all persons in both groups after six weeks. We find a mean resting heart rate of 83 bpm for group 1, with a standard deviation of 9.0, and a mean resting heart rate of 73 bpm for group 2, with a standard deviation of 7.0.

   Given these results, we must estimate—at a certain confidence level—a range of values that aims to capture any difference in means between these two groups.

Hypothesis testing and configuration #2

PURPOSE

a.   One reason we apply hypothesis testing to configuration #2 is to detect any difference between the means of two independent groups that differ based on some attribute, such as gender identity. If a difference is found, we then calculate the probability of finding a difference of that size between the means.

b.   A second reason we apply hypothesis testing to configuration #2 is to detect any difference between the means of two independent groups that differ based on some exposure, such as caffeine consumption. If a difference is found, we then calculate the probability of finding a difference of that size between the means.

c. A third reason we apply hypothesis testing to configuration #2 is to detect any difference between the means of two populations that differ in attribute or exposure based on data from population 1 and data from a representative sample from population 2. If a difference is found, we then calculate the probability of finding a difference of that size between the means.

EXAMPLE

a. There are 200 high-school long-distance runners in Mandela County. Of these, 110 identify as cis males and 90 as cis females. We want to know if there is any difference between the mean resting heart rates of our cis-male and cis-female runners. We recruit a random sample of 40 cis-male and 40 cis-female high-school long-distance runners. We find a mean resting heart rate of 70 bpm for cis males, with a standard deviation of 9.0, and 76 bpm for cis females, with a standard deviation of 7.0.

Given these results, we must determine the probability of finding a difference of this size between the means of these two groups.

b. There are 200 high-school long-distance runners in Mandela County. We are concerned that caffeine consumption may be elevating the resting heart rates of our runners. We recruit a random sample of 80 high-school long-distance runners and randomly assign 40 to group 1 and 40 to group 2. Note that group 1 and group 2 differ based on an exposure, as opposed to an attribute in example A.

Over six weeks, group 1 consumes three caffeine beverages per day and group 2 consumes no caffeine beverages. We record the resting heart rate for all persons in both groups after six weeks. We find a mean resting heart rate of 83 bpm for group 1, with a standard deviation of 9.0, and a mean resting heart rate of 73 bpm for group 2, with a standard deviation of 7.0.

Given these results, we must determine the probability of finding a difference of this size between the means of these two groups.

c. There are 200 high-school long-distance runners in Lumumba County. We have limited health data for these runners. It happens that we have statewide data indicating that four years earlier the mean resting heart rate for all high-school long-distance runners was 70 bpm. We want to know if the current mean resting heart rate for all high-school long-distance runners in Lumumba County differs from the earlier statewide data.

Given this, we hypothesize that the current mean resting heart rate for all high-school long-distance runners in Lumumba County is 70 bpm. We then recruit a random sample of 40 high-school long-distance runners and find a mean resting heart rate for this sample of 73 bpm, with a standard deviation of 8.0.

Thus, we have data for two populations. The mean resting heart rate for population 1 is 70 bpm. The mean resting heart rate for a sample from population 2 is 73 bpm.

Given these results, we must determine the probability of finding a difference of this size between the means of these two populations.

Configuration #3

Goal: To assess the mean of the differences between scores either (a) for the same person before and after some exposure or (b) for matched pairs of persons from two dependent groups before and after some exposure for one of the two groups.

outcome variable: continuous
number and relation of groups: one group (before/after design) or two dependent
                                           groups (matched pairs)
number of independent variables: one
biostatistical tool or tests: estimation equation; pair-sample *t*-test

Confidence interval estimation and configuration #3

Purpose

The reason we apply confidence interval estimation to configuration #3 is to assess the impact of some exposure on some continuous outcome. We compare two dependent groups that are as identical as possible. One group is exposed to some risk factor and the other is not. For this purpose, there are two scenarios.

One scenario is a before-and-after study. In this study, we compare a group of individuals with themselves before and after some exposure. Each participant is matched with her/himself for a before-and-after comparison.

A second scenario is a matched-pairs study. In this study, we recruit one set of participants who will receive an exposure. This is group 1. We then recruit a second set of participants for group 2 who receive no exposure. Those in group 2 are chosen so that the attributes of each person match the attributes of a person in group 1. These attributes include personal characteristics, such as age, race, zip code, etc.

Example

a. (This example illustrates a before-and-after study.) There are reports from Nyerere County of improved cardiovascular health among its student athletes. We recruit 40 high-school long-distance runners from across Nyerere County to detect if long-distance running impacts a student's resting heart rate. First, we measure the resting heart rate for each runner before the track season. Second, each runner receives an exposure. In this case, the exposure is all those activities comprising the track season.

Third, we measure the resting heart rate for each runner after the exposure. Fourth, we calculate the differences between each runner's resting heart rate before and after the track season. Fifth, we calculate the *mean of these differences between the before-and-after* resting heart rates. We find a mean of these differences of −8.3 bpm, with a standard deviation of 18.0. (Note that a negative value suggests that the exposure decreases the resting heart rate.)

Given these results, we must estimate—at a certain confidence level—a range of values that aims to capture the true *mean of these differences* for the resting heart rates before and after the track season.

b. (This example illustrates a matched-pairs study.) There are reports from Nyerere County of improved cardiovascular health among its student athletes. First, we recruit 40 high-school long-distance runners from across Nyerere County to detect if long-distance running impacts a student's resting heart rate. This is group 1. We collect data for three attributes for each person (gender identity, age, and body mass index) and one exposure (caffeine consumption level).

Second, we recruit another 40 high-school students from across Nyerere County. This is group 2. No member of group 2 participates in sports and the attributes and exposures of each person in group 2 otherwise match the attributes and exposures of a person in group 1. Each person in each group thus has a matched pair. We have 80 participants and 40 matched pairs.

Third, we record the resting heart rate for each person in both groups before and after the track season. Fourth, we find the difference between the resting heart rate before and after the track season for each person in both groups. Fifth, we subtract the value of the difference we found in step 4 for each person in group 2 from the value of the difference for their matched pair in group 1. This results in 40 scores that represent the difference between any change in resting heart rates between our 40 matched pairs. Sixth, we find a mean for these 40 scores of –4.0 bpm, with a standard deviation of 10.0. (Again, note that a negative value suggests that the exposure decreases the resting heart rate.)

Illustration of steps 5 and 6:

Isabella is in group 1 and Shaquana is her matched pair in group 2. The resting heart rate for Isabella before the track season was 70 bpm. For Shaquana it was also 70 bpm. After the track season, the resting heart rate for Isabella was 60 bpm. This is a difference of –10.0. The resting heart rate of Shaquana at the end of the track season was still 70 bpm. This is a difference of 0.0. We subtract Shaquana's score from Isabella's score (–10.0 – 0.0) and find a difference of –10.0. We repeat this for each matched pair. This produces 40 differences. We then find the mean for these 40 differences.

Given these results, we must estimate—at a certain confidence level—a range of values that aims to capture the true *mean of the differences between the before-and-after scores* for the matched pairs in group 1 and group 2.

Hypothesis testing and configuration #3

PURPOSE

The reason we apply hypothesis testing to configuration #3 is to assess the impact of some exposure on some continuous outcome. We compare two dependent groups that are as identical as possible. One group is exposed to some risk factor and the other is not. For this purpose, there are two scenarios. These are the same scenarios presented above for confidence interval estimation, a before-and-after study and a matched-pairs study.

EXAMPLE

a. (This example illustrates a before-and-after study.) There are reports from Nyerere County of improved cardiovascular health among its student athletes. We recruit 40 high-school long-distance runners from across Nyerere County to detect if long-distance running impacts a student's resting heart rate. First, we measure the resting heart rate for each runner before the track season. Second, each runner receives an exposure. In this case, the exposure is all those activities comprising the track season.

   Third, we measure the resting heart rate for each runner after the exposure. Fourth, we calculate the differences between each runner's resting heart rate before and after the track season. Fifth, we calculate the *mean of these differences between the before-and-after* resting heart rates. We find a mean of these differences of –8.3 bpm, with a standard deviation of 18.0. (Note that a negative value suggests that the exposure decreases the resting heart rate.)

Given these results, we must determine the probability of finding a *mean of these differences* of this size for the resting heart rates before and after the track season.

b. (This example illustrates a matched-pairs study.) There are reports from Nyerere County of improved cardiovascular health among its student athletes. First, we recruit 40 high-school long-distance runners from across Nyerere County to detect if long-distance running impacts a student's resting heart rate. This is group 1. We collect data for three attributes for each person (gender identity, age, and body mass index) and one exposure (caffeine consumption level).

Second, we recruit another 40 high-school students from across Nyerere County. This is group 2. No member of group 2 participates in sports and the attributes and exposures of each person in group 2 otherwise match the attributes and exposures of a person in group 1. Each person in each group thus has a matched pair. We have 80 participants and 40 matched pairs.

Third, we record the resting heart rate for each person in both groups before and after the track season. Fourth, we find the difference between the resting heart rate before and after the track season for each person in both groups. Fifth, we subtract the value of the difference we found in step 4 for each person in group 2 from the value of the difference for their matched pair in group 1. This results in 40 scores that represent the difference between any change in resting heart rates between our 40 matched pairs. Sixth, we find a mean for these 40 scores of −4.0 bpm, with a standard deviation of 10.0. (Again, note that a negative value suggests that the exposure decreases the resting heart rate.)

Illustration of steps 5 and 6:

Isabella is in group 1 and Shaquana is her matched pair in group 2. The resting heart rate for Isabella before the track season was 70 bpm. For Shaquana it was also 70 bpm. After the track season, the resting heart rate for Isabella was 60 bpm. This is a difference of −10.0. The resting heart rate of Shaquana at the end of the track season was still 70 bpm. This is a difference of 0.0. We subtract Shaquana's score from Isabella's score (−10.0 − 0.0) and find a difference of −10.0. We repeat this for each matched pair. This produces 40 differences. We then find the mean for these 40 differences.

Given these results, we must determine the probability of finding a *mean of the differences between the before-and-after scores* of this size for the matched pairs in group 1 and group 2.

Configuration #4

Goal: To compare the means of three or more independent groups for some continuous outcome variable based on a difference in attribute or exposure.

(Configuration #4 and configuration #9 (examples a and b) are similar in form and differ only regarding the type of outcome variable. The examples for both configurations are, therefore, alike for purposes of comparison.)

outcome variable: continuous
number and relation of groups: three or more independent groups
number of independent variables: one independent variable
biostatistical tool or test: analysis of variance (ANOVA)

Confidence interval estimation and configuration #4

Given more than two groups, we cannot apply confidence interval estimation to configuration #4.

Hypothesis testing and configuration #4

PURPOSE

a. One reason we apply hypothesis testing to configuration #4 is to assess any difference in means between three or more independent groups that differ based on some attribute, such as blood type. If a difference is found, we then calculate the probability of finding a difference of this size between the means of the groups.

b. A second reason we apply hypothesis testing to configuration #4 is to assess any difference in means between three or more independent groups that differ based on some exposure, such as caffeine consumption. If a difference is found, we then calculate the probability of finding a difference of this size between the means of the groups.

EXAMPLE

a. There are 200 high-school long-distance runners in Machel County. We are curious about a possible relationship between blood type and the resting heart rate of long-distance runners. Given this interest, we compare the mean resting heart rates for three groups of runners based on the three most common blood types in the population. Our groups are group A, group B, and group O. (We combine the positive and negative subgroups for each of these that—along with AB positive and negative—form the eight blood types.)

   We then recruit 15 runners for each group and record the resting heart rates for all 45 runners. We find that group A has a mean resting heart rate of 83 bpm; group B, 77 bpm; and group O, 73 bpm. (Note that we do not require the standard deviation in this example.)

   Given these results, we must determine the probability of finding differences of this size between the mean resting heart rates of these three groups.

b. There are 200 high-school long-distance runners in Machel County. We are concerned that caffeine consumption might be impacting the resting heart rate of our runners. We recruit a random sample of 45 high-school long-distance runners and randomly assign 15 to group 1, 15 to group 2, and 15 to group 3.

   Over a six-week period, group 1 will consume three or more daily caffeine beverages. Group 2 will consume one to two daily caffeine beverages. Group 3 will consume no caffeine beverages. After six weeks, we record the resting heart rate of all participants. We find that group 1 has a mean resting heart rate of 83 bpm; group 2, 77 bpm; and group 3, 73 bpm. (Note again that we do not require the standard deviation in this example.)

   Given these results, we must determine the probability of finding differences of this size between the mean resting heart rates of these three groups.

Configuration #5

Goal: To compare the means of two independent groups for some continuous outcome variable based on differences in multiple attributes and/or exposures.

outcome variable:	continuous
number and relation of groups:	two independent groups
number of independent variables:	three or more independent variables
biostatistical tool or test:	linear regression

Configuration #5 requires multiple linear regression. Thus, for details regarding the conceptual content of configuration #5 you may review the earlier discussion of linear regression in Chapter 2. The technical consideration of configuration #5 (and linear regression) in Chapter 7 is based on the discussion in Chapter 2.

Configuration #6

Goal: To estimate a population proportion for some dichotomous variable based on a sample proportion.

   (Configurations #1 and #6 are similar in form and differ only regarding the type of outcome variable. The examples for both configurations are, therefore, alike for purposes of comparison.)

outcome variable:	dichotomous
number and relation of groups:	one group
number of independent variables:	one independent variable
biostatistical tool or test:	estimation equation; one-sample t-test

Confidence interval estimation and configuration #6

PURPOSE

We apply confidence interval estimation to configuration #6 to discover an unknown population proportion based on a sample proportion. For this, we must estimate—at a certain confidence level—a range of values that aims to capture the true population proportion.

EXAMPLE

There are 200 high-school long-distance runners in Lumumba County. We have limited general health data for these runners. We want to know the proportion of all high-school long-distance runners in Lumumba County with a resting heart rate of 83 bpm or greater. For this, we recruit a random sample of 40 high-school long-distance runners and find 10 runners with a resting heart rate of 83 bpm or greater. This is a proportion of 0.25.

   Given these results, we must estimate—at a certain confidence level—a range of values that aims to capture the true proportion of high-school long-distance runners in Lumumba County with a resting heart rate of 83 bpm or greater.

HYPOTHESIS TESTING AND CONFIGURATION #6

We cannot apply hypothesis testing to this scenario without more data to construct a null and alternative hypotheses.

Configuration #7

Goal: To compare the proportions of two independent groups for some dichotomous outcome variable based on a difference in attribute or exposure.

(Configuration #2 and configuration #7 are similar in form and differ only regarding the type of outcome variable. The examples for both configurations are, therefore, alike—except for operation 7.0—for purposes of comparison. Recall that operation 7.0 is similar to example C for configuration #2 and hypothesis testing along with example C for configuration #9.)

outcome variable: dichotomous
number and relation of groups: two independent groups
number of independent variables: one
biostatistical tool or test: risk difference, risk ratio, odds ratio

There are two points to clarify regarding configuration #7. First, configuration #7 includes four distinct operations to demonstrate its three distinct measures. These are operation 7.0 and operation 7.1 for risk difference, operation 7.2 for risk ratio, and operation 7.3 for odds ratio.

Second, the terms "risk ratio" and "relative risk" refer to the same concept. We prefer "risk ratio" to better emphasize that both the risk ratio and the odds ratio are actual ratios, while the risk difference is not. The risk difference is an absolute difference. This matters because the properties of a ratio differ from the properties of an absolute difference, as we shall see.

Hypothesis testing and configuration #7 with operation 7.0 (risk difference)

Goal: To calculate the risk difference between the proportions of two independent populations for some dichotomous outcome variable based on a difference in attribute or exposure.

PURPOSE

We apply hypothesis testing to configuration #7 (operation 7.0) to detect any risk difference between the proportions of two populations that differ based on some attribute or exposure when we rely on data from first population 1 and data from a sample from population 2. If a difference is found, we then determine the probability of finding a difference of that size between the proportions.

For hypothesis testing, a risk difference of 0.0 indicates there is no difference between the proportions of two groups.

EXAMPLE

There are 200 high-school long-distance runners in Lumumba County. We have limited general health data for these runners. It happens that we have statewide data indicating that four years earlier the proportion of all high-school long-distance runners with a resting heart rate of 83 bpm or greater was 0.25. We want to know if the current proportion of all high-school long-distance runners in Lumumba County differs from the earlier statewide data.

Given this, we hypothesize that the proportion of all current high-school long-distance runners in Lumumba County with a resting heart rate of 83 bpm is 0.25. We then recruit a random sample of 40 high-school long-distance runners and find a proportion of 0.22 for those with a resting heart rate of 83 bpm or greater.

Thus, we have data for two populations. The proportion of those with a resting heart rate above 83 bpm for population 1 is 0.25. The proportion of those with a resting heart rate above 83 bpm for population 2 is 0.22.

Given these results, we must determine the probability of finding a difference of this size between the proportions of these two populations.

Configuration #7: operation 7.1 and risk difference

Goal: To calculate the risk difference between the proportions of two independent groups for some dichotomous outcome variable based on a difference in attribute or exposure.

outcome variable:	dichotomous
number and relation of groups:	two independent groups
number of independent variables:	one
biostatistical tool or test:	risk difference

Confidence interval estimation and configuration #7 with operation 7.1 (risk difference)

PURPOSE

a. One reason we apply confidence interval estimation to configuration #7 (operation 7.1) is to detect any risk difference between the proportions of two independent groups that differ based on some attribute, such as gender identity. For this, we estimate—at a certain confidence level—a range of values that aims to capture the true risk difference between the two groups, based on any difference in their proportions.

Note that a risk difference of 0.0 indicates no difference between the proportions of the two groups. Therefore, if the estimated confidence interval includes 0.0, we cannot rule out that there is no risk difference between the proportions of the two groups.

b. A second reason we apply confidence interval estimation to configuration #7 (operation 7.1) is to detect any risk difference between the proportions of two independent groups that differ based on some exposure, such as caffeine consumption. For this, we estimate—at a certain confidence level—a range of values that aims to capture the true risk difference between the two groups, based on any difference in their proportions.

Note that a risk difference of 0.0 indicates no difference between the proportions of the two groups. Therefore, if the estimated confidence interval includes 0.0, we cannot rule out that there is no risk difference between the proportions of the two groups.

EXAMPLE

a. There are 200 high-school long-distance runners in Mandela County. Of these, 110 identify as cis males and 90 as cis females. We want to know if there is any difference between the proportion of cis-male runners and the proportion of cis-female runners with a resting heart rate of 83 bpm. We recruit a random sample of 40 cis-male and 40 cis-female high-school long-distance runners. We find that eight cis males (or 20%) and 12 cis females (or 30%) have a resting heart rate of 83 bpm or greater.

Given these findings, we must estimate—at a certain confidence level—a range of values that aims to capture the true risk difference between group 1 and group 2 regarding the proportion of persons with a resting heart rate of 83 bpm or greater.

b. There are 200 high-school long-distance runners in Mandela County. We are concerned that caffeine consumption may be elevating the resting heart rate of our runners. We recruit a random sample of 80 high-school long-distance runners and randomly assign 40 to group 1 and 40 to group 2.

   Over six weeks, group 1 consumes three caffeine beverages per day and group 2 consumes no caffeine beverages. We record the resting heart rate for all persons in both groups after the six weeks and find that 16 of those in group 1 (or 40%) and 10 of those in group 2 (or 25%) have resting heart rates of 83 bpm or greater.

   Given these results, we must estimate—at a certain confidence level—a range of values that aims to capture the true risk difference between group 1 and group 2 regarding the proportion of persons with a resting heart rate of 83 bpm or greater.

Hypothesis testing and configuration #7 with operation 7.1 (risk difference)

Purpose

a. One reason we apply hypothesis testing to configuration #7 (operation 7.1) is to detect any risk difference between the proportions of two independent groups that differ based on some attribute, such as gender identity. If a difference is found, we then determine the probability of finding a risk difference of that size.

   For hypothesis testing, a risk difference of 0.0 indicates there is no difference between the proportions of two groups.

b. A second reason we apply hypothesis testing to configuration #7 (operation 7.1) is to detect any risk difference between the proportions of two independent groups that differ based on some exposure, such as caffeine. If a difference is found, we then determine the probability of finding a risk difference of that size.

   For hypothesis testing, a risk difference of 0.0 indicates there is no difference between the proportions of two groups.

Example

a. There are 200 high-school long-distance runners in Mandela County. Of these, 110 identify as cis males and 90 as cis females. We want to know if there is any difference between the proportion of cis-male runners and the proportion of cis-female runners with a resting heart rate of 83 bpm or greater. We recruit a random sample of 40 cis-male and 40 cis-female high-school long-distance runners. We find that eight cis males (or 20%) and 12 cis females (or 30%) have a resting heart rate of 83 bpm or greater.

   Given these results, we calculate the risk difference. We then determine the probability of finding a risk difference of this size between group 1 and group 2 regarding the proportion of persons with a resting heart rate of 83 bpm or greater.

b. There are 200 high-school long-distance runners in Mandela County. We are concerned that caffeine consumption may be elevating the resting heart rate of our runners. We recruit a random sample of 80 high-school long-distance runners and randomly assign 40 to group 1 and 40 to group 2.

   Over six weeks, group 1 consumes three caffeine beverages per day and group 2 consumes no caffeine beverages. We record the resting heart rate for all persons in both groups after the six weeks and find that 16 of those in group 1 (or 40%) and 10 of those in group 2 (or 25%) have resting heart rates of 83 bpm or greater.

Given these results, we calculate the risk difference. We then determine the probability of finding a risk difference of this size between group 1 and group 2 regarding the proportion of persons with a resting heart rate of 83 bpm or greater.

Configuration #7: operation 7.2 and risk ratio

Goal: To calculate the risk ratio as a ratio of the probabilities between two independent groups regarding some dichotomous outcome variable based on a difference in attribute or exposure.

outcome variable: dichotomous
number and relation of groups: two independent groups
number of independent variables: one
biostatistical tool or test: risk ratio

Confidence interval estimation and configuration #7 with operation 7.2 (risk ratio)

PURPOSE

a. One reason we use confidence interval estimation to apply the risk ratio to configuration #7 (operation 7.2) is to determine the risk ratio between two independent groups that differ based on some attribute, such as gender identity. The risk ratio is the ratio between the probability of an event occurring and the probability of an event NOT occurring for the members of a particular group.

We then estimate—at a certain confidence level—a range of values that aims to capture the true risk ratio. A risk ratio of 1.0 (or 1:1) indicates no difference between the risk ratios of the two groups. Therefore, if the estimated confidence interval includes a risk ratio of 1.0 (or 1:1), we cannot rule out no difference between the risk ratios of the two groups.

b. A second reason we use confidence interval estimation to apply the risk ratio to configuration #7 (operation 7.2) is to determine the risk ratio between two independent groups that differ based on some exposure, such as caffeine. The risk ratio is the ratio between the probability of an event occurring and the probability of an event NOT occurring for the members of a particular group.

We then estimate—at a certain confidence level—a range of values that aims to capture the true risk ratio. A risk ratio of 1.0 (or 1:1) indicates no difference between the risk ratios of the two groups. Therefore, if the estimated confidence interval includes a risk ratio of 1.0 (or 1:1), we cannot rule out no difference between the risk ratios of the two groups.

EXAMPLE

a. There are 200 high-school long-distance runners in Mandela County. Of these, 110 identify as cis males and 90 as cis females. We want to know if there is any difference between the proportion of cis-male runners and the proportion of cis-female runners with a resting heart rate of 83 bpm or greater. We recruit a random sample of 40 cis-male and 40 cis-female high-school long-distance runners. We find that eight cis males (or 20%) and 12 cis females (or 30%) have a resting heart rate of 83 bpm or greater.

Given these findings, we must estimate—at a certain confidence level—a range of values that aims to capture the true risk ratio between group 1 and group 2 regarding the proportion of persons with a resting heart rate of 83 bpm or greater.

b. There are 200 high-school long-distance runners in Mandela County. We are concerned that caffeine consumption may be elevating the resting heart rate of our runners. We recruit a random sample of 80 high-school long-distance runners and randomly assign 40 to group 1 and 40 to group 2.

Over six weeks, group 1 consumes three caffeine beverages per day and group 2 consumes no caffeine beverages. We record the resting heart rate for all persons in both groups after the six weeks and find that 16 of those in group 1 (or 40%) and 10 of those in group 2 (or 25%) have resting heart rates of 83 bpm or greater.

Given these results, we must estimate—at a certain confidence level—a range of values that aims to capture the true risk ratio between group 1 and group 2 regarding the proportion of persons with a resting heart rate of 83 bpm or greater.

Hypothesis testing and configuration #7 with operation 7.2 (risk ratio)

PURPOSE

a. One reason we use hypothesis testing to apply the risk ratio to configuration #7 (operation 7.2) is to determine the risk ratio between two independent groups that differ based on some attribute, such as gender identity. The risk ratio is the ratio between the probability of an event occurring and the probability of an event NOT occurring for the members of a particular group.

For hypothesis testing, a risk ratio of 1.0 (or 1:1) indicates that there is no difference between the risk for the two groups.

b. A second reason we use hypothesis testing to apply the risk ratio to configuration #7 (operation 7.2) is to determine the risk ratio between two independent groups that differ based on some exposure, such as caffeine. The risk ratio is the ratio between the probability of an event occurring and the probability of an event NOT occurring for the members of a particular group.

For hypothesis testing, a risk ratio of 1.0 (or 1:1) indicates that there is no difference between the risk for the two groups.

EXAMPLE

a. There are 200 high-school long-distance runners in Mandela County. Of these, 110 identify as cis males and 90 as cis females. We want to know if there is any difference between the proportion of cis-male runners and the proportion of cis-female runners with a resting heart rate of 83 bpm or greater. We recruit a random sample of 40 cis-male and 40 cis-female high-school long-distance runners. We find that eight cis males (or 20%) and 12 cis females (or 30%) have a resting heart rate of 83 bpm or greater.

Given these results, we calculate the risk ratio. We then determine the probability of finding a risk ratio of this size between the proportion of cis-male runners and the proportion of cis-female runners with a resting heart rate greater than 83 bpm.

b. There are 200 high-school long-distance runners in Mandela County. We are concerned that caffeine consumption may be elevating the resting heart rate of our runners. We recruit a random sample of 80 high-school long-distance runners and randomly assign 40 to group 1 and 40 to group 2.

Over six weeks, group 1 consumes three caffeine beverages per day and group 2 consumes no caffeine beverages. We record the resting heart rate for all persons in both groups after the six weeks and find that 16 of those in group 1 (or 40%) and 10 of those in group 2 (or 25%) have resting heart rates of 83 bpm or greater.

Given these results, we calculate the risk ratio. We then determine the probability of finding a risk ratio of this size between the proportion of group 1 and the proportion of group 2 with a resting heart rate greater than 83 bpm.

Configuration #7: operation 7.3 and odds ratio

Goal: To calculate the odds ratio as a ratio of the odds between two independent groups regarding some dichotomous outcome variable based on a difference in attribute or exposure.

outcome variable: dichotomous
number and relation of groups: two independent groups
number of independent variables: one
biostatistical tool or test: odds ratio

Confidence interval estimation and configuration #7 with operation 7.3 (odds ratio)

PURPOSE

One reason we use confidence interval estimation to apply the odds ratio to configuration #7 (operation 7.3) is when use of a risk ratio is not optimal. Examples of this include logistic regression and a case-control study. For a case-control study, the odds ratio is a ratio between (a) the odds of exposure to some risk factor for those with a certain condition (cases) with (b) the odds of exposure to the same risk factor for those without that condition (controls). The odds ratio in this example would indicate whether or not the cases had greater odds of exposure to the risk factor than the controls.

We thus estimate—at a certain confidence level—a range of values that aims to capture the true odds ratio. An odds ratio of 1.0 (or 1:1) indicates no difference between the odds of the two groups. Therefore, if the estimated confidence interval includes an odds ratio of 1.0 (or 1:1), we cannot rule out no difference between the odds of the two groups.

EXAMPLE

To better illustrate the use of the odds ratio, for this example, we slightly alter the previous example measuring the impact of caffeine consumption on the resting heart rate. Here, we elevate the dichotomous variable—the proportion of runners with a resting heart rate of 83 bpm or greater—to 95 bpm or greater. This provides a relatively rare resting heart rate.

There are 200 high-school long-distance runners in Mandela County. We are concerned that caffeine consumption may be elevating the resting heart rate of our runners. We recruit a random sample of 80 high-school long-distance runners and randomly assign 40 to group 1 and 40 to group 2.

Over six weeks, group 1 consumes three caffeine beverages per day and group 2 consumes no caffeine beverages. We record the resting heart rate for all persons in both groups after six weeks and find that 14 of those in group 1 (or 35%) and four of those in group 2 (or 10%) have resting heart rates of 95 bpm or greater.

Given these results, we must estimate—at a certain confidence level—a range of values that aims to capture the true odds ratio between group 1 and group 2 regarding the proportion of persons with a resting heart rate of 95 bpm or greater.

Hypothesis testing and configuration #7 with operation 7.3 (odds ratio)

PURPOSE

One reason we use hypothesis testing to apply the odds ratio to configuration #7 (operation 7.3) is when use of a risk ratio is not optimal. Examples of this include logistic regression and a case-control study. For a case-control study, the odds ratio is a ratio between (a) the odds of exposure to some risk factor for those with a certain condition (cases) with (b) the odds of exposure to the same risk factor for those without that condition (controls). The odds ratio in this example would indicate whether or not the cases had greater odds of exposure to the risk factor than the controls.

For hypothesis testing, an odds ratio of 1.0 (or 1:1) indicates that there is no difference between the odds for the two groups.

EXAMPLE

There are 200 high-school long-distance runners in Mandela County. We are concerned that caffeine consumption may be elevating the resting heart rates of our runners. We recruit a random sample of 80 high-school long-distance runners and randomly assign 40 to group 1 and 40 to group 2.

Over six weeks, group 1 consumes three caffeine beverages per day and group 2 consumes no caffeine beverages. We record the resting heart rate for all persons in both groups after six weeks and find that 14 of those in group 1 (or 35%) and four of those in group 2 (or 10%) have resting heart rates of 95 bpm or greater.

Given these results, we calculate the odds ratio. We then determine the probability of finding an odds ratio of this size between the proportion of group 1 and the proportion of group 2 with a resting heart rate greater than 95 bpm.

Configuration #8

Goal: To compare the proportions of two independent groups for some dichotomous outcome variable based on differences in multiple attributes and/or exposures.

outcome variable:	dichotomous
number and relation of groups:	two independent groups
number of independent variables:	three or more independent variables
biostatistical tool or test:	logistic regression

Configuration #8 requires multiple logistic regression. Thus, for details regarding the conceptual content of configuration #8 you may review the earlier discussion of logistic regression in Chapter 2. The technical consideration of configuration #8 (and logistic regression) in Chapter 7 is based on the discussion in Chapter 2.

Configuration #9

Goal: To compare two or more independent groups regarding the distribution of cases across multiple response options for an ordinal or categorical outcome variable. Groups differ based on an attribute or exposure.

(Configurations #4 and #9 are similar in form and differ only regarding the type of outcome variable. The examples for both configurations are, therefore, alike for purposes of comparison. The one exception is example C which aligns with configuration #2, example C, and configuration #7, operation 7.0, for reasons previously detailed.)

outcome variable:　　　　　　　　　　　categorical (with multiple response options)
number and relation of groups:　　　　two or more independent groups
number of independent variables:　　　one
biostatistical tool or test:　　　　　　chi-square test of independence

Confidence interval estimation and configuration #9

Given more than two groups and/or the inclusion of ordinal or categorical outcome variables, we cannot apply confidence interval estimation to configuration #9.

Hypothesis testing and configuration #9

PURPOSE

a.　One reason we apply hypothesis testing to configuration #9 is to calculate any differences in the distribution of cases across multiple response options (such as low, moderate, elevated, and very high resting heart rates) for two or more independent groups that differ based on some attribute. If a difference is found, we then determine the probability of finding differences of this size between groups for the distribution of cases.

b.　A second reason we apply hypothesis testing to configuration #9 is to calculate any differences in the distribution of cases across multiple response options (such as low, moderate, elevated, and very high resting heart rates) for two or more independent groups that differ based on some exposure. If a difference is found, we then determine the probability of finding differences of this size between groups for the distribution of cases.

c.　A third reason we apply hypothesis testing to configuration #9 is to calculate any differences in the distribution of cases across multiple response options (such as low, moderate, elevated, and very high resting heart rates) for two populations that differ based on some attribute or exposure. This comparison is based on data from the first population and data from a representative sample from the second population. If a difference is found, we then determine the probability of finding differences of this size between populations for the distribution of cases.

EXAMPLE

a.　There are 300 high-school long-distance runners in Machel County. We suspect an attribute (blood type) may be impacting a runner's resting heart rate. We create four ordinal categories for resting heart rates. These are: low (50 bpm or lower), moderate (51–82 bpm), elevated (83–99 bpm), and very high (100 bpm or higher). We create three groups of runners based on the three most common blood groups in the population (A, B, and O).

　　Our groups are thus group A, group B, and group O. (We combine the positive and negative subgroups for each of these that—along with AB positive and negative—form the eight blood types.) We then recruit 50 high-school long-distance runners for each blood group, record each participant's resting heart rate, and catalogue her or him according to our ordinal categories. Table 4.2 provides the distribution of runners across ordinal categories based on group membership.

Table 4.2 Distribution of blood types across levels of resting heart rates, n = 150

	Low rate	Moderate rate	Elevated rate	Very high rate	Total
Group A	9	26	8	7	50
Group B	14	21	7	8	50
Group O	10	22	12	6	50
Total	33	69	27	21	150

Table 4.3 Distribution of levels of caffeine consumption across levels of resting heart rates, n = 150

	Low rate	Moderate rate	Elevated rate	Very high rate	Totals
Group 1	0	9	29	12	50
Group 2	8	28	12	2	50
Group 3	12	33	4	1	50
Total	20	70	46	15	

Given these results, we must determine the probability of finding differences of this size in the distribution of responses across ordinal categories for the three groups that differ by blood type.

b.   There are 300 high-school long-distance runners in Machel County. We suspect an exposure (caffeine consumption) may be impacting the resting heart rate of our runners. We create four ordinal categories for resting heart rates. These are: low (50 bpm or lower), moderate (51–82 bpm), elevated (83–99 bpm), and very high (100 bpm or higher). We recruit a random sample of 150 high-school long-distance runners and randomly assign these 150 runners to three groups of 50 persons each.

Group 1 will consume three or more daily caffeine beverages. Group 2 will consume one to two daily caffeine beverages. Group 3 will consume no caffeine beverages. After six weeks, we record each participant's resting heart rate and catalogue her or him according to our ordinal categories for resting heart rates. Table 4.3 provides the distribution of runners across our ordinal categories based on group membership.

Given these results, we must determine the probability of finding differences of this size in the distribution of responses across ordinal categories for the three groups that differ by level of caffeine consumption.

c.   There are 200 high-school long-distance runners in Lumumba County. We want to know how many runners have resting heart rates that are low (50 bpm or lower), moderate (51–82 bpm), or high (83 bpm or greater). Statewide data from two years earlier indicate that the distribution among all high-school long-distance runners was 20% low, 40% moderate, and 40% high.

We hypothesize that the distribution for all current high-school long-distance runners in Lumumba County is similarly 20% low, 40% moderate, and 40% high. We then recruit a random sample of 40 high-school long-distance runners and find that the distribution for this sample is 4 (10%) low, 18 (45%) moderate, and 18 (45%) high.

Thus, we have data for two populations. Population 1 has a distribution of resting heart rates of 20% low, 40% moderate, and 40% high. Population 2, based on sample data, has a distribution of resting heart rates of 10% low, 45% moderate, and 45% high.

Given these results, we must determine the probability of finding differences of this size between population 1 and population 2 regarding the distribution of responses across ordinal categories.

Lessons to be wrung from our nine configurations

If we return now to the four elements distinguishing one configuration from another, we can draw out some further implications for biostatistical analysis and its mathematical premises. Again, these elements are:

- the type of outcome variable;
- the number of groups;
- the type of relationship between groups (dependent or independent); and
- the number of causal (or independent) variables.

The first element is the type of outcome variable—continuous, dichotomous, ordinal, or categorical. Let us explore the nature of these types of variables a bit more closely. In particular, it helps to distinguish between the logical nature of what each is and the practical utility of the role each serves. Note incidentally that the four scales (nominal, ordinal, interval, and ratio)—which we need not revisit here—are merely contrivances that allow these four types of variables to realize their practical utility *vis-à-vis* the mathematical rationale of biostatistical analysis. Our entry point for this distinction between logical nature and practical utility is the concept of measurement.

Measurement is a feature of each type of outcome variable and can thus help to demonstrate the logical nature and practical utility of each in comparative fashion. (Even qualitative things generate outcome variables that can be measured, such as nominal categories that are counted.) To illustrate, we explore the logical nature and practical utility of continuous variables *vis-à-vis* their measurement. A continuous outcome variable, for example a person's height, possesses a value that lies along a continuum of numbers that are (theoretically) infinitely divisible.

A person two meters tall also stands 200 centimeters, 2,000 millimeters, or even 0.002 kilometers tall. And were we so inclined, we could continue to infinitely reduce (or increase) these increments of length to describe this two-meter tall person. Infinity, in this sense, is a mathematical concept.

The question is whether the use of infinity here is merely a mathematical property aiding in the interpretation of a variable (the height of a person) or is it an actual property of the variable itself. Upon further inspection, infinity would seem less the property of any specific variable—or even a *mathematical property* aiding our interpretation of a variable—and more a description of the (mathematical) relationships between certain types of things.

To clarify, let us distinguish between the concepts of "mathematical" and "quantitative." "Mathematical" connotes a body of rules and operations applied to phenomena that have been rendered quantitative. A mathematical property is any principle or axiom that follows from these rules and operations, such as "non-divisibility" as a property of integers. The term "quantitative" connotes phenomena whose qualitative features have been converted to countable units of measure. In this way, "a tall person" becomes "a person two meters in length." Once the qualitative features of some phenomenon are converted to quantitative units of measure, we are able to apply mathematical properties—such as, perhaps, infinity—to that thing.

Measurement then is the application of relational tools to quantifiable things via mathematical rules and operations. For instance, a measurement may indicate that two sticks stand in relation to a tape measure, such that the first stick is six inches longer than the second stick. The two sticks are thus mediated by the tape measure. The measurement itself, as a property, does not belong to either stick alone—*it would be nonsensical if it did*.

This would be the equivalent of saying a cup of coffee costs 5,000 *pesos* in a certain country when we do not know the "measure" of a *peso*. If we do not know the measure of a *peso vis-à-vis* some currency whose measure we do know, we cannot make sense of 5,000 *pesos*. The measure, therefore—and its properties (like infinity)—belong neither to the first or second stick, nor to the tape measure itself. The measure is an expression of the relationship between the two sticks, as quantitative things.

Thus, the flat statement that a person stands two meters tall is actually meaningless. Rather, we can only (mean to) say that, after first converting a person's quality of "tallness" into quantitative, countable units and then juxtaposing this "tallness" with the "tallness" of a second person via some common unit of measure, the height of the first person is two meters. If we were to periodically change this common unit of measure, the only thing that would *not* change would be the relation—that is, the ratio—between the tallness of the first person and the tallness of the second person. That is why the property of two meters expresses—or "belongs to"—the *relationship* between the heights of two people and not the actual height of either person.

On the one hand, the fact that infinity is a relational property that is given expression through measurement—and not an inherent property of that which we measure (or of the measurement itself)—makes it possible to universally apply such concepts within biostatistical analysis. However, the confusion between a relational property and an inherent property contributes significantly to the mystification of measurement more generally within biostatistical analysis. This is because the reductive frame encourages us to view these as *properties* of specific variables. This, in fact, reflects the practical utility of how we tend to think of both measurement and variables and this is what necessitates the occasional willful suspension of disbelief.

For the limited purpose of applying biostatistical tools and techniques to health and medicine this is arguably fine. But if we persist beyond this purpose in misconstruing the nature of measurement—as an inherent property rather than an expression of relationships—we will fail to understand the fundamental role of quantitative measurement (its practical utility) as a technique for imposing a reductive mathematical order on the world of health and medicine. (This is further explored in Chapter 10.)

As a generic instrument of measurement, it is the logical nature of each type of variable to express the quantifiable relationships between phenomena whose content conforms with the conceptual precepts of either continuous, dichotomous, ordinal, or categorical variables. However, as an instrument of measurement within biostatistical analysis, it is the practical utility of each type of variable to adhere itself as the property of certain phenomena (*vis-à-vis* other phenomena) whose (discrete) content conforms with the conceptual precepts of either continuous, dichotomous, ordinal, or categorical variables.

From this arrangement troubling contradictions often surface among these four "distinct" variables that appear to reveal less about differences among phenomena across health and medicine and more about the stresses and strains of ramrodding qualitative phenomena into quantitative schemata. The strained efforts to conceptually distinguish between dichotomous, ordinal, and categorical variables is emblematic of this. It is true that, if so inclined, we could contrive a separate measure for each of these. But it is equally true that each is most clearly a variation on a categorical (or nominal) measure. Table 4.4 contrasts dichotomous, ordinal, and categorical response options to "describe your health."

Each set of response options, by any ordinary understanding, represents categories. In other words, a dichotomous variable, in fact, is a type of categorical variable with two categorical options. Likewise, an ordinal variable is a type of categorical variable with at least three options—to distinguish it from a dichotomous variable—with a rank order of categories. A categorical variable is then a type of categorical variable with at least three options and NO rank order. Configurations #6, #7, and #9 are quite revealing in this regard.

Table 4.4 Response options for dichotomous, ordinal, and categorical variables to "describe your health"

Dichotomous	Good	Bad		
Ordinal	Very poor	Poor	Good	Very good
Categorical	A waterfall	A car engine	A tree in a forest	A swan on a lake

Configuration #9 (example C) works with data taken from a sample in which our outcome variable is a distribution of ordinal responses. These responses indicate the number of persons with a low, moderate, or high resting heart rate. This is akin to configuration #6 that indicates—in dichotomous fashion—the proportion of persons with (or without) a resting heart rate of 83 bpm or greater. An outcome variable pertaining to a distribution of responses across multiple categorical options is thus logically equivalent to a distribution of responses across two categorical options, such as yes/no. In fact, this is the reason that configuration #9 requires *three* or more response options! There is otherwise no way to distinguish between these and configurations #6 and #7, with dichotomous variables.

Examples A and B for configuration #9 further illustrate this shared logic between configurations #6 and #9. Example A has four groups that differ based on an attribute (blood type). Example B has four groups that differ based on an exposure (the level of caffeine consumption). In both cases, our outcome variable is a distribution of ordinal responses (for each group) that indicates the number of persons with a low, moderate, elevated, or very high resting heart rate. Our results for both examples are the percentages of persons in each group with a low, moderate, elevated, or very high resting heart rate. This allows us to assess any differences between groups with regard to the percentages of persons with a low, moderate, elevated, or very high resting heart rate.

Note further how dichotomous outcome variables are actually treated as *a single outcome* (yes) and not two outcomes (yes or no). This is because the outcome of interest is the probability of a single outcome (yes). Similarly, each of the multiple response options for configuration #9 is effectively treated as a single option. Again, this is because each option—low, moderate, elevated, or very high resting heart rate—is treated as the probability of "yes" for each. However, because these options are mutually exclusive, across all four options there can only be one "yes" response for each person. Therefore, *even the combination of four (discrete) binary response options is treated as a single outcome* for each person.

This betrays a curious affinity between those configurations with dichotomous, ordinal, and categorical outcome variables (#6, #7, and #9). As we will be seen in Chapter 10, this "affinity," in fact, reflects a discomforting conceptual slippage between qualitative and quantitative phenomena across health and medicine. The contortions deployed by biostatistical analysis to paper over this slippage, for the sake of treating qualitative phenomena as though they were quantitative, only exacerbate the absurdity of this contrivance. At times, we indeed find ourselves severely tested by the limits of our willful suspension of disbelief.

The second element distinguishing between configurations is the number of groups that we compare. The number of groups also determines whether or not we are able to use confidence interval estimation and hypothesis testing. Both are available for studies with one or two groups and a continuous or dichotomous outcome variable. However, only hypothesis testing applies to studies with three or more comparison groups. Again, for this reason, confidence interval estimation applies to only five of the nine configurations. Hypothesis testing applies to seven of the nine configurations.

In addition, it is helpful to keep in mind technical distinctions between a group, a sample, and a population. A "group" refers generically to any collection of persons, large or small.

Thus, a group may be the entire population, a sample drawn from the population, or a subgroup within either the population or a sample. Configurations #1 and #6 each feature both a sample and a population. However, this is treated as one "group" (the sample), not two. All other configurations have at least two groups that may or may not include a sample from a known population. Though popular use of these terms may not adhere to such distinctions, it is good to keep in mind these technical differences between groups, samples, and populations.

The third distinguishing element between configurations is the dependence or independence of groups. As with our outcome variables, it is important to recognize that the terms "dependence" and "independence" are not properties of a group. They are descriptions of the relationships between groups. In addition, note that a dependent or independent relationship *between groups* differs from a dependent or independent relationship *between variables*. As discussed in Chapter 2, a reductive frame assumes that variables are independent and a holistic frame assumes that variables are inter-related, that is, dependent.

This distinction of dependent or independent groups may itself seem trivial. After all, there is *only one* configuration (#3) with dependent relationships between groups. All others either compare groups whose relationships are independent or work with single samples that do not compare groups (configurations #1 and #6). However, this one exception is itself telling on two counts. First, the rarity of dependent relationships between groups spotlights the full scale of the transformation brought on by reconfiguring the subject matter of health and medicine to conform with the mathematical rules of biostatistical analysis. Again, independent relationships between variables and between groups are the hallmark of reductive frames.

Second, with respect to groups, the principal distinction between independent relationships and dependent relationships is the form of data that each generates. Thus, in the case of independent relationships, we compare the mean (or proportion) for different groups that differ based on some attribute or exposure. Configurations #2 and #7 are examples. In the case of dependent relationships between groups, we compare the *mean of the differences for each pairing of individuals* from both groups that differ based on some exposure. Configuration #3 is an example.

The fourth distinguishing element between configurations is the number of independent (or causal) variables. Note that no configuration has more than one dependent (or outcome) variable. All but two of the nine configurations have a single independent variable. (Configurations #1 and #6 technically do not have independent variables.) Five configurations conduct bivariate analysis (#2, #3, #4, #7, #9). These configurations assess the relationship between one causal (or independent) variable and one outcome (or dependent) variable.

Two configurations conduct univariate analysis (#1, #6). These configurations describe a single variable within a sample or population. Two configurations conduct multiple regression analysis (#5, #8). These configurations simultaneously assess the relationships between multiple causal (or independent) variables and a single outcome (or dependent) variable.

Final warning

Now we must prepare to set sail for some fairly rough seas. The pressures to succumb to the dazzling allure of biostatistical techniques will be great. Take courage over the next few chapters, as there are two fearsome dangers and not all may make it to the other shore.

The first danger is the failure to sustain one's willful suspension of disbelief long enough to fully grasp biostatistical tools and techniques on their own terms. A premature return to disbelief will leave one cut off from the reductive conceptual premises and mathematical rationale rendering a person unreachable and unable to master the depths of biostatistical analysis. You will be left adrift, unable to strategically incorporate essential insights from biostatistical analysis.

At the other extreme, the danger is to become lost in the entrancing mélange of precision, certainty, and mysticism that is biostatistical analysis. The next three chapters are well apt to amaze and mesmerize the uninitiated, as we walk through the minutiae of tools and techniques devised quite seductively for each configuration. Steel yourself accordingly.

Chapter 5

Configurations for Biostatistical Analysis
Technical Steps (1)

In Chapter 4 we reviewed the conceptual premises of the nine configurations that cover the broad ambit of univariate and bivariate analysis. Multivariable analysis—specifically, linear and logistic regression—was addressed in like fashion in Chapter 2. We now walk through the technical steps for analyzing the data generated by each of these configurations.

Given the level of detail that a review of the technical steps forces upon us, we have distributed our discussion of the nine configurations across three chapters. Thus, the present chapter takes up the first four configurations, Chapter 6 moves to configurations #6, #7, and #9, and Chapter 7 finishes up with regression analysis and configurations #5 and #8.

Both confidence interval estimation and hypothesis testing use equations to compare a given statistical measure of interest, such as a mean or proportion, between groups. In the case of confidence interval estimation, these are **estimation equations** that generate estimated confidence intervals. A confidence interval aims to capture the true value for some measure of interest, at a given confidence level. For hypothesis testing, these are **statistical tests** that generate test statistics. A test statistic, in combination with a p-value, then determines the statistical significance of our findings regarding some measure of interest.

Researchers, therefore, select an "estimation equation" to generate estimated confidence intervals and they select a "statistical test" to generate a test statistic when carrying out hypothesis testing. See Table 5.1.

Table 5.1 is for handy reference. For an explanation of the symbols and notation in Table 5.1 see the individual equations and tests as they are presented in Chapters 5, 6, and 7.

Reviewing these estimation equations and statistical tests side by side allows us, first, to illustrate certain exaggerated notions about the complexity of biostatistical analysis and, second, to highlight the outsized importance of a small number of key statistical measures. Notice, for example, that for all of these tests, the level of math does not go much beyond basic algebra. The one exception is the role of logarithms for configuration #7 (operations 7.2 and 7.3) and configuration #8. This exception points to certain unique qualities of binomial distributions associated with dichotomous outcomes, such as the risk ratio or odds ratio. These qualities are detailed in Chapters 6 and 7.

Notice that there are actually only four statistical measures that account for about 80% of all values in these estimation equations and statistical tests. These are the sample size, the standard deviation, the z-value (or t-value), and either the mean or proportion. This helps keep matters in perspective and greatly qualifies the alleged complexity. Thus, not only are we working with nothing more sophisticated than a handful of tools we learned in junior high school, but this reliance on a small number of measures further reduces the number of unique technical steps via the repetition of many of these operations.

That said, it is also true that—in the real world—one rarely ever needs to memorize the technical steps for these equations and tests. Statistical software programs execute these

DOI: 10.4324/9781003316985-5

Table 5.1 Estimation equations and statistical tests for configurations, by confidence interval estimation or hypothesis testing

Configuration	Confidence interval estimation and estimation equations		Hypothesis testing and statistical tests	
	$n \geq 30$	$n < 30$	$n \geq 30$	$n < 30$
#1	$\bar{X} \pm z\dfrac{s}{\sqrt{n}}$	$\bar{X} \pm t\dfrac{s}{\sqrt{n}}$	N/A	N/A
#2	$(\bar{X}_1 - \bar{X}_2) \pm z(S_p)\sqrt{\dfrac{1}{n_1} + \dfrac{1}{n_2}}$	$(\bar{X}_1 - \bar{X}_2) \pm t(S_p)\sqrt{\dfrac{1}{n_1} + \dfrac{1}{n_2}}$	$z = \dfrac{\bar{X}_1 - \bar{X}_2}{S_p\sqrt{\dfrac{1}{n_1} + \dfrac{1}{n_2}}}$	$t = \dfrac{\bar{X}_1 - \bar{X}_2}{S_p\sqrt{\dfrac{1}{n_1} + \dfrac{1}{n_2}}}$
#2 Example C	N/A	N/A	$z = \dfrac{\bar{X} - \mu_0}{s/\sqrt{n}}$	$t = \dfrac{\bar{X} - \mu_0}{s/\sqrt{n}}$
#3	$\bar{X}_d \pm (z)\dfrac{s_d}{\sqrt{n}}$	$\bar{X}_d \pm (z)\dfrac{s_d}{\sqrt{n}}$	$z = \dfrac{\bar{X}_d - \mu_d}{s_d/\sqrt{n}}$	$t = \dfrac{\bar{X}_d - \mu_d}{s_d/\sqrt{n}}$
#4	N/A		$F = \dfrac{\sum \dfrac{(\bar{X}_i - \bar{X})^2}{n_i} \Big/ (k-1)}{\sum\sum (X - \bar{X}_i)^2 \Big/ (N-k)}$	
#5	N/A		$\hat{y} = b_0 + b_1 x_1 + b_2 x_2 + \ldots b_p x_p$	
#6	$\hat{p} \pm z\sqrt{\dfrac{\hat{p}(1.0 - \hat{p})}{n}}$		N/A	
#7.0	N/A		$z = \dfrac{\hat{p} - p_0}{\sqrt{\dfrac{p_0(1.0 - p_0)}{n}}}$	
#7.1	$(\hat{p}_1 - \hat{p}_2) \pm z\sqrt{\dfrac{\hat{p}_1(1.0 - \hat{p}_1)}{n_1} + \dfrac{\hat{p}_2(1.0 - \hat{p}_2)}{n_2}}$		$z = \dfrac{\hat{p}_1 - \hat{p}_2}{\sqrt{\hat{p}(1.0 - \hat{p}) \times \left(1.0/n_1 + 1.0/n_2\right)}}$	
#7.2	$\ln(\widehat{RR}) \pm z\sqrt{\dfrac{(n_1 - x_1)/x_1}{n_1} + \dfrac{(n_2 - x_2)/x_2}{n_2}}$		$\chi^2 = \sum_{(r*c)} \dfrac{(O - E)^2}{E}$	
#7.3	$\ln(\widehat{OR}) \pm z\sqrt{\dfrac{1}{x_1} + \dfrac{1}{(n_1 - x_1)} + \dfrac{1}{x_2} + \dfrac{1}{(n_2 - x_2)}}$		$\chi^2 = \sum_{(r*c)} \dfrac{(O - E)^2}{E}$	
#8	N/A		$\ln\left(\dfrac{\hat{p}}{1.0 - \hat{p}}\right) = \alpha + b_1 x_1 + b_2 x_2 + \ldots b_p x_p$	
#9	N/A		$\chi^2 = \sum_{(r*c)} \dfrac{(O - E)^2}{E}$	
#9 Example C	N/A		$\chi^2 = \sum_k \dfrac{(O - E)^2}{E}$	

Table 5.2 Elements of the nine configurations

	Outcome variable	Number of groups	Relation of groups	Independent variables	Confidence intervals	Hypothesis testing	Type of analysis
#1	Continuous	1	–	1	Yes	No	Univariate
#2	Continuous	2	Independent	1	Yes	Yes	Bivariate
#3	Continuous	1 or 2	Dependent	1	Yes	Yes	Bivariate
#4	Continuous	3+	Independent	1	No	Yes	ANOVA
#5	Continuous	2+	Independent	3+	No	Yes	Regression
#6	Dichotomous	1	–	1	Yes	No	Univariate
#7	Dichotomous	2	Independent	1	Yes	Yes	Bivariate
#8	Dichotomous	2+	Independent	3+	No	Yes	Regression
#9	Ordinal or categorical	2+	Independent	1	No	Yes	Chi square

steps with lightning speed and require compliant biostatisticians—reduced to typists—to simply import their data and check off a series of boxes. Consequently, conducting biostatistical analysis with such statistical programs is not merely rote but over time becomes an exercise in opaque obedience. Indeed, a good portion of lower-level statistics courses is dedicated largely to training students in operating statistical programs.

Given the demands of upper-level statistical courses, however, these lower-level courses are often the best opportunity for conceptual exploration and for a grounding in the nitty gritty of these technical steps—and their consequences. Without this grounding, the significance of the underlying descriptive statistics (such as the mean or standard deviation) can become detached from their more fundamental repercussions. These we discuss in Chapter 10.

To further set things up and for reference, we reprint Table 4.1 as Table 5.2, laying out the elements of our nine configurations.

Before jumping in just yet there are a few further items to spell out by way of orientation. To begin, there are three concepts essential for carrying out a number of these steps. These are the standard normal distribution, z-values, and t-values. Each of these are developed more fully in Chapter 9. For now, it is well enough to understand the basics of each. The standard normal distribution is a distribution of values with a mean of 0.0 and standard deviations to the right of the mean that are labeled 1.0, 2.0, and so on. To the left of the mean we find their negative equivalents, -1.0, -2.0, etc.

Exactly one half of all cases lie above or below the mean—meaning to the right and left—and its bell-shaped curve is perfectly symmetrical. This shape and the uniform distances between standard deviations make possible many of the technical steps discussed in this chapter.

z-Values allow us to convert any value along the standard normal distribution to a standard value that fits that distribution. For this, it does not matter if the original value is measured in kilos, centimeters, or decibels. In this way, we are able to compare qualitatively unlike things, such as the weight of a jet, the height of a mouse, or the volume of a shriek.

Importantly, the standard normal distribution assures that a 95% confidence level includes all cases that fall within two standard deviations above and below the mean when using confidence interval estimation. A z-value of 1.96 happens to correspond with this 95% confidence level that contains all cases within two standard deviations of the mean. By our good fortune, a 95% confidence level—or a 5% significance level for hypothesis testing—is very popular with biostatisticians. Consequently, we will see a lot of number 1.96!

When our sample size is smaller than 30, t-values allow us to perform the same operations as z-values—though the distribution of t-values does not follow the standard normal distribution. Thus, notwithstanding that the assumptions producing t-values differ from those producing z-values, each is otherwise applied in identical fashion.

We now walk through the technical steps for analyzing the data generated by each of these configurations.

Configuration #1

Goal: To estimate a population mean for some continuous variable based on a sample mean.

Confidence interval estimation and configuration #1

Example

There are 200 high-school long-distance runners in Lumumba County. We have limited health data for these runners. We want to know the mean resting heart rate for all high-school long-distance runners in Lumumba County. For this, we recruit a random sample of 40 high-school long-distance runners and find a mean resting heart rate of 73 bpm for this sample, with a standard deviation of 8.0.

Given these results, we must estimate—at a certain confidence level—a range of values that aims to capture the true mean resting heart rate for all high-school long-distance runners in Lumumba County.

Technical steps

We begin by choosing a 95% confidence level. Because our sample is greater than 30, we use an estimation equation with z-values. If our sample had fewer than 30 people, we would use an estimation equation with t-values. We find the z-value at a 95% confidence level (1.96) in Table A.1 in the Appendix.

With a sample greater than 30, our estimation equation is:

$$\bar{X} \pm z\frac{s}{\sqrt{n}}$$

$\bar{X}$ is the sample mean and this is read "x-bar"
s is the standard deviation
n is the sample size

We substitute the values from our example and find:

$$\bar{X} \pm z\frac{s}{\sqrt{n}} \rightarrow 73 \pm 1.96\frac{8.0}{\sqrt{40}} = 73 \pm 2.481\,(70.51, 75.48)$$

Thus, we estimate—at a 95% confidence level—that the true population mean is between 70.51 and 75.48 bpm.

Now notice what happens if we increase the sample size to 4,000, or if we decrease the sample size to 10. We first increase the sample size from 40 to 4,000, while retaining the same confidence level (95%), sample mean (73 bpm), and standard deviation (8.0). We find:

$$\bar{X} \pm z\frac{s}{\sqrt{n}} \rightarrow 73 \pm 1.96\frac{8.0}{\sqrt{4000}} = 73 \pm 0.247 \ (72.75, 73.25)$$

Thus, we now estimate—at a 95% confidence level—that the true population mean is between 72.75 and 73.25 bpm. This is a smaller estimated confidence interval than that with a sample size of 40.

Notice in this example that we chose a z-value of ± 1.96. The plus/minus sign indicates that we do not know if the sample mean is larger or smaller than the population mean.

Commonly, our interest is whether the mean of one group is either larger or smaller than the mean of another group. There are three distinct tests for this. If our interest is whether the mean of one group is larger than the mean of another group, we use an "upper-tailed" test. If our interest is whether the mean of one group is smaller than the mean of another group, we use a "lower-tailed" test. If our interest is a difference in means of any kind, larger or smaller, we use a "two-tailed" test.

Each of these tests requires a certain critical value of z to assert the statistical significance of the results. For both a 95% confidence level in the case of estimation equations, and a 5% significance level in the case of statistical tests and hypothesis testing, these critical values are:

- z-values above 1.645 for upper-tailed tests;
- z-values below −1.645 for lower-tailed tests; and
- z-values either above 1.96 or below −1.96 for two-tailed tests.

The same notion also applies to estimation equations and statistical tests that employ t-values. However, these values must also address degrees of freedom. For example, for our results to be statistically significant with 10 degrees of freedom and a 95% confidence level, or a 5% significance level, the critical values of t are:

- t-values above 1.812 for upper-tailed tests;
- t-values below −1.812 for lower-tailed tests; and
- t-values either above 2.228 or below −2.228 for two-tailed tests.

In general, this distinction between upper, lower, and two-tailed tests applies more commonly to hypothesis testing than confidence interval estimation. This follows from the need to state a specific hypothesis regarding the nature of the difference between the means of different groups, as we will see.

Continuing with our example we next decrease the sample size to 10. Again, the confidence level (95%), sample mean (73 bpm), and standard deviation (8.0) remain the same. With a sample size below 30, we rely on t-values rather than z-values.

To determine the t-value we find the degrees of freedom (df) and, given this, we find the t-value in Table A.2 in the Appendix. The degrees of freedom = $n - 1$. This is $10 - 1 = 9$. From the table, we find that the t-value associated with nine degrees of freedom and a 95% confidence level is 2.262.

$$\bar{X} \pm t\frac{s}{\sqrt{n}} \rightarrow 73 \pm 2.262\frac{8.0}{\sqrt{10}} = 73 \pm 5.727 \ (67.27, 78.73)$$

Table 5.3 List of tables of distributions in the Appendix

Table A.1: Standard normal distribution and probabilities of z-values
Table A.2: *t* Distribution and critical values of *t*
Table A.3: Chi-square distributions and critical values of chi-square
Table A.4: *F* distribution and critical values of *F*
Table A.5: Standard normal distribution and z-values for percentiles
Table A.6: Standard normal distribution and z-values for confidence intervals

Table 5.4 Effect of changes to sample size, standard deviation, and mean on estimated confidence intervals

Mean	Standard deviation	Sample size	Confidence intervals
73	8.0	40	2.481 (70.51, 75.48)
73	8.0	4000	0.247 (72.75, 73.25)
73	8.0	10	5.722 (67.28, 78.72)
73	8.0	40	2.479 (70.52, 75.48)
73	1.0	40	0.310 (72.59, 73.31)
73	18	40	5.582 (67.42, 78.58)
73	8.0	40	2.479 (70.52, 75.48)
53	8.0	40	2.479 (50.52, 55.48)
93	8.0	40	2.479 (90.52, 95.48)

Thus, we estimate—at a 95% confidence level—that the true population mean is between 67.27 and 78.73 bpm. This is a larger estimated confidence interval than that with a sample size of 40.

A brief explanation of Table A.2 (a *t* distribution table) referred to above—and "distributions" tables more generally—is in order here. In the Appendix to this book there are six tables of distributions (see Table 5.3 for a list of these tables). Each distribution provides the probability of finding certain values.

The basic idea is simple. If we find a certain value in a distribution that has a very low probability of occurring then there is a very high likelihood that this value is significantly different from the mean of that distribution. Throughout Chapters 5, 6, and 7 we refer to Tables A.1 through A.6 to indicate where we found a certain value based on a distribution.

This is sufficient for now. The underlying rationale for a distribution is detailed in Chapter 9.

Table 5.4 indicates how altering the sample size, the standard deviation, and the mean affects the estimated confidence intervals. Notice that increasing the sample size to 4,000, or reducing the standard deviation to 1.0, results in the smallest estimated confidence interval. As a general rule, either increasing the sample size or decreasing the standard deviation reduces the estimated confidence interval. In addition, altering the mean, while retaining the same sample size and standard deviation, does *not* change the size of the estimated confidence interval.

Hypothesis testing and configuration #1

We cannot apply hypothesis testing to this scenario, insofar as we do not have sufficient data to construct a null and alternative hypotheses.

Configuration #2

Goal: To compare the means of two independent groups for some continuous outcome variable based on a difference in attribute or exposure.

Confidence interval estimation and configuration #2

Example A

There are 200 high-school long-distance runners in Mandela County. Of these, 110 identify as cis males and 90 as cis females. We want to know if there is any difference between the mean resting heart rates of our cis-male and cis-female runners. We recruit a random sample of 40 cis-male and 40 cis-female high-school long-distance runners. We find a mean resting heart rate of 70 bpm for cis males, with a standard deviation of 9.0, and 76 bpm for cis females, with a standard deviation of 7.0.

Given these results, we must estimate—at a certain confidence level—a range of values that aims to capture any difference in means between these two groups.

Technical steps

Our technical steps now grow slightly more complex.

The estimation equation is reasonably short. Again, if the sample size is 30 or greater, we rely on z-values. If the sample size is less than 30, we rely on t-values. Thus, we have:

$$\left(\bar{X}_1 - \bar{X}_2\right) \pm z(S_p)\sqrt{\frac{1}{n_1} + \frac{1}{n_2}} \quad OR \quad \left(\bar{X}_1 - \bar{X}_2\right) \pm t(S_p)\sqrt{\frac{1}{n_1} + \frac{1}{n_2}}$$

Notice that the only difference between these two estimation equations is the use of either a critical value of z or a critical value of t. This is the case for each of the estimation equations (and statistical tests) associated with configurations #1, #2, and #3.

To further clarify, this difference follows from assumptions about the z-distribution and t-distribution. Each of these is a distribution of sample means. The z-distribution is a distribution of sample means that we would expect to find with samples taken from a population that conforms to the standard normal distribution. Again, this applies to sample sizes of 40 or greater. This is taken up in greater detail in Chapter 9.

The t-distribution is a distribution of sample means from some population mean that does NOT conform to the normal distribution. The variability—meaning uncertainty—among t-values is thus greater than that among z-values.

The sample size for our example is 40. So we use the estimation equation with z-values. Given a 95% confidence level, we know the critical value of z will be ± 1.96. (Again, for confidence interval estimation, a 95% confidence level will always result in a critical value of z of ± 1.96, unless we specify that we are expecting an increase or decrease in values.) After we plug in the values from our example, we thus have:

$$\left(\overline{X}_1 - \overline{X}_2\right) \pm z(S_p)\sqrt{\frac{1}{n_1} + \frac{1}{n_2}} \rightarrow (70 - 76) \pm 1.96\,(S_p)\sqrt{\frac{1}{40} + \frac{1}{40}}$$

At this point, we still have many moving pieces. In fact, before we can proceed at all we must account for a potentially devastating mismatch between the variability of each sample. If the difference in variability between our two samples is too great, our results may be doomed.

To assure compatibility we rely on a simple guideline. We are good to go if the ratio of our two sample variances $\left(\dfrac{s_1^2}{s_2^2}\right)$ is between 0.5 and 2.0.

In our case, we know that the standard deviation for sample 1 is 9.0 and the standard deviation for sample 2 is 7.0. If we multiply the standard deviation by itself—or square each of these—we have the variance. Thus:

$$\frac{s_1^2}{s_2^2} \rightarrow \frac{9^2}{7^2} = \frac{81}{49} = 1.65$$

The ratio between variances (1.65) is indeed safely between 0.5 and 2.0. Now let us identify further parts of the estimation equation:

$\overline{X}_1 - \overline{X}_2$ are the sample means for the outcome of interest from the two independent samples z (or t) are values from the z (or t) distribution tables based on the confidence level n_1, n_2 are the sample sizes

S_p is the pooled estimate of the common standard deviation for both samples ... hold on, the what?

This pooled estimate is the weighted average of the standard deviations in the two samples. In other words, this is a "common" standard deviation for both samples after accounting for any differences in the sample size and the magnitude of the two standard deviations. Assuring that the ratio of variances $\left(\dfrac{s_1^2}{s_2^2}\right)$ is between 0.5 and 2.0 is a further check on the validity of this value.

We now must find the value of S_p. This requires the following equation which we calculate with the data from our example:

$$S_p = \sqrt{\frac{\left(n_1 - 1.0\right)s_1^2 + \left(n_2 - 1.0\right)s_2^2}{n_1 + n_2 - 2}} \rightarrow S_p = \sqrt{\frac{(40 - 1.0)81 + (40 - 1.0)49}{40 + 40 - 2}} = 8.06$$

We can now complete the original estimation equation:

$$\left(\overline{X}_1 - \overline{X}_2\right) \pm z(S_p)\sqrt{\frac{1}{n_1} + \frac{1}{n_2}} \rightarrow (70 - 76) \pm 1.96(8.06)\sqrt{\frac{1}{40} + \frac{1}{40}} = -6 \pm 3.53(-9.53, -2.47)$$

Thus, we estimate—at a 95% confidence level—that the true difference in the mean resting heart rates of cis-male and cis-female high-school long-distance runners is between −9.53 and −2.47. (Note that these negative values indicate that the second sample mean is greater than the first sample mean.)

Note that $S_p\sqrt{\dfrac{1}{n_1}+\dfrac{1}{n_2}}$ provides something called the "standard error of the difference in means"—that is, the "standard error" of $(\overline{X}_1 - \overline{X}_2)$.

There are actually two further references to a standard error in this chapter (and in Chapter 6). In fact, the standard error plays some role in virtually all estimation equations and statistical tests. To clarify, a reference to the "standard error" is most often an abbreviation for the "standard error of the mean." This type of standard error applies to a specific sample and is discussed further in Chapter 9. In the present chapter (and Chapter 6), however, we have three separate references to three separate types of standard error—*none of which* is the standard error of the mean.

As noted, the first type is the "standard error of the *difference in means*." We encounter this in the technical steps for both confidence interval estimation and hypothesis testing for configuration #2.

The second type is the "standard error of the *point estimate*." We encounter this in the technical steps for both confidence interval estimation and hypothesis testing for configuration #3. The point estimate is a best approximation of the true value for a statistical measure, such as a mean. For confidence interval estimation, this serves as the "middle" value within an interval range.

The third type is the "standard error of the *difference in proportions*." We encounter this in the technical steps for confidence interval estimation and hypothesis testing for configuration #6.

In each case, we derive some statistical measure for a sample, such as a mean. But imagine that we had drawn a different sample, or that we were to continue to draw further samples from the same population. Each time, we would derive a slightly different value for the mean. The standard error provides an estimation of the variability in the values derived for the means (or other statistical measures) from many different samples.

This then has a direct impact on different aspects of estimation equations and statistical tests. For example, for configurations #2, #3, and #6 it helps us to determine the margin of error when using confidence interval estimation.

Before moving to Example B, just for fun, let's re-run Example A after reducing both sample sizes to 10 and employing a *t*-test instead of a *z*-test.

The standard deviations remain the same, and so the ratio between these remains 1.65—allowing us to proceed.

For degrees of freedom we find: $(10 + 10) - 2 = 18$. Given 18 degrees of freedom, a two-tailed test, and a 95% confidence level, our critical value of t is 2.101. This we find in Table A.2.

We calculate S_p as follows:

$$S_p = \sqrt{\frac{(n_1 - 1.0)s_1^2 + (n_2 - 1.0)s_2^2}{n_1 + n_2 - 2}} \rightarrow S_p = \sqrt{\frac{(10 - 1.0)81 + (10 - 1.0)49}{10 + 10 - 2}} = 8.06$$

We thus have:

$$(\overline{X}_1 - \overline{X}_2) \pm t(S_p)\sqrt{\frac{1}{n_1}+\frac{1}{n_2}} \rightarrow (70 - 76) \pm 2.101(8.06)\sqrt{\frac{1}{10}+\frac{1}{10}} = -6 \pm 7.57(-13.57, 1.57)$$

Thus, we estimate—at a 95% confidence level—that the true difference in mean resting heart rates for cis-male and cis-female high-school long-distance runners is between −13.57

and 1.57. We have an absurdly large interval, indicating that the small sample size has made our results all but useless—notwithstanding that all other values remain the same. In addition, the interval itself includes the value 0.0 indicating "no statistically significant difference" between samples.

Example B

There are 200 high-school long-distance runners in Mandela County. We are concerned that caffeine consumption may be elevating the resting heart rate of our runners. We recruit a random sample of 80 high-school long-distance runners and randomly assign 40 to group 1 and 40 to group 2.

Over six weeks, group 1 consumes three caffeine beverages per day and group 2 consumes no caffeine beverages. We record the resting heart rate for all persons in both groups after six weeks. We find a mean resting heart rate of 83 bpm for group 1, with a standard deviation of 9.0, and a mean resting heart rate of 73 bpm for group 2, with a standard deviation of 7.0.

Given these results, we must estimate—at a certain confidence level—a range of values that aims to capture any difference in means between these two groups.

Technical steps

To begin, notice that the only substantive difference between Example A and Example B is that A explores a difference in attribute (gender identity) and B a difference in exposure (caffeine consumption). These are otherwise conceptually identical scenarios, comparing two independent groups on a continuous variable. Therefore, we proceed here in the same manner as Example A.

Recognizing this similarity of form and difference in substance can help clarify the technical steps all the better. All that differs is the mean resting heart rate for each group.

Given two samples of 40 persons each, we turn to the same estimation equation as Example A with z-values:

$$\left(\bar{X}_1 - \bar{X}_2\right) \pm z(S_p)\sqrt{\frac{1}{n_1} + \frac{1}{n_2}}$$

We thus reconfirm the compatibility of our two standard deviations: $\frac{9^2}{7^2} = 1.65$. This falls well within the range of 0.5 and 2.0.

We choose a 95% confidence interval, which yields a critical z-value of ± 1.96. Hence:

$$\left(\bar{X}_1 - \bar{X}_2\right) \pm z(S_p)\sqrt{\frac{1}{n_1} + \frac{1}{n_2}} \rightarrow (83 - 73) \pm 1.96(S_p)\sqrt{\frac{1}{40} + \frac{1}{40}}$$

We calculate (the same) S_p:

$$S_p = \sqrt{\frac{\left(n_1 - 1.0\right)s_1^2 + \left(n_2 - 1.0\right)s_2^2}{n_1 + n_2 - 2}} \rightarrow S_p = \sqrt{\frac{\left(40 - 1\right)81 + \left(40 - 1\right)49}{40 + 40 - 2}} = 8.06$$

We then plug in our final numbers and discover:

$$(83-73)\pm1.96(8.06)\sqrt{\frac{1}{40}+\frac{1}{40}}=10\pm3.53\,(6.47,13.53)$$

Thus, we estimate—at a 95% confidence level—that the true difference in mean resting heart rates for high-school long-distance runners who consume three or more caffeine beverages daily and those who abstain is between 6.47 and 13.53 bpm.

Hypothesis testing and configuration #2

Example A

There are 200 high-school long-distance runners in Mandela County. Of these, 110 identify as cis males and 90 as cis females. We want to know if there is any difference between the mean resting heart rates of our cis-male and cis-female runners. We recruit a random sample of 40 cis-male and 40 cis-female high-school long-distance runners. We find a mean resting heart rate of 70 bpm for cis males, with a standard deviation of 9.0, and 76 bpm for cis females, with a standard deviation of 7.0.

Given these results, we must determine the probability of finding a difference of this size between the means of these two groups.

Technical steps

We have seen that, for configuration #2, confidence interval estimation generates a range of values that aim to capture the true difference between the means of two groups. Hypothesis testing, meanwhile, assesses whether the size of any observed difference between the means of two groups is statistically significant. This difference between means is a single value (the point estimate) that represents our best approximation of the true difference.

For confidence interval estimation, the point estimate plus or minus the margin of error provides the estimated interval range that captures the true difference between the means of two groups. For hypothesis testing, the probability of finding a point estimate of that size determines its statistical significance. If there is a high probability of finding a difference of that size, this is NOT considered statistically significant. If there is a very low probability of finding a difference of that size, this will likely be considered statistically significant.

For this purpose we must choose a specific significance level as our threshold for declaring a finding to be significant. We choose a significance level of 5% for this. To determine if the probability of a finding is less than 5%, we follow five steps. *Note that we follow these same five steps whenever conducting hypothesis testing.*

1. We choose a null hypothesis, an alternative hypothesis, and a significance level.
2. We select a statistical test.
3. We set criteria for a decision rule based on this statistical test.
4. We calculate the statistical test and produce a test statistic.
5. We assess the findings.
    a. If the statistical test indicates that we do not reject the null hypothesis, then there is no significant difference.
    b. If the statistical test indicates that we reject the null hypothesis, then this suggests a significant difference and we find the *p*-value to determine the probability of finding a difference of this size; again, the "p" in *p*-value is short for "probability."

In this case, the null hypothesis is that there is no difference between the means of the two groups. The alternative hypothesis is that there is some difference between the means of these two groups.

We choose a 5% significance level. This can be written $\alpha = 0.05$. The symbol α is the Greek letter "alpha."

> A quick word about the Greeks. There is a certain infatuation among biostatisticians for the Greek alphabet. Because it is rather unusual for students (outside Greece) to have much knowledge of Greek letters, we prefer to state things more plainly in the local language. However, it is important that students recognize certain conventions within biostatistical analysis that rely on arcane traditions, such as a fetish for Greek letters. There are three Greek letters, in particular, to keep in mind:
>
> μ – Greek letter mu that represents the population mean;
> σ – Greek letter sigma that represents the population standard deviation; and
> α – Greek letter alpha that represents the significance level.

To clarify, both confidence interval estimation and hypothesis testing generate z-values (or t-values). Confidence interval estimation uses these to provide a value that helps determine the size of an interval range. Hypothesis testing uses these to provide a criterion (a test threshold) for determining the significance of some difference between means. A test threshold is also referred to as a critical value of z (or t).

Given two samples of 40 persons each, we choose a z-test. For samples of fewer than 30 persons, we have the t-test.

$$z = \frac{\bar{X}_1 - \bar{X}_2}{S_p \sqrt{\frac{1}{n_1} + \frac{1}{n_2}}} \quad \text{or} \quad t = \frac{\bar{X}_1 - \bar{X}_2}{S_p \sqrt{\frac{1}{n_1} + \frac{1}{n_2}}}$$

Before advancing, we confirm the compatibility of the variability of our two samples. This requires that the ratio between the two squared standard deviations is at least 0.5 and no greater than 2.0. We calculate this as follows:

$$\frac{s_1}{s_2} \rightarrow \frac{9^2}{7^2} = \frac{81}{49} = 1.65$$

Thus, our ratio (1.65) falls between 0.05 and 2.0 and we proceed.

Because we are interested in any difference—either greater than or less than—we have a two-tailed z-test at a 5% significance level. Therefore, the critical value of z is ± 1.96. This can be found in Table A.1.

The decision rule is thus to reject the null hypothesis if: $[z \le -1.960]$ or $[z \ge 1.960]$.

This tells us that there is a less than 5% probability of finding a z-value either less than -1.96 or greater than 1.96.

CALCULATE STATISTICAL TEST

There are two steps to calculate the statistical test. First, we must determine the value of "S_p."

$$S_p = \sqrt{\frac{(n_1 - 1.0)s_1^2 + (n_2 - 1.0)s_2^2}{n_1 + n_2 - 2}} \rightarrow S_p = \sqrt{\frac{(40 - 1)81 + (40 - 1)49}{40 + 40 - 2}} = 8.06$$

Second, we must plug the S_p value (8.06)—along with the other values from our example—into the z-test to find the value of z.

$$z = \frac{\bar{X}_1 - \bar{X}_2}{S_p\sqrt{\dfrac{1}{n_1} + \dfrac{1}{n_2}}} \rightarrow z = \frac{70 - 76}{1.802} = 3.30$$

ASSESSMENT OF FINDINGS

Thus, we reject the null hypothesis because -3.30 is less than -1.960. This indicates that a difference of 6 bpm between the mean resting heart rates of cis-male and cis-female high-school long-distance runners is a large enough difference—with $\alpha = 0.05$—to meaningfully distinguish between these two groups.

We now turn to the p-value as a measure of the strength of the significance of this finding. *To clarify, we know that our z-value is statistically significant at* $\alpha = 0.05$. Our goal now is to see how much stronger it may be than 0.05—meaning how much smaller the probability of finding a z-value of -3.30 might be.

For this, we make use of Table A.1 and we find a probability of 0.000967 associated with a z-value of -3.30. Thus, our p-value is approximately 0.0009. This is considerably below 0.05. So this is considered a very strong result. Again, any p-value below 0.05 is treated as statistically significant.

To transform any z-value into a p-value we first find the z-value in Table A.1. This indicates the probability for finding any specific z-value within the standard normal distribution. Note that our z-value in this example is negative. In later examples, with a positive z-value, we will see that we must subtract the probability that we find in Table A.1 from 1.0 to derive the p-value.

Example B

There are 200 high-school long-distance runners in Mandela County. We are concerned that caffeine consumption may be elevating the resting heart rates of our runners. We recruit a random sample of 80 high-school long-distance runners and randomly assign 40 to group 1 and 40 to group 2.

Over six weeks, group 1 consumes three caffeine beverages per day and group 2 consumes no caffeine beverages. We record the resting heart rate for all persons in both groups after six weeks. We find a mean resting heart rate of 83 bpm for group 1, with a standard deviation of 9.0, and a mean resting heart rate of 73 bpm for group 2, with a standard deviation of 7.0.

Given these results, we must determine the probability of finding a difference of this size between the means of these two groups.

Technical steps

Again, we shift from a difference in attribute (gender identity) to a difference in exposure (caffeine consumption). The technical steps are identical. In addition, the sample size and standard deviations are the same as the previous example, while the difference in means between groups increases from 6 bpm to 10 bpm.

We follow the same five steps for hypothesis testing.

HYPOTHESES AND SIGNIFICANCE LEVEL

The null hypothesis is that there is no difference between the means of the two groups. The alternative hypothesis is that there is some difference between the means of these two groups.

We choose a 5% significance level, or $\alpha = 0.05$.

STATISTICAL TEST

Again, our choice is between a z-test and a t-test. Because our samples are both greater than 30, we choose a z-test.

$$z = \frac{\bar{X}_1 - \bar{X}_2}{S_p \sqrt{\frac{1}{n_1} + \frac{1}{n_2}}}$$

To proceed we first confirm the compatibility of the variability of our two samples. Again, this requires that the ratio between the two squared standard deviations is at least 0.5 and no greater than 2.0. We calculate this as follows:

$$\frac{s_1}{s_2} \rightarrow \frac{9^2}{7^2} = \frac{81}{49} = 1.65$$

Voila!

CRITERIA FOR DECISION RULE

Because we are interested in any difference—either greater than or less than—we have a two-tailed z-test at a 5% significance level. Therefore, the critical value of z is ±1.96. This can be found in Table A.1.

The decision rule is thus to reject the null hypothesis if: $[z \leq -1.960]$ or $[z \geq 1.960]$.

CALCULATE STATISTICAL TEST

There are two steps to calculate the statistical test. First, we must determine the value of S_p.

$$S_p = \sqrt{\frac{(n_1 - 1.0)s_1^2 + (n_2 - 1.0)s_2^2}{n_1 + n_2 - 2}} \rightarrow S_p = \sqrt{\frac{(40 - 1)81 + (40 - 1)49}{40 + 40 - 2}} = 8.06$$

Second, we plug the S_p value (8.06)—along with our other values from our example—into our z-test to find the value of z.

$$z = \frac{\overline{X}_1 - \overline{X}_2}{S_p\sqrt{\dfrac{1}{n_1} + \dfrac{1}{n_2}}} \quad \rightarrow \quad z = \frac{73 - 83}{1.902} = -5.55$$

ASSESSMENT OF FINDINGS

Thus, again we reject the null hypothesis because −5.55 is less than −1.960. This indicates that a difference of 10 bpm between the mean resting heart rates of caffeine consumers and non-consumers is a large enough difference—with $\alpha = 0.05$—to meaningfully distinguish between these two groups.

Given this, we must calculate the p-value to see how much stronger this may be than 0.05. Because distribution tables for z-values generally run between 3.0 and −3.0, we must consult a statistical program, such as Excel, to derive a p-value for −5.55. In this way, we find a quite robust p-value of 0.00001.

Example C

There are 200 high-school long-distance runners in Lumumba County. We have limited health data for these runners. It happens that we have statewide data indicating that four years earlier the mean resting heart rate for all high-school long-distance runners was 70 bpm. We want to know if the current mean resting heart rate for all high-school long-distance runners in Lumumba County differs from the earlier statewide data.

Given this, we hypothesize that the current mean resting heart rate for all high-school long-distance runners in Lumumba County is 70 bpm. We then recruit a random sample of 40 high-school long-distance runners and find a mean resting heart rate for this sample of 73 bpm, with a standard deviation of 8.0.

Thus, we have data for two populations. The mean resting heart rate for population 1 is 70 bpm. The mean resting heart rate for a sample from population 2 is 73 bpm.

Given these results, we must determine the probability of finding a difference of this size between the means of these two populations.

Technical steps

Recall that hypothesis testing determines the probability of finding a value of a certain size. In this case, we are comparing the mean resting heart rate of population 1 (70 bpm) with the mean resting heart rate of population 2, based on the mean resting heart rate of a sample from population 2 (73 bpm). We want to know if the size of this difference between mean resting heart rates is large enough to be a statistically significant difference.

With that in mind, we return to the five steps of hypothesis testing.

HYPOTHESES AND SIGNIFICANCE LEVEL

In this case, our null hypothesis is that the mean resting heart rate of population 1 and the mean resting heart rate of population 2 are the same. Our alternative hypothesis is that the mean resting heart rate of population 1 is not the same as that of population 2.

We choose a 5% significance level, or $\alpha = 0,05$.

STATISTICAL TEST

Our sample size is greater than 30, therefore, our statistical test is a z-test: $z = \dfrac{\bar{X} - \mu_0}{s / \sqrt{n}}$

- $\bar{X}$ is the sample mean—in this case, 73 bpm;
- μ_0 refers to the mean of the null hypothesis—in this case, 70 bpm;
- s is the sample standard deviation; and
- n is the sample size.

CRITERIA FOR DECISION RULE

Our sample is greater than 30 and the alternative hypothesis is that the current population mean is *greater than* the prior population mean. Therefore, we have an upper-tailed z-test at a 5% significance level.

Given an upper-tailed z-test with $\alpha = 0.5$, we refer to Table A.1 and discover that the critical value of z is 1.645. Our decision rule is thus to reject the null hypothesis if $z \geq 1.645$.

This tells us that there is a less than 5% probability of finding a z-value larger than 1.654.

CALCULATE STATISTICAL TEST

To calculate the z-statistical test, we plug the values from our example into the equation.

$$z = \frac{\bar{X} - \mu_0}{s / \sqrt{n}} \rightarrow \frac{73 - 70}{8.0 / \sqrt{40}} = 2.371$$

ASSESS FINDINGS

We reject the null hypothesis because 2.371 is greater than 1.645, the critical value of z. Thus, a sample of 40, with a mean resting heart rate of 73 bpm and a standard deviation of 8.0, provides statistically significant evidence that the mean resting heart rate of population 1 is not the same as that of population 2, with $\alpha = 0.05$.

We now turn to the p-value as a measure of the strength of the significance of this finding. For this, we make use of Table A.1 and we find a probability of 0.991 associated with a z-value of 2.371.

We thus calculate $1.0 - 0.991 = 0.009$. This gives us a p-value of approximately 0.009. This is considerably below 0.05. So this is considered a very strong result. Again, any p-value below 0.05 is treated as statistically significant. Remember that when a z-value is positive, we must subtract the probability we find in Table A.1 from 1.0.

Let us now repeat these five steps for the same example after reducing the sample size to 10 and keeping the same significance level (5%), sample mean (73), population mean (70), and standard deviation (8.0).

HYPOTHESES AND SIGNIFICANCE LEVEL

These hypotheses are identical to the situation with the prior example with a sample of 40. Thus, our null hypothesis is that the mean resting heart rate of population 1 and the mean resting heart rate of population 2 are the same. Our alternative hypothesis is that the mean resting heart rate of population 1 is not the same as that of population 2.

We choose a 5% significance level, or $\alpha = 0.05$.

STATISTICAL TEST

This time, our sample size is less than 30, therefore, our statistical test is a t-test: $t = \dfrac{\bar{X} - \mu_0}{s / \sqrt{n}}$

CRITERIA FOR DECISION RULE

The alternative hypothesis is that the current population mean is greater than the prior population mean. Therefore, we have an upper-tailed t-test at a 5% significance level.
We determine that our degrees of freedom $(n - 1)$ are: $10 - 1 = 9$.
We now refer to Table A.2 and discover that—given an upper-tailed test with nine degrees of freedom and $\alpha = 0.5$—the critical value of t is 1.83.
Our decision rule is thus that we will reject the null hypothesis if: $t \geq 1.83$.
Thus, there is a less than 5% probability of finding a t-value greater than 1.83.

CALCULATE STATISTICAL TEST

To calculate the statistical test, we plug the values from our example into the equation—after changing the sample size to 10.

$$t = \frac{\bar{X} - \mu_0}{s / \sqrt{n}} \rightarrow \frac{73 - 70}{8.0 / \sqrt{10}} = 1.185$$

ASSESSMENT OF FINDINGS

We do NOT reject the null hypothesis because 1.185 is NOT greater than 1.83. Thus, a sample of 10 with a mean resting heart rate of 73 bpm and a standard deviation of 8.0 does not provide evidence of a difference between the means of population 1 and population 2—based on sample data for population 2—with $\alpha = 0.05$.
Incidentally, you may be wondering why it is that a confidence level is set at 95% and a significance level is set at 5%, or $\alpha = 0.05$. To unravel this, let us use the example of comparing a sample mean and population mean. The confidence level applies to confidence interval estimation. For example, the question might be how confident we are that the true population mean falls within an estimated confidence interval that is based on a sample mean. Meanwhile, the significance level applies to hypothesis testing. The same question for this would be whether the difference between the sample mean and the population mean is large enough to indicate a true (or significant) difference.
A 95% confidence level assures us that—if we took 100 samples—95 of those samples would produce an interval range that contained the true mean. This would indicate that a sample mean is *at most* two standard deviations from the actual population mean. Hence, the sample mean is **within** two standard deviations, where *95% of all cases* reside for the standard normal distribution.
A 5% significance level assures us that the probability for finding a difference of a certain size between a sample mean and population mean is 5% or less. This indicates that the sample mean is *at least* two standard deviations from the population mean. Hence, the sample mean is **beyond** two standard deviations, where *5% or fewer of all cases* reside for the standard normal distribution.

Configuration #3

Goal: To assess the mean of the differences between scores either (a) for the same person before and after some exposure or (b) for matched pairs of persons from two dependent groups before and after some exposure for one of the two groups.

Confidence interval estimation and configuration #3

Example A

(This example illustrates a before-and-after study.) There are reports from Nyerere County of improved cardiovascular health among its student athletes. We recruit 40 high-school long-distance runners from across Nyerere County to detect if long-distance running impacts a student's resting heart rate. First, we measure the resting heart rate for each runner before the track season. Second, each runner receives an exposure. In this case, the exposure is all those activities comprising the track season.

Third, we measure the resting heart rate for each runner after the exposure. Fourth, we calculate the differences between each runner's resting heart rate before and after the track season. Fifth, we calculate the *mean of these differences between the before-and-after* resting heart rates. We find a mean of these differences of –8.3 bpm, with a standard deviation of 18.0. (Note that a negative value suggests that the exposure decreases the resting heart rate.)

Given these results, we must estimate—at a certain confidence level—a range of values that aims to capture the true *mean of these differences* for the resting heart rates before and after the track season.

Technical steps

To begin, we must specify our unit of observation. The unit of observation identifies the persons from whom we will collect data. The unit of analysis identifies the population (or group) about whom we will draw conclusions. For example, commonly a sample is the unit of observation, and the population from which the sample was taken is the unit of analysis.

For studies with one sample, such as configuration #1, or with two independent samples, such as configuration #2, the unit of observation is the individual participant. In study designs with either one before-and-after sample or two dependent (matched-pair) samples, the unit of observation is the difference between the pre/post scores for each individual or paired match—*not each score, meaning not always each individual.*

Imagine we have 100 participants in a before-and-after study. For each participant who is "paired" with her- or himself, there is one score prior to an exposure and one score after an exposure. Each participant, therefore, records a score prior to the exposure and each participant records a score after. We have 100 self-paired matches that produce 200 scores. After we subtract the second score from the first, we have 100 differences between scores. Thus, in this case, the unit of observation is the 100 participants paired with themselves, $n = 100$.

Imagine that we again have 100 participants. This time, however, 50 of these participants in group 1 (the experimental group) are matched with 50 participants in group 2 (the control group) based on certain shared attributes. Each participant in both groups records a score prior to some exposure for group 1 and each participant in both groups again records a score after that exposure. We have 50 paired matches and 200 observations. Notice, however, that now we have a further step.

After we collect our data (200 observations), we first subtract the second score from the first score for each of the 100 participants. This produces 100 "difference scores" for all participants. Next, we must subtract the difference score of each participant in group 2 from the difference score of her or his paired match in group 1. This produces 50 difference scores for each matched pair. Thus, in this case—though we again have 100 participants—the unit of observation is the 50 paired matches, and so, $n = 50$.

Let's now walk through Example A. To do so, we will need three numbers:

- n the sample size, or the number of paired matches;
- $\bar{X}_d$ the mean of the differences between scores; and
- s_d the standard deviation of the differences between scores.

A brief illustration with partial data will illustrate how we generate the measures of $\bar{X}_d$ and s_d. See Tables 5.5 and 5.6.

We continue with Example A. Our data for Example A are based on the full sample of 40 students:

$$n = 40; \quad \bar{X}_d = -8.3; \quad s_d = 18.0$$

The formula for finding the confidence interval again distinguishes between z-values for samples of 30 or more and t-values for samples of fewer than 30.

$$\bar{X}_d \pm (z)\frac{s_d}{\sqrt{n}} \quad \text{OR} \quad \bar{X}_d \pm (t)\frac{s_d}{\sqrt{n}}$$

Table 5.5 Partial data for Example A and confidence interval estimation for configuration #3 and the mean of the differences between scores

Runner	Heart rate before	Heart rate after	Difference
1	82	80	−2
2	86	83	−3
3	75	65	−10
4	80	60	−20
5	95	73	−22
6	83	82	−1
			$\bar{X}_d = -9.7$

Table 5.6 Partial data for Example A and confidence interval estimation for configuration #3 and the standard deviation of the differences between scores

Runner	Difference	Difference − $\bar{X}_d$ (−9.7)	(Difference − $\bar{X}_d$)^2
1	−2	7.7	59.29
2	−3	6.7	44.89
3	−10	−0.3	0.09
4	−20	−10.3	106.09
5	−22	−12.3	151.29
6	−1	8.5	75.69
		Variance of differences = 87.46	
		Thus, $s_d = \sqrt{87.46} = 9.35$	

Given our sample size of 40, we choose an estimation equation with z-values. Given a 95% confidence level, our z-value is ± 1.96. After plugging in the numbers from our example, we then have:

$$\bar{X}_d \pm (z)\frac{s_d}{\sqrt{n}} \rightarrow -8.3 \pm (1.96)\frac{18.0}{\sqrt{40}} = -8.3 \pm 5.582(-13.882, -2.718)$$

Thus, we estimate—at a 95% confidence level—that the mean difference for the resting heart rate between measure one (before the track season) and measure two (after the track season) is a value between -13.882 and -2.718 bpm. A negative value in this case indicates that the exposure—the track season—was associated with a reduction in the resting heart rate.

Note that $\frac{s_d}{\sqrt{n}}$ yields the standard error of the point estimate—or $SE(\bar{X}_d)$. This was discussed above.

Example B

(This example illustrates a matched-pairs study.) There are reports from Nyerere County of improved cardiovascular health among its student athletes. First, we recruit 40 high-school long-distance runners from across Nyerere County to detect if long-distance running impacts a student's resting heart rate. This is group 1.

We collect data for three attributes for each person (gender identity, age, and body mass index) and one exposure (caffeine consumption level).

Second, we recruit another 40 high-school students from across Nyerere County. This is group 2. No member of group 2 participates in sports and the attributes and exposures of each person in group 2 otherwise match the attributes and exposures of a person in group 1. Each person in each group thus has a matched pair. We have 80 participants and 40 matched pairs.

Third, we record the resting heart rate for each person in both groups before and after the track season. Fourth, we find the difference between the resting heart rate before and after the track season for each person in both groups. Fifth, we subtract the value of the difference we found in step four for each person in group 2 from the value of the difference for their matched pair in group 1. This results in 40 scores that represent the difference between any change in resting heart rates between our 40 matched pairs. Sixth, we find a mean for these 40 scores of -4.0 bpm, with a standard deviation of 10.0. (Again, note that a negative value suggests that the exposure decreases the resting heart rate.)

Illustration of steps 5 and 6:

Isabella is in group 1 and Shaquana is her matched pair in group 2. The resting heart rate for Isabella before the track season was 70 bpm. For Shaquana it was also 70 bpm. After the track season, the resting heart rate for Isabella was 60 bpm. This is a difference of -10.0. The resting heart rate of Shaquana at the end of the track season was still 70 bpm. This is a difference of 0.0. We subtract Shaquana's score from Isabella's score $(-10.0 - 0.0)$ and find a difference of -10.0. We repeat this for each matched pair. This produces 40 differences. We then find the mean for these 40 differences.

Given these results, we must estimate—at a certain confidence level—a range of values that aims to capture the true *mean of the differences between the before-and-after scores* for the matched pairs in group 1 and group 2.

Technical steps

The steps here will be very similar to Example A. Because there are two groups we will perform these steps twice and we will then need one additional step.

Notice that for Example B we have 80 participants and 40 matched pairs. Therefore, $n = 40$. Our data for this example are:

$$n = 40; \quad \bar{X}_d = -4.0; \quad s_d = 10.0$$

Given that $n = 40$, we choose an estimation equation with z-values. Given a 95% confidence level, our z-value is ± 1.96. After plugging in the values from our example, we then have:

$$\bar{X}_d \pm (z)\frac{s_d}{\sqrt{n}} \rightarrow -4.0 \pm (1.96)\frac{10.0}{\sqrt{40}} = -4.0 \pm 3.1\,(-7.1, -0.9)$$

Thus, we estimate—at a 95% confidence level—that the mean difference for the resting heart rate between group 1 (with exposure) and group 2 (without exposure) is a value between −7.1 and −0.9 bpm.

Hypothesis testing and configuration #3

Example A

(This example illustrates a before-and-after study.) There are reports from Nyerere County of improved cardiovascular health among its student athletes. We recruit 40 high-school long-distance runners from across Nyerere County to detect if long-distance running impacts a student's resting heart rate. First, we measure the resting heart rate for each runner before the track season. Second, each runner receives an exposure. In this case, the exposure is all those activities comprising the track season.

Third, we measure the resting heart rate for each runner after the exposure. Fourth, we calculate the differences between each runner's resting heart rate before and after the track season. Fifth, we calculate the *mean of these differences between the before-and-after* resting heart rates. We find a mean of these differences of −8.3 bpm, with a standard deviation of 18.0. (Note that a negative value suggests that the exposure decreases the resting heart rate.)

Given these results, we must determine the probability of finding a *mean of these differences* of this size for the resting heart rates before and after the track season.

Technical steps

Notice that we have the exact same scenario that we had for Example A for confidence interval estimation and configuration #3.

Again, we have 40 high-school long-distance runners performing a before-and-after test and our data are:

$$n = 40; \quad \bar{X}_d = -8.3; \quad s_d = 18.0$$

We derive $\bar{X}_d = -8.3$ and $s_d = 18.0$ in the same manner as Example A for confidence interval estimation. (So we do not need to repeat Tables 5.5 and 5.6.)

We then follow the familiar five steps for hypothesis testing.

The null hypothesis is that the mean difference (μ_d) is zero. This is the equivalent of saying that, on average, there is no difference between a runner's resting heart rate before and after the track season. The alternative hypothesis is that the mean difference (μ_d) is NOT zero.

We choose a 5% significance level, or $\alpha = 0.05$.

STATISTICAL TEST

Given a sample of 40 persons, we choose a z-test.

$$z = \frac{\bar{X}_d - \mu_d}{s_d / \sqrt{n}}$$

As a reminder:

- n sample size, or the number of paired matches;
- $\bar{X}_d$ mean of the differences between scores (for sample);
- μ_d mean of the differences between scores (for population); and
- s_d standard deviation of the differences between scores.

For the purposes of this statistical test, the value of μ_d is set at zero. This is because the null hypothesis is that there is no difference.

CRITERIA FOR DECISION RULE

Because we are interested in any difference—either greater than or less than—we have a two-tailed z-test at a 5% significance level. The critical value for z is thus ± 1.96. This can be found in Table A.1.

The decision rule is to reject the null hypothesis if [$z \leq -1.960$] or [$z \geq 1.960$]

CALCULATE STATISTICAL TEST

We now have all the data that we need to calculate the z-value for this scenario.

$$z = \frac{\bar{X}_d - \mu_d}{s_d / \sqrt{n}} \rightarrow z = \frac{-8.3 - 0.0}{18.0 / \sqrt{40}} = -2.91$$

ASSESSMENT OF FINDINGS

We reject the null hypothesis because -2.91 is less than -1.96.

This indicates that the size of the mean difference for the resting heart rate between measure one (before the track season) and measure two (after the track season) is large enough—with $\alpha = 0.05$—to meaningfully distinguish between the before-and-after scores for these 40 participants.

To further specify our p-value we turn to Table A.1 and find that a z-value of -2.91 corresponds with a probability of 0.0018. This is our p-value.

Example B

(This example illustrates a matched-pairs study.) There are reports from Nyerere County of improved cardiovascular health among its student athletes. First, we recruit 40 high-school long-distance runners from across Nyerere County to detect if long-distance running impacts a student's resting heart rate. This is group 1. We collect data for three attributes for each person (gender identity, age, and body mass index) and one exposure (caffeine consumption level).

Second, we recruit another 40 high-school students from across Nyerere County. This is group 2. No member of group 2 participates in sports and the attributes and exposures of each person in group 2 otherwise match the attributes and exposures of a person in group 1. Each person in each group thus has a matched pair. We have 80 participants and 40 matched pairs.

Third, we record the resting heart rate for each person in both groups before and after the track season. Fourth, we find the difference between the resting heart rate before and after the track season for each person in both groups. Fifth, we subtract the value of the difference we found in step 4 for each person in group 2 from the value of the difference for their matched pair in group 1. This results in 40 scores that represent the difference between any change in resting heart rates between our 40 matched pairs. Sixth, we find a mean for these 40 scores of –4.0 bpm, with a standard deviation of 10.0. (Again, note that a negative value suggests that the exposure decreases the resting heart rate.)

Illustration of steps 5 and 6:

> Isabella is in group 1 and Shaquana is her matched pair in group 2. The resting heart rate for Isabella before the track season was 70 bpm. For Shaquana it was also 70 bpm. After the track season, the resting heart rate for Isabella was 60 bpm. This is a difference of –10.0. The resting heart rate of Shaquana at the end of the track season was still 70 bpm. This is a difference of 0.0. We subtract Shaquana's score from Isabella's score (–10.0 – 0.0) and find a difference of –10.0. We repeat this for each matched pair. This produces 40 differences. We then find the mean for these 40 differences.
>
> Given these results, we must determine the probability of finding a *mean of the differences between the before-and-after scores* of this size for the matched pairs in group 1 and group 2.

Technical steps

Here again, most of the steps are identical with those for Example A. Because there are two groups, we must repeat certain steps for both groups and there is an extra step at the end to compare the two groups.

We continue with Example B based on the data from the example. We have 80 participants and 40 matched pairs. Therefore, $n = 40$.

$$n = 40; \quad \overline{X}_d = -4.0; \quad s_d = 10.0$$

Hypotheses and significance level

The null hypothesis is that the mean difference (μ_d) between group 1 and group 2 is zero. The alternative hypothesis is that the mean difference (μ_d) is NOT zero.

We choose a 5% significance level, or $\alpha = 0.05$.

STATISTICAL TEST

Given a sample of 40 persons, we choose a z-test.

$$z = \frac{\bar{X}_d - \mu_d}{s_d / \sqrt{n}}$$

For the purposes of this statistical test, μ_d is again set at zero.

CRITERIA FOR DECISION RULE

Because we are interested in any difference—either greater than or less than—we have a two-tailed z-test at a 5% significance level. The critical value of z is ± 1.96. This can be found in Table A.1.

The decision rule is to reject the null hypothesis if $[z \leq -1.960]$ or $[z \geq 1.960]$.

CALCULATE STATISTICAL TEST

We now have all the data that we need to calculate the z-value for this scenario.

$$z = \frac{\bar{X}_d - \mu_d}{s_d / \sqrt{n}} \rightarrow z = \frac{-4.0 - 0.0}{10 / \sqrt{40}} = -2.528$$

ASSESSMENT OF FINDINGS

We reject the null hypothesis because -2.528 is less than -1.96.

This indicates that the size of the mean difference for the resting heart rate between measure one (before the track season) and measure two (after the track season) for group 1 and group 2 is large enough—with $\alpha = 0.05$—to meaningfully distinguish between these two groups.

We again turn to Table A.1 and find that a z-value of -2.528 corresponds with a probability of approximately 0.0059. This is our p-value.

Configuration #4

Goal: To compare the means of three or more independent groups for some continuous outcome variable based on a difference in attribute or exposure.

Confidence interval estimation and configuration #4

Given more than two groups, we cannot apply confidence interval estimation to configuration #4.

Hypothesis testing and configuration #4

Example A

There are 200 high-school long-distance runners in Machel County. We are curious about a possible relationship between blood type and the resting heart rate of long-distance runners.

Given this interest, we compare the mean resting heart rates for three groups of runners based on the three most common blood types in the sample. Our groups are group A, group B, and group O. (We combine the positive and negative subgroups for each of these that—along with AB positive and negative—form the eight blood types.)

We then recruit 10 runners for each group and record the resting heart rates for all 30 runners. We find that group A has a mean resting heart rate of 83 bpm; group B, 77 bpm; and group O, 73 bpm. (Note that we do not require the standard deviation in this example.)

Given these results, we must determine the probability of finding differences of this size between the mean resting heart rates of these three groups.

Technical steps

The statistical test that we use to assess these differences is the analysis of variance, or ANOVA. In particular, we are performing a "one-way" ANOVA here. A one-way ANOVA has one causal (or independent) variable, such as blood type. A two-way ANOVA has two causal (or independent) variables.

The ANOVA requires that we first gather sample sizes, sample means, and sample standard deviations for all our comparison groups. See Tables 5.7 and 5.8.

In our case, these values are presented in Table 5.8.

The null hypothesis for an ANOVA analysis is that there are no differences between group means. The alternative hypothesis is that there is at least one difference between group means.

Our first challenge is the F test that is associated with ANOVA. Initially, our impression is complexity.

$$F = \frac{\sum_{ni} (\bar{X}_1 - \bar{X})^2 / (k-1.0)}{\sum\sum (x - \bar{X}_1)^2 / (N-k)}$$

This is actually equivalent to: $F = \dfrac{\text{between-groups variance}}{\text{within-groups variance}}$

Table 5.7 Table of statistics for ANOVA

	Group 1	Group 2	Group 3
Sample size	n_1	n_2	n_3
Sample mean	$\bar{X}_1$	$\bar{X}_2$	$\bar{X}_3$
Sample standard deviation	s_1	s_2	s_3

Table 5.8 Statistics for Example A for ANOVA, $n = 30$

	Group A	Group B	Group O
Sample size	10	10	10
Sample mean	83	77	73
Sample standard deviation	11.0	7.0	8.0

Given this apparent complexity, we must take a moment to break down this statistical test into its simpler parts. To begin, notice that the right side of the equation is a ratio, with a numerator and denominator. The numerator measures the variance *between* groups. This we call the "mean square between" (or MS_B). The denominator measures the variance *within* each group. This we call the "mean square within" (or MS_W).

It may be that three groups have an identical mean of 73 bpm. Thus, between-group variance is zero. However, the standard deviations of these same three groups may be 10.0, 5.0, and 2.0. Thus, the within-group variance is considerable. The identical means, therefore, seems to be pure chance. The purpose of the F test is to assess the ratio between (a) the between-group variance and (b) the within-group variance. Doing so will help determine if our similar means are similar by chance or if they represent an actual similarity between the three groups.

The F test, therefore, tells us whether differences among the sample means are larger than would be expected by pure chance. There are two key criteria for the decision rule for the F test—the significance level and the degrees of freedom.

Per usual, we set our significance level at 95%.

There are then two measures of degrees of freedom—df_1 (for the numerator) and df_2 (for the denominator).

With these, we can create a table of summary statistics to compute the F statistic. See Table 5.9.

There are many symbols here to account for. Let's take these one at a time.

k is the number of groups.
N is the number of observations (adding the observations from all groups).
n_i is the size of each group.
SS_b is the "sum of squares of between-group differences."

This refers to the values in the numerator. This is computed by summing the squared differences between each group mean ($\overline{X}_i$) and the overall mean ($\overline{X}$) for all groups. For this, the squared differences are weighted by the sample sizes of each group. (This is the meaning of n_i.)

SS_w is the "sum of squares of within-group differences."

This refers to the values in the denominator. This is computed by summing the squared differences between each observation in group (X) and its group mean ($\overline{X}_i$).

Note that the double summa ($\Sigma\Sigma$) indicates that we first sum the squared differences within each group and we then sum these totals across groups to produce a single value.

Note further that the sum of squares of within-group differences (SS_W) is sometimes referred to as the sum of squares of errors, or SS_E.

Table 5.9 Table of summary statistics for ANOVA

Source of variation	Sum of squares	Degrees of freedom	Mean squares	F
Numerator (between groups)	$SS_b = \Sigma n_i(\overline{X}_i - \overline{X})^2$	$k - 1$	$MS_b = \dfrac{SS_b}{k - 1.0}$	$F = \dfrac{MS_b}{MS_w}$
Denominator (within groups)	$SS_w = \Sigma\Sigma(X - \overline{X}_i)^2$	$N - k$	$MS_w = \dfrac{SS_w}{N - k}$	
Total	$SS_T = \Sigma\Sigma(X - \overline{X})^2$	$N - 1$		

SS_T is the total sum of squares—SS_B and SS_W.

This is computed by summing the squared differences between each observation (X) and the overall sample mean ($\bar{X}$). When all data for all groups are pooled into a single sample, SS_T is the numerator for calculating the sample variance.

Note that SS_T does not contribute to the F statistic directly. However, $SS_T = SS_B + SS_W$. Therefore, if we know the values of any two of these three (SS_B, SS_W, SS_T), we can deduce the value of the third element.

MS_b is the mean sum of squares of between-group differences. This again refers to values in the numerator.

MS_w is the mean sum of squares of within-group differences. This again refers to values in the denominator.

MS_b / MS_w is a ratio between:

- The mean sum of squares of between-group differences
- The mean sum of squares of within-group differences

Hence, our ratio between the numerator (between groups) and the denominator (within groups) is sustained throughout the computation of the F test.

Lastly, because large values of the F statistic indicate significant differences between means, the critical value of F requires an upper-tailed test.

This overview allows us to now run through the five steps of hypothesis testing for Example A.

We first construct our table of statistics for ANOVA. For this, we have Table 5.10.

HYPOTHESES AND SIGNIFICANCE LEVEL

Again, the null hypothesis for ANOVA is that there are no differences between group means. The alternative hypothesis is that at least one group's mean differs from the other groups' means.

We choose a 5% significance level, or $\alpha = 0.05$.

STATISTICAL TEST

The statistical test for a one-way ANOVA is the F test:

$$F = \frac{\sum_{ni}(\bar{X}_1 - \bar{X})^2 \Big/ (k-1.0)}{\sum\sum(x - \bar{X}_1)^2 \Big/ (N-k)} \quad \text{or} \quad F = \frac{MS_b}{MS_w}$$

Table 5.10 Statistics for Example A for ANOVA, $n = 30$

	Group A	Group B	Group O
Sample size	10	10	10
Sample mean	83	77	73
Sample standard deviation	11.0	7.0	8.0

CRITERIA FOR DECISION RULE

To determine the critical value of F, we calculate the degrees of freedom for: $df_1 = (k - 1)$ and $df_2 = (N - k)$.

For our example: $df_1 = 3 - 1 = 2$ AND $df_2 = 30 - 3 = 27$.

Given this, we turn to Table A.4 for the critical value of F and find 3.35. Again, this is an upper-tailed test.

Thus, our decision rule is to reject the null hypothesis if: $F \geq 3.35$

CALCULATE STATISTICAL TEST

To calculate our F statistic, we need further data that we gather into four tables: Tables 5.11, 5.12, 5.13, and 5.14.

Now the final three steps.

First, we calculate SS_b.

$$SS_b = \sum n_j \left(\bar{X}_i - \bar{X} \right)^2$$

We know the sample mean for each group ($\bar{X}_j$) from Table 5.10. We divide the sum of these by the number of groups (three) to derive the mean for all 30 participants.

$$\frac{83 + 77 + 73}{3} = 77.7$$

Table 5.11 Statistics for resting heart rates, by blood type, $n = 30$

Group	Sample size	Group mean
Group 1 (type A)	10	83
Group 2 (type B)	10	77
Group 3 (type O)	10	73

Table 5.12 Deviations from mean resting heart rate (group 1), $n = 10$

Runner	Heart rate	$(X - 83)$	$(X - 83)^2$
1	83	0	0
2	82	−1	1
3	88	5	25
4	81	−2	4
5	85	2	4
6	87	4	16
7	79	−4	16
8	83	0	0
9	78	−5	25
10	84	1	1
Total	830		92

Table 5.13 Deviations from mean resting heart rate (group 2), $n = 10$

Runner	Heart rate	$(X - 77)$	$(X - 77)^2$
1	77	0	0
2	87	10	100
3	72	−5	25
4	79	2	4
5	80	3	9
6	74	−3	9
7	82	5	25
8	75	−2	4
9	77	0	0
10	67	−10	100
Total	770		276

Table 5.14 Deviations from mean resting heart rate (group 3), $n = 10$

Runner	Heart rate	$(X - 73)$	$(X - 73)^2$
1	73	0	0
2	79	6	36
3	84	11	121
4	73	0	0
5	67	−6	36
6	66	−7	49
7	80	7	49
8	74	1	1
9	62	−11	121
10	72	−1	1
Total	730		414

Thus, we have:

$$SS_b = [10(83 - 77.7)^2 + 10(77 - 77.7)^2 + 10(73 - 77.7)^2] =$$
$$[280.9 + 4.9 + 220.9] = 506.7$$

Second, we calculate SS_w based on the same four tables of data: Tables 5.11 through 5.14.

$$SS_w = \Sigma\Sigma\left(X - \bar{X}_i\right)^2$$

Thus, $SS_w = 92 + 276 + 414 = 782$

Third, we construct our table of summary statistics for ANOVA and derive an F statistic. See Table 5.15.

ASSESSMENT OF FINDINGS

We reject the null hypothesis because 8.75 is greater than 3.24.

Table 5.15 Example A summary statistics for ANOVA

Source of variation	Sum of squares	Degrees of freedom	Mean square	F
Numerator (between groups)	506.7	3 – 1 = 2	$\dfrac{506.7}{2}$	$\dfrac{253.4}{28.96} = 8.75$
Denominator (within groups)	782	30 – 3 = 27	$\dfrac{782}{27}$	
Total	1,272.7	30 – 1 = 29		

We have statistically significant evidence—with $\alpha = 0.05$—that there is a difference between the mean resting heart rates among the three groups that differ by blood type.

As a general rule, it becomes very complex to approximate p-values for ANOVA by hand. We thus rely on statistical software programs to provide an exact p-value. In this case, Excel finds $p = 0.0011$.

Example B

There are 200 high-school long-distance runners in Machel County. We are concerned that caffeine consumption might be impacting the resting heart rate of our runners. We recruit a random sample of 18 high-school long-distance runners and randomly assign six to group 1, six to group 2, and six to group 3. Note that these three groups will differ based on an exposure (caffeine consumption) and not an attribute, such as blood type in Example A.

Over a six-week period, group 1 will consume three or more daily caffeine beverages. Group 2 will consume one to two daily caffeine beverages. Group 3 will consume no caffeine beverages. After six weeks, we record the resting heart rate of all participants. We find that group 1 has a mean resting heart rate of 83 bpm; group 2, 77 bpm; and group 3, 73 bpm. (Note again that we do not require the standard deviation in this example.)

Given these results, we must determine the probability of finding differences of this size between the mean resting heart rates of these three groups.

Technical steps

Before turning to Example B, note that the basic elements of Example A and Example B are identical except for two considerations. First, the difference between the three groups in Example A was an attribute (blood type). In Example B, this difference is an exposure (caffeine consumption). Second, the size of each group in Example A is 10. The size of each group in Example B is six. With those differences in mind, we proceed to our table of summary statistics for ANOVA. See Table 5.16.

Table 5.16 Statistics for Example B for ANOVA, $n = 18$

	Group 1	Group 2	Group 3
Sample size	6	6	6
Sample mean	83	77	73
Sample standard deviation	10.0	8.2	8.2

The null hypothesis is that there are no differences between group means. The alternative hypothesis is that at least one group's mean differs from the other groups' means.

We choose a 5% significance level, or $\alpha = 0.05$.

STATISTICAL TEST

The statistical test for our one-way ANOVA is the F test:

$$F = \frac{\sum \frac{(\bar{X}_i - \bar{X})^2}{ni}}{\sum\sum \frac{(X - \bar{X}_1)^2}{(N-k)}} \Big/ (k - 1.0) \quad \text{or} \quad F = \frac{MS_b}{MS_w}$$

CRITERIA FOR DECISION RULE

To determine the critical value of F, we calculate the degrees of freedom for: $df_1 = (k - 1)$ and $df_2 = (N - k)$.

For our example: $df_1 = 3 - 1 = 2$ AND $df_2 = 18 - 3 = 15$

Based on this, we turn to Table A.4 for the critical value of F and find 2.69. Again, this is an upper-tailed test.

Thus, our decision rule is to reject the null hypothesis if: $F \geq 2.69$.

CALCULATE STATISTICAL TEST

To calculate our F statistic we need further data that we gather into four tables: Tables 5.17, 5.18, 5.19, and 5.20.

Table 5.17 Statistics for resting heart rate, by daily caffeine consumption, $n = 18$

Group	Sample size	Group mean
Group 1 (3 or more caffeine beverages)	6	83
Group 2 (1 or 2 caffeine beverages)	6	77
Group 3 (no caffeine beverages)	6	73

Table 5.18 Deviations from mean resting heart rate (group 1), $n = 6$

Runner	Heart rate	$(X - 83)$	$(X - 83)^2$
1	68	−15	225
2	82	−1	1
3	88	5	25
4	78	−5	25
5	84	1	1
6	98	15	225
Total	498		502

Table 5.19 Deviations from mean resting heart rate (group 2), n = 6

Runner	Heart rate	(X – 77)	(X – 77)²
1	81	4	16
2	65	–12	144
3	80	3	9
4	74	–3	9
5	89	12	144
6	73	–4	16
Total	462		338

Table 5.20 Deviations from mean resting heart rate (group 3), n = 6

Runner	Heart rate	(X – 73)	(X – 73)²
1	83	10	100
2	75	2	4
3	71	–2	4
4	65	–8	64
5	81	8	64
6	63	–10	100
Total	438		336

Now, the final three steps.

First, we calculate SS_b.

$$SS_b = \sum n_j \left(\bar{X}_i - \bar{X} \right)^2$$

We know the sample mean for each group ($\bar{X}_j$) from Table 5.16. We divide the sum of these by the number of groups (three) to derive the mean for all 18 participants.

$$\frac{83 + 77 + 73}{3} = 77.7$$

Thus, we have:

$$SS_b = [6(83 - 77.7)^2 + 6(77 - 77.7)^2 + 6(73 - 77.7)^2] = [168.5 + 2.9 + 132.5]$$
$$= 303.9$$

Second, we calculate SS_w based on the same four tables of data, Tables 5.17 through 5.20.

$$SS_w = \sum \sum \left(X - \bar{X}_i \right)^2$$

Thus, $SS_w = 502 + 338 + 336 = 1,176$

Third, we construct our table of summary statistics for ANOVA and derive an F statistic. See Table 5.21.

Table 5.21 Example B summary statistics for ANOVA

Source of variation	Sum of squares	Degrees of freedom	Mean squares	F
Numerator (between groups)	303.9	$3 - 1 = 2$	$\dfrac{303.9}{2}$	$\dfrac{151.9}{78.4} = 1.94$
Denominator (within groups)	1,176	$18 - 3 = 15$	$\dfrac{1176}{15}$	
Total	1,479.9	$18 - 1 = 17$		

ASSESSMENT OF FINDINGS

We do NOT reject the null hypothesis because 1.94 is less than 3.24.

We do not have statistically significant evidence—with $\alpha = 0.05$—that there is a difference between the mean resting heart rates among the three groups that differ by level of caffeine consumption.

Recall that the only measurement difference between Example A (which was statistically significant) and Example B is the sample size for the three groups, $n = 10$ and $n = 6$, respectively.

Configuration #5

Goal: To compare the means of two independent groups for some continuous outcome variable based on differences in multiple attributes and/or exposures.

See Chapter 7 for these technical steps.

We proceed now to Chapter 6 and configurations #6, #7, and #9.

Configurations for Biostatistical Analysis
Technical Steps (2)

Chapter 5 detailed the technical steps for the first four configurations, all of which had continuous outcome variables. In this chapter we detail the technical steps for configurations #6, #7, and #9. These include those configurations with dichotomous, ordinal, or categorical outcome variables.

For convenient reference, we reprint the tables for the 10 configurations (Table 4.1, presented here as Table 6.1) and for the estimation equations and statistical tests associated with each of these (Table 5.1, presented here as Table 6.2).

We continue now with our configurations.

Configuration #6

Goal: To estimate a population proportion for some dichotomous variable based on a sample proportion.

Confidence interval estimation and configuration #6

Example

There are 200 high-school long-distance runners in Lumumba County. We have limited general health data for these runners. We want to know the proportion of all high-school long-distance runners in Lumumba County with a resting heart rate of 83 bpm or higher. For this, we recruit a random sample of 40 high-school long-distance runners and find 10 runners with a resting heart rate of 83 bpm or greater. This is a proportion of 0.25.

Given these results, we must estimate—at a certain confidence level—a range of values that aims to capture the true proportion of high-school long-distance runners in Lumumba County with a resting heart rate of 83 bpm or greater.

Technical steps

When addressing this same scenario in configuration #1, with a continuous outcome variable, we were trying to find an unknown population mean. Here, with a dichotomous outcome variable, we want to find an unknown population proportion. Specifically, our interest is the proportion of the population with a resting heart rate of 83 bpm or greater, given the data for our sample.

There are five steps to this process. (To clarify, these are NOT the five steps of hypothesis testing.)

DOI: 10.4324/9781003316985-6

Table 6.1 Comparison of nine configurations

Configuration	Four basic features of biostatistical research				Confidence intervals	Hypothesis testing
	Type of outcome variable	Number of groups	Relation of groups	Number of independent variables		
#1	Continuous	1	–	1	Yes	No
#2	Continuous	2	Independent	1	Yes	Yes
#3	Continuous	1 or 2	Dependent	1	Yes	Yes
#4	Continuous	3+	Independent	1	No	Yes
#5	Continuous	2+	Independent	3+	No	Yes
#6	Dichotomous	1	–	1	Yes	No
#7	Dichotomous	2	Independent	1	Yes	Yes
#8	Dichotomous	2+	Independent	3+	No	Yes
#9	Ordinal or categorical	2+	Independent	1	No	Yes

Table 6.2 Estimation equations and statistical tests for configurations, by confidence interval estimation or hypothesis testing

Configuration	Confidence interval estimation and estimation equations		Hypothesis testing and statistical tests	
	$n \geq 30$	$n < 30$	$n \geq 30$	$n < 30$
#1	$\bar{X} \pm z \dfrac{s}{\sqrt{n}}$	$\bar{X} \pm t \dfrac{s}{\sqrt{n}}$	N/A	N/A
#2 examples A, B	$(\bar{X}_1 - \bar{X}_2) \pm z(S_p)\sqrt{\dfrac{1}{n_1}+\dfrac{1}{n_2}}$	$(\bar{X}_1 - \bar{X}_2) \pm t(S_p)\sqrt{\dfrac{1}{n_1}+\dfrac{1}{n_2}}$	$z = \dfrac{\bar{X}_1 - \bar{X}_2}{S_p\sqrt{\dfrac{1}{n_1}+\dfrac{1}{n_2}}}$	$t = \dfrac{\bar{X}_1 - \bar{X}_2}{S_p\sqrt{\dfrac{1}{n_1}+\dfrac{1}{n_2}}}$
#2 example C	N/A	N/A	$z = \dfrac{\bar{X} - \mu_0}{s / \sqrt{n}}$	$t = \dfrac{\bar{X} - \mu_0}{s / \sqrt{n}}$
#3	$\bar{X}_d \pm (z)\dfrac{s_d}{\sqrt{n}}$	$\bar{X}_d \pm (z)\dfrac{s_d}{\sqrt{n}}$	$z = \dfrac{\bar{X}_d - \mu_d}{s_d / \sqrt{n}}$	$t = \dfrac{\bar{X}_d - \mu_d}{s_d / \sqrt{n}}$
#4	N/A		$F = \dfrac{\sum_{ni}\dfrac{(\bar{x}_i - \bar{x})^2}{(k-1)}}{\sum\sum\dfrac{(x - \bar{x}_i)^2}{(N-k)}}$	
#5	N/A		$\hat{y} = b_0 + b_1 x_1 + b_2 x_2 + \ldots b_p x_p$	
#6	$\hat{p} \pm z\sqrt{\dfrac{\hat{p}(1.0-\hat{p})}{n}}$		N/A	

(continued)

Table 6.2 Cont.

Configuration	Confidence interval estimation and estimation equations	Hypothesis testing and statistical tests
#7.0	N/A	$z = \dfrac{\hat{p} - p_0}{\sqrt{\dfrac{p_0 (1.0 - p_0)}{n}}}$
#7.1	$(\hat{p}_1 - \hat{p}_2) \pm z \sqrt{\dfrac{\hat{p}_1 (1.0 - \hat{p}_1)}{n_1} + \dfrac{\hat{p}_2 (1.0 - \hat{p}_2)}{n_2}}$	$z = \dfrac{\hat{p}_1 - \hat{p}_2}{\sqrt{\hat{p}(1.0 - \hat{p}) \times \left(1.0/n_1 + 1.0/n_2\right)}}$
#7.2	$\ln(\widehat{RR}) \pm z \sqrt{\dfrac{(n_1 - x_1)/x_1}{n_1} + \dfrac{(n_2 - x_2)/x_2}{n_2}}$	$\chi^2 = \Sigma_{(r*c)} \dfrac{(O - E)^2}{E}$
#7.3	$\ln(\widehat{OR}) \pm z \sqrt{\dfrac{1}{x_1} + \dfrac{1}{(n_1 - x_1)} + \dfrac{1}{x_2} + \dfrac{1}{(n_2 - x_2)}}$	$\chi^2 = \Sigma_{(r*c)} \dfrac{(O - E)^2}{E}$
#8	N/A	$\ln\left(\dfrac{\hat{p}}{1.0 - \hat{p}}\right) = \alpha + b_1 x_1 + b_2 x_2 + \ldots b_p x_p$
#9 examples A, B	N/A	$\chi^2 = \Sigma_{(r*c)} \dfrac{(O - E)^2}{E}$
#9 example C	N/A	$\chi^2 = \Sigma_k \dfrac{(O - E)^2}{E}$

First, we record—as yes/no—whether or not each member of the sample has a resting heart rate of 83 bpm or greater. From this, we generate a ratio of "successes" *vis-à-vis* the sample size. Importantly, "success" does not always mean a positive outcome. It is simply an outcome that we are interested in documenting. Thus:

$$\hat{p} = \frac{x}{n} \;\rightarrow\; \hat{p} = \frac{10}{40} = 0.25$$

Note that the symbol $\hat{p}$ is the sample proportion. This is pronounced "p-hat." The symbol p with no "hat" represents the population proportion.

Second, we confirm that there are *at least* five successes and *at least* five non-successes. If so, then our sample size is large enough to use the z-values associated with the standard normal distribution. To determine this, naturally, we have a formula:

$$\min[n(\hat{p}), n(1.0 - \hat{p})] \geq 5 \;\rightarrow\; \min[40(0.25), 40(1.0 - 0.25)] \geq 5 \;\rightarrow\; \min[10, 30] = 10$$

The abbreviation "min" is short for minimum.

The formula thus generates two values—$n(\hat{p})$ and $n(1.0 - \hat{p})$—both of which are greater than 5 in this case, allowing us to continue.

Third, We choose a confidence level—of course, 95%—and then we find a z-value based on this. We know from previous examples that a 95% confidence level has a z-value of ± 1.96.

Fourth, we calculate the standard error of the difference in proportions:

$$\sqrt{\frac{\hat{p}(1.0 - \hat{p})}{n}} \rightarrow \sqrt{\frac{0.25(1.0 - 0.25)}{40}} = 0.068$$

Again, this tells us how greatly the "difference in proportions" would vary between samples if we continued to draw more samples from the same population. The standard error in this case is moderately small (0.068). Thus, we would expect minimal variation from the results of further samples compared to this sample.

Fifth, we calculate the margin of error:

$$\hat{p} \pm z\sqrt{\frac{\hat{p}(1.0 - \hat{p})}{n}} \rightarrow 0.25 \pm 1.96\sqrt{\frac{0.25(1.0 - 0.25)}{40}} = 0.25 \pm 0.133\,(0.119, 0.383)$$

Notice that the margin of error is the z-value (1.96) times the standard error of the difference in proportions (0.068). The smaller the standard error, the smaller the margin of error. The smaller the margin of error, the more precise our findings.

Thus, we estimate—at a 95% confidence level—that the true population proportion for persons with a resting heart rate of 83 bpm or greater is between 11.7% and 38.3%. This suggests a fairly large interval. Our sample data, therefore, do not result in a very precise understanding of the true proportion.

However, as with configuration #1, if we increase the sample size from 40 to 4,000, the estimated confidence interval again shrinks appreciably.

$$\hat{p} \pm z\sqrt{\frac{\hat{p}(1.0 - \hat{p})}{n}} \rightarrow 0.25 \pm 1.96\sqrt{\frac{0.25(1.0 - 0.25)}{4000}} = 0.25 \pm 0.0134\,(0.237, 0.263)$$

Now, we estimate—at a 95% confidence level—that the true population proportion for persons with a resting heart rate of 83 bpm or greater is between 23.7% and 26.3%.

Hypothesis testing and configuration #6

We cannot apply hypothesis testing to this scenario, insofar as we do not have sufficient data to construct null and alternative hypotheses.

Configuration #7: some preliminaries for consideration of the risk difference, risk ratio, odds ratio

Goal: To compare the proportions of two independent groups for some dichotomous outcome variable based on a difference in attribute or exposure.

As we have seen, it is very common within biostatistical analysis to compare two independent groups regarding the presence or absence of some attribute or exposure. For example, we might ask about the presence or absence of asthma among third-graders versus fourth-graders or the presence or absence of infection after surgery among heart transplant patients with a new antibiotic versus patients with a current antibiotic. As noted, in cases such as these with dichotomous outcomes, our analysis compares the proportions of successes in each group.

There are three methods for comparing proportions in this manner. These—the risk difference, the risk ratio, and the odds ratio—warrant special attention. Each has its unique utility and technical steps. Here we briefly revisit and summarize key aspects of these three measures.

The risk difference is the absolute difference between the proportions of success for the members of group 1 and the members of group 2. A risk difference of 0.0, therefore, indicates that there is no difference between the proportions of success for the two groups.

The risk ratio is a ratio between the probability of an event occurring for the members of group 1 and the probability of the same event occurring for the members of group 2. A risk ratio of 1.0 (or 1:1), therefore, indicates that there is no difference between the probabilities of an event occurring for the members of either group.

The odds ratio is the ratio between the odds of an event occurring for an individual in group 1 and the odds of the same event occurring for an individual in group 2. An odds ratio of 1.0 (or 1:1), therefore, indicates that there is no difference between the odds of the event occurring for an individual in either group.

There is a subtle yet important distinction between the risk ratio and the odds ratio that can easily get lost. Each is a ratio between two groups. However, the risk ratio is a ratio between the probable proportion of persons in group 1 who will experience a certain event and the probable proportion of persons in group 2 who will experience a certain event. The odds ratio is a ratio between the odds that an individual in group 1 will experience a certain event and the odds that an individual in group 2 will experience a certain event.

The difference here is certainly nuanced. And, indeed, most often the risk ratio and odds ratio tend to be almost identical. Hence, we can generally reserve the use of the odds ratio for special occasions, such as logistic regression or case-control studies. This we explore below.

See Table 6.3 for the null and alternative hypotheses that are attached to the risk difference, risk ratio, and odds ratio for hypothesis testing.

For confidence interval estimation, we have three separate estimation equations for the risk difference, risk ratio, and odds ratio. For hypothesis testing, we have one statistical test for the risk difference and one statistical test for the risk ratio and odds ratio. This is detailed in Table 5.1 (re-presented here as Table 6.2) for risk difference (#7.1), risk ratio (#7.2), and odds ratio (#7.3).

While the goal of configuration #7 distinguishes it as a singular configuration, for greater clarity, we designate risk difference as operation 7.1, risk ratio as operation 7.2, and odds ratio as operation 7.3.

Before proceeding with these three operations however, we must briefly revisit a common situation pertaining to configuration #7 that we encountered with configuration #2 (with continuous outcome variables) and that we will later encounter with configuration #9 (with ordinal or categorical outcome variables).

Table 6.3 Null hypothesis and alternative hypothesis for the risk difference, risk ratio, and odds ratio

	Null hypothesis	Alternative hypothesis
Risk difference	The risk difference is 0.0	The risk difference is NOT 0.0
Risk ratio	The risk ratio is 1.0 (or 1:1)	The risk ratio is NOT 1.0 (or 1:1)
Odds ratio	The odds ratio is 1.0 (or 1:1)	The odds ratio is NOT 1.0 (or 1:1)

The situation arises when we compare a proportion for two populations based on data for population 1 and data for a sample from population 2. We designate this operation 7.0 to set it apart and we illustrate it with an example for hypothesis testing and risk difference. For comparison, see configuration #2, Example C, and configuration #9, Example C.

Configuration #7: operation 7.0

Hypothesis testing and operation 7.0

Example

There are 200 high-school long-distance runners in Lumumba County. We have limited general health data for these runners. It happens that we have statewide data indicating that four years earlier the proportion of all high-school long-distance runners with a resting heart rate of 83 bpm or greater was 0.25. We want to know if the current proportion of all high-school long-distance runners in Lumumba County differs from the earlier statewide data.

Given this, we hypothesize that the proportion of all current high-school long-distance runners in Lumumba County with a resting heart rate of 83 bpm is 0.25. We then recruit a random sample of 40 high-school long-distance runners and find a proportion of 0.22 for those with a resting heart rate of 83 bpm or greater.

Thus, we have data for two populations. The proportion of those with a resting heart rate above 83 bpm for population 1 is 0.25. The proportion of those with a resting heart rate above 83 bpm for population 2 is 0.22, based on sample data.

Given these results, we calculate the risk difference. We then determine the probability of finding a risk difference of this size between population 1 and population 2, regarding the proportion of persons with a heart rate above 83 bpm.

Technical steps

As noted, this example is akin to Example C for configuration #2 and hypothesis testing. We merely shift from a measure of the mean to a measure of the proportion. (It is also similar to Example C for configuration #9.)

Our task is to compare (a) the proportion of successes in a sample from population 1 with (b) a known proportion of successes from population 2. The known proportion is generally derived from a past study, as in this example.

From our sample, we know $\hat{p} = 0.25$. From past data, we know $p_0 = 0.22$. The notation "p_0" refers to a known population proportion that is associated with the null hypothesis.

The question is simply this. If the true population proportion of population 2 is 0.22, what is the probability of finding a sample of 40 persons with a proportion of 0.25 at a 5% significance level? If the probability is less than 5% then our results will indicate that this sample most likely was not taken from a population whose true proportion was 0.22. Therefore, we will have evidence that the proportion for population 1 differs from the proportion for population 2. This would mean that there is a very low probability that the risk difference between population 1 and population 2 is 0.0.

Now our five steps for hypothesis testing.

HYPOTHESES AND SIGNIFICANCE LEVEL

Our null hypothesis is that the population proportion for persons with a resting heart rate above 83 bpm remains 0.22. Thus, the risk difference is 0.0. Our alternative hypothesis is that the population proportion for persons with a resting heart rate above 83 bpm is greater than 0.22. Thus, the risk difference is not 0.0.

We choose a 5% significance level, or $\alpha = 0.05$.

STATISTICAL TEST

We have two steps to set up our statistical test.

The statistical test for hypothesis testing pertaining to the difference in proportions for the risk difference relies on a z-distribution (Table A.1). This is also true for the estimation equation and confidence interval estimation. There is no alternative statistical test (or estimation equation) based on a t-distribution for smaller groups.

Thus, to proceed we must have at least five successes and at least five non-successes in each sample. To confirm this, we calculate:

$$\min[n(p_0),\ n(1.0 - p_0)] \geq 5$$

Each of these two values must be at least five. For this example, we find:

$$\min[40(0.22),\ 40(1.0 - 0.22)] = \min[8.8,\ 31.2] = 8.8$$

Thus, given that $8.8 \geq 5$, we can use the z-test to assess the null hypothesis.

Second, given this, we turn to the z-test.

$$z = \frac{\hat{p} - p_0}{\sqrt{\dfrac{p_0\left(1.0 - p_0\right)}{n}}}$$

CRITERIA FOR DECISION RULE

Because we anticipate that the sample proportion is greater than the population proportion, this is an upper-tailed test at a 5% significance level. Given this, the critical value of z that we find in Table A.1 is 1.645.

Our decision rule is thus to reject the null hypothesis if: $z \geq 1.645$.

CALCULATE STATISTICAL TEST

We now plug our numbers into the z-test:

$$z = \frac{\hat{p} - p_0}{\sqrt{\dfrac{p_0\left(1.0 - p_0\right)}{n}}} \rightarrow \frac{0.25 - 0.22}{\sqrt{\dfrac{0.22(1.0 - 0.22)}{40}}} = 0.458$$

We find a z-value of 0.458.

ASSESSMENT OF FINDINGS

We thus do NOT reject the null hypothesis because 0.458 is not greater than 1.645. We do not have statistically significant evidence, at $\alpha = 0.05$, that the risk difference is not 0.0.

Hence, our results do not support the claim that the proportion of persons with a resting heart rate above 83 bpm for population 2 is greater than 0.22.

Now we continue with further examples of risk difference, risk ratio, and odds ratio.

Configuration #7: operation 7.1 and risk difference

Confidence interval estimation and operation 7.1 and risk difference

Example A

There are 200 high-school long-distance runners in Mandela County. Of these, 110 identify as cis males and 90 as cis females. We want to know if there is any difference between the proportion of cis-male runners and the proportion of cis-female runners with a resting heart rate of 83 bpm. We recruit a random sample of 40 cis-male and 40 cis-female high-school long-distance runners. We find that eight cis males (or 20%) and 12 cis females (or 30%) have a resting heart rate of 83 bpm or greater.

Given these findings, we must estimate—at a certain confidence level—a range of values that aims to capture the true risk difference between group 1 and group 2 regarding the proportion of persons with a resting heart rate of 83 bpm or greater.

Technical steps

Again, because there is no alternative estimation equation (or statistical test based on a t-distribution for smaller groups), we need at least five successes and at least five non-successes in each sample. To confirm this, we calculate:

$$\min[n_1(\hat{p}_1), n_1(1.0 - \hat{p}_1), n_2(\hat{p}_2), n_2(1.0 - \hat{p}_2) \geq 5$$

Each of these four values must be at least five. For Example A, we find:

$$\min[40(0.2), 40(1.0 - 0.2), 40(0.3), 40(1.0 - 0.3)] \geq 5 \rightarrow \min[8, 32, 12, 28] = 8$$

The minimum value we find (eight) is greater than five. So we have at least five successes and five non-successes for each and we are good to go.

To begin, we create a table to identify the point estimate for each group. Again, the point estimate is our best guess—based on the available data—about the actual proportion of persons with a resting heart rate above 83 bpm in the population from which each group was taken based on the available data.

For this purpose, we provide a generic two-by-two frequency table and a two-by-two frequency table with data from Example A. See Tables 6.4 and 6.5.

The point estimate for cis-male high-school long-distance runners is: $\dfrac{8}{40} = 0.2$.

The point estimate for cis-female high-school long-distance runners is: $\dfrac{12}{40} = 0.3$.

Given these point estimates, we calculate the difference in the proportion of runners with a resting heart rate above 83 bpm between group 1 and group 2. We choose a 95% confidence level, which tells us again that our z-value is ± 1.96. The estimation equation for this is:

Table 6.4 Two-by-two frequency table

	With condition	Without condition	Total
Group 1 (with exposure)	a	b	a + b
Group 2 (without exposure)	c	d	c + d
Total	a + c	b + d	

(a + b) – the total number of persons with exposure
(c + d) – the total number of persons without exposure
(a + c) – the total number of persons with condition
(b + d) – the total number of persons without condition

Table 6.5 Two-by-two frequency table for gender identity and resting heart rate, $n = 40$

	Heart rate ≥ 83 bpm	Heart rate < 83 bpm	Total
Cis male	8	32	40
Cis female	12	28	40
Total	20	60	

$$\left(\hat{p}_1 - \hat{p}_2\right) \pm z \sqrt{\frac{\hat{p}_1\left(1.0 - \hat{p}_1\right)}{n_1} + \frac{\hat{p}_2\left(1.0 - \hat{p}_2\right)}{n_2}}$$

Thus, we have:

$$(0.2 - 0.3) \pm 1.96 \sqrt{\frac{0.2(1 - 0.2)}{40} + \frac{0.3(1 - 0.3)}{40}} = -0.1 \pm 0.18(-0.28, 0.089)$$

We estimate—at a 95% confidence level—that the true difference in proportions between group 1 and group 2 is between and −28.6% and 8.6%.

Because a risk difference of 0.0—indicating no difference between proportions—falls within this estimated confidence interval, we cannot rule out no risk difference between group 1 and group 2 with respect to the proportion of people with a resting heart rate above 83 bpm.

Example B

There are 200 high-school long-distance runners in Mandela County. We are concerned that caffeine consumption may be elevating the resting heart rate of our runners. We recruit a random sample of 80 high-school long-distance runners and randomly assign 40 to group 1 and 40 to group 2.

Over six weeks, group 1 consumes three caffeine beverages per day and group 2 consumes no caffeine beverages. We record the resting heart rate for all persons in both groups after the six weeks and find that 16 of those in group 1 (or 40%) and 10 of those in group 2 (or 25%) have resting heart rates of 83 bpm or greater.

Given these results, we must estimate—at a certain confidence level—a range of values that aims to capture the true risk difference between group 1 and group 2 regarding the proportion of persons with a resting heart rate of 83 bpm or greater.

Technical steps

To begin, we must again establish that we have at least five successes and at least five non-successes in each sample. To confirm that this, we calculate:

$$\min[n_1(\hat{p}_1), n_1(1.0-\hat{p}_1), n_2(\hat{p}_2), n_2(1.0-\hat{p}_2)] \geq 5$$

Thus, each of these four values must be five or greater. For Example B we find:

$$\min[40(0.4), 40(1.0-0.4), 40(0.25), 40(1.0-0.25)] \geq 5 = \min[16, 24, 10, 30] = 10$$

The minimum value we find (10) is greater than five. So we have at least five successes and five non-successes and we push on.

To begin, we create a two-by-two frequency table to identify the point estimate for each group. See Table 6.6.

The point estimate for those consuming caffeine is: $\dfrac{16}{40} = 0.4$.

The point estimate for those not consuming caffeine is: $\dfrac{10}{40} = 0.25$.

Given these point estimates, we calculate the difference between the proportions of runners with a resting heart rate above 83 bpm in group 1 and group 2. We set a 95% confidence level, giving us a z-value of ±1.96. Again, the estimation equation for this is:

$$\left(\hat{p}_1-\hat{p}_2\right) \pm z\sqrt{\frac{\hat{p}_1\left(1.0-\hat{p}_1\right)}{n_1}+\frac{\hat{p}_2\left(1.0-\hat{p}_2\right)}{n_2}}$$

Thus, we have:

$$(0.4-0.25) \pm 1.96\sqrt{\frac{0.4(1.0-0.4)}{40}+\frac{0.25(1.0-0.25)}{40}} = 0.15 \pm 0.203\,(-0.053, 0.353)$$

We estimate—at a 95% confidence level—that the true difference between the proportions for group 1 and group 2 is between −5.3% and 35.3%.

Because a risk difference of 0.0—indicating no difference between proportions—again falls within this estimated confidence interval, we cannot rule out no risk difference between group 1 and group 2, with respect to the proportion of people with a resting heart rate above 83 bpm.

Notice something interesting about these two examples. In Example A, the absolute difference between the proportions for group 1 and 2 is 0.1 (0.2 − 0.3). In Example B, this is 0.15 (0.4 − 0.25). In light of these absolute differences, our question was whether we could

Table 6.6 Two-by-two frequency table for caffeine consumption and resting heart rate, $n = 80$

	Heart rate ≥ 83 bpm	Heart rate < 83 bpm	Total
Caffeine	16	24	40
No caffeine	10	30	40
Total	26	54	

rule out the possibility of no true risk difference between the two groups—*given the sample sizes and given a 95% confidence level*. In fact, these values (sample size and confidence level) are often as consequential as the actual absolute difference between group 1 and group 2.

For instance, see what happens if we increase the sample size of each group in Example B from 40 to 4,000, while retaining the same absolute difference (0.15) and a 95% confidence level. Suddenly, the same absolute difference between the proportions in group 1 and group 2 produces an estimated confidence interval of 12.98% to 17.02%. Certainly, a profound contrast with our previous estimated confidence interval of −5.3% to 35.3%!

Hypothesis testing and operation 7.1 and risk difference

Example A

There are 200 high-school long-distance runners in Mandela County. Of these, 110 identify as cis males and 90 as cis females. We want to know if there is any difference between the proportion of cis-male runners and the proportion of cis-female runners with a resting heart rate of 83 bpm or greater. We recruit a random sample of 40 cis-male and 40 cis-female high-school long-distance runners. We find that eight cis males (or 20%) and 12 cis females (or 30%) have a resting heart rate of 83 bpm or greater.

Given these results, we calculate the risk difference. We then determine the probability of finding a risk difference of this size between group 1 and group 2 regarding the proportion of persons with a resting heart rate of 83 bpm or greater.

Technical steps

Before initiating the five steps of hypothesis testing, we must find the proportions for our two groups—cis-male and cis-female high-school long-distance runners. See Table 6.7. Not surprisingly, this replicates our previous numbers.

The point estimate for cis-male high-school long-distance runners is: $\frac{8}{40} = 0.2$.

The point estimate for cis-female high-school long-distance runners is: $\frac{12}{40} = 0.3$.

Given these point estimates, we calculate the risk difference between the proportions of runners with a resting heart rate above 83 bpm for group 1 and group 2. For this, we follow the five steps of hypothesis testing.

HYPOTHESES AND SIGNIFICANCE LEVEL

The null hypothesis is that the proportions for each group are equal. Thus, the risk difference is 0.0. The alternative hypothesis is that the proportions for each group are not equal. Thus, the risk difference is not 0.0.

We choose a 5% significance level, or $\alpha = 0.05$.

Table 6.7 Two-by-two frequency table for gender identity and resting heart rate, $n = 80$

	Heart rate ≥ 83 bpm	Heart rate < 83 bpm	Total
Cis male	8	32	40
Cis female	12	28	40
Total	20	60	

STATISTICAL TEST

Before moving to our statistical test, we must again demonstrate that we have at least five successes and five non-successes.

$$\min[n_1(\hat{p}_1), n_1(1.0 - \hat{p}_1), n_2(\hat{p}_2), n_2(1.0 - \hat{p}_2)] \geq 5$$

Thus, each of these four values must be equal to or greater than five. For Example A we find:

$$\min[40(0.2), 40(1.0 - 0.2), 40(0.3), 40(1.0 - 0.3)] \geq 5 = \min[8, 32, 12, 28] = 8$$

Eight is greater than five. So we have at least five successes and five non-successes and we are free to use the following z-test.

$$z = \frac{\hat{p}_1 - \hat{p}_2}{\sqrt{\hat{p}(1.0 - \hat{p}) \times \left(\frac{1.0}{n_1} + \frac{1.0}{n_2}\right)}}$$

Take care with the pieces of this equation. Trickery lurks within this otherwise straightforward equation. DO NOT BE FOOLED!

Previously, we distinguished $\hat{p}$ from p, by explaining that the former represented the proportion for a sample and the latter represented the proportion for a population. This statistical test introduces a new wrinkle.

$\hat{p}_1$ and $\hat{p}_2$ (in the numerator) = the proportion for group 1 and group 2.

$\hat{p}$ (in the denominator) = the overall proportion of successes; we know this because $\hat{p}$ is not given a specific group designation such as $\hat{p}_1$ or $\hat{p}_2$.

CRITERIA FOR DECISION RULE

Because we are interested in any difference—whether greater than or less than—we want a two-tailed z-test at a 5% significance level. The critical value for z is 1.96. This is found in Table A.1—though by now the number is likely memorized.

Thus, the decision rule is to reject the null hypothesis if $[z \leq -1.960]$ or $[z \geq 1.960]$.

CALCULATE STATISTICAL TEST

Now we calculate: $z = \dfrac{\hat{p}_1 - \hat{p}_2}{\sqrt{\hat{p}(1.0 - \hat{p}) \times \left(\frac{1.0}{n_1} + \frac{1.0}{n_2}\right)}}$

$$\hat{p}_1 = \frac{x_1}{n_1}$$

$$\hat{p}_2 = \frac{x_2}{n_2}$$

$$\hat{p} = \frac{x_1 + x_2}{n_1 + n_2}$$

x = the number of successes

We already know the value of $\hat{p}_1$ and $\hat{p}_2$. These are the point estimates for cis males (0.2) and cis females (0.3). We thus face down two further calculations.

First, we have:

$$\hat{p} = \frac{x_1 + x_2}{n_1 + n_2} \rightarrow \frac{8+12}{40+40} = \frac{20}{80} = 0.25$$

Second, we have:

$$z = \frac{\hat{p}_1 - \hat{p}_2}{\sqrt{\hat{p}(1.0 - \hat{p}) \times \left(\frac{1.0}{n_1} + \frac{1.0}{n_2}\right)}} \rightarrow \frac{0.2 - 0.3}{\sqrt{0.25(0.75) \times \left(\frac{1.0}{40} + \frac{1.0}{40}\right)}} = \frac{-0.1}{0.097} = -1.031$$

ASSESSMENT OF FINDINGS

We do NOT reject the null hypothesis because −1.031 is neither less than −1.960, nor greater than 1.960. We do not have statistically significant evidence, at $\alpha = 0.05$, that the risk difference between group 1 and group 2 is not 0.0, regarding the proportion of persons with a resting heart rate of 83 bpm or greater.

Example B

There are 200 high-school long-distance runners in Mandela County. We are concerned that caffeine consumption may be elevating the resting heart rate of our runners. We recruit a random sample of 80 high-school long-distance runners and randomly assign 40 to group 1 and 40 to group 2.

Over six weeks, group 1 consumes three caffeine beverages per day and group 2 consumes no caffeine beverages. We record the resting heart rate for all persons in both groups after the six weeks and find that 16 of those in group 1 (or 40%) and 10 of those in group 2 (or 25%) have resting heart rates of 83 bpm or greater.

Given these results, we calculate the risk difference. We then determine the probability of finding a risk difference of this size between group 1 and group 2 regarding the proportion of persons with a resting heart rate of 83 bpm or greater.

Technical steps

Again, we begin by finding the proportions for our two groups—caffeine consumers and non-consumers among high-school long-distance runners. See Table 6.8. These are the point estimates.

Table 6.8 Two-by-two frequency table for caffeine consumption and resting heart rate, $n = 80$

	Heart rate ≥ 83 bpm	Heart rate < 83 bpm	Total
Caffeine	16	24	40
No caffeine	10	30	40
Total	26	54	

The point estimate for those consuming caffeine is thus: $\hat{p}_1 = \dfrac{16}{40} = 0.4$.

The point estimate for those not consuming caffeine is thus: $\hat{p}_2 = \dfrac{10}{40} = 0.25$.

Given these proportions, we calculate the risk difference between the proportions of runners with a resting heart rate above 83 bpm in group 1 and group 2. For this, we follow the five steps for hypothesis testing.

HYPOTHESES AND SIGNIFICANCE LEVEL

The null hypothesis is that the proportions for each group are equal. Thus, the risk difference is 0.0. The alternative hypothesis is that the proportions for each group are not equal. Thus, the risk difference is not 0.0.

We choose a 5% significance level, or $\alpha = 0.05$.

STATISTICAL TEST

Before moving to our statistical test, we must again demonstrate that we have at least five successes and five non-successes.

$$\min[n_1(\hat{p}_1), n_1(1.0 - \hat{p}_1), n_2(\hat{p}_2), n_2(1.0 - \hat{p}_2)] \geq 5$$

Thus, each of these four values must be equal to or greater than 5. For Example B this is:

$$\min[40(0.4), 40(1.0 - 0.4), 40(0.25), 40(1.0 - 0.25)] \geq 5 = \min[16, 24, 10, 30] = 10$$

Ten is greater than five. So we have at least five successes and five non-successes and we are free to use the following z-test.

$$z = \frac{\hat{p}_1 - \hat{p}_2}{\sqrt{\hat{p}(1.0 - \hat{p}) \times \left(1.0 \middle/ n_1 + 1.0 \middle/ n_2 \right)}}$$

Again, bear in mind that:
$\hat{p}_1$ and $\hat{p}_2$ (in the numerator) = the proportions for group 1 and group 2.
$\hat{p}$ (in the denominator) = the overall proportion of successes.

CRITERIA FOR DECISION RULE

Because we are interested in any difference—whether greater than or less than—we want a two-tailed z-test, at a 5% significance level. The critical value for z is 1.96. This is found in Table A.1.

Thus, the decision rule is to reject the null hypothesis if $[z \leq -1.960]$ or $[z \geq 1.960]$.

CALCULATE STATISTICAL TEST

Now we calculate $z = \dfrac{\hat{p}_1 - \hat{p}_2}{\sqrt{\hat{p}(1.0 - \hat{p}) \times \left(1.0 \middle/ n_1 + 1.0 \middle/ n_2 \right)}}$

$$\hat{p}_1 = \frac{x_1}{n_1}$$

$$\hat{p}_2 = \frac{x_2}{n_2}$$

$$\hat{p} = \frac{x_1 + x_2}{n_1 + n_2}$$

$x =$ the number of successes

We again face two calculations.
First, we have:

$$\hat{p} = \frac{x_1 + x_2}{n_1 + n_2} = \frac{10+16}{40+40} = \frac{26}{80} = 0.325$$

Second we have:

$$z = \frac{\hat{p}_1 - \hat{p}_2}{\sqrt{\hat{p}(1.0 - \hat{p}) \times \left(\frac{1.0}{n_1} + \frac{1.0}{n_2}\right)}} \rightarrow \frac{0.4 - 0.25}{\sqrt{0.325(0.675) \times \left(\frac{1}{40} + \frac{1}{40}\right)}} = \frac{0.15}{0.105} = 1.43$$

ASSESSMENT OF FINDINGS

We do not reject the null hypothesis because 1.43 is neither less than −1.960, nor greater than 1.960. We do not have statistically significant evidence at $\alpha = 0.05$ that the risk difference between group 1 and 2 is not 0.0, regarding the proportion of persons with a resting heart rate of 83 bpm or greater.

It will be recalled that in Example B above for confidence interval estimation and risk difference we had the same values as in this example. And, likewise, we could not rule out no difference between proportions because the estimated confidence interval included the null value of 0.0. However, after raising the sample size for each group from 40 to 4,000 we magically found a most agreeable estimated confidence interval of 12.98% to 17.02%.

Repeating the same trick here, we generate a rather large z-value of 14.3! A value of invincible statistical significance for the same absolute difference of 0.15 between the proportions for group 1 and group 2, with a p-value < 00001.

Configuration #7: operation 7.2 and risk ratio

Confidence interval estimation and operation 7.2 and risk ratio

Example A

There are 200 high-school long-distance runners in Mandela County. Of these, 110 identify as cis males and 90 as cis females. We want to know if there is any difference between the proportion of cis-male runners and the proportion of cis-female runners with a resting heart rate of 83 bpm or greater. We recruit a random sample of 40 cis-male and 40 cis-female high-school long-distance runners. We find that eight cis males (or 20%) and 12 cis females (or 30%) have a resting heart rate of 83 bpm or greater.

Given these findings, we must estimate—at a certain confidence level—a range of values that aims to capture the true risk ratio between group 1 and group 2 regarding the proportion of persons with a resting heart rate of 83 bpm or greater.

Technical steps

We begin with a fair warning. We have been largely able to avoid an abundance of symbolic notation up to now. Here we will need to work a bit more than usual with this notation to better follow the presentation.

A risk ratio is a ratio of proportions for two groups or populations: $\dfrac{p_1}{p_2}$.

Our interest here is the risk ratio between two populations.

A risk ratio between two populations is written: $\text{RR} = \dfrac{p_1}{p_2}$.

Our interest is also the risk ratio between two groups and this is written: $\widehat{\text{RR}} = \dfrac{\hat{p}_1}{\hat{p}_2}$.

Remember, the "hat" $(\hat{p})$ indicates a measure for a group (or sample). No hat indicates a measure of a population. In Example A, our point estimate for the risk ratio is: $\widehat{\text{RR}} = \dfrac{0.2}{0.3}$.

We now hit a snag. Until this point, the rules of the standard normal distribution (or a binomial distribution) have served us well. So well, in fact, that we have even held off any detailed conversation about these distributions, which we take up with gusto in Chapter 9. However, the risk ratio (as well as the odds ratio) does not follow the rules when it comes to these distributions—regardless of sample size.

Fortunately, a natural log (ln) does follow the standard normal distribution and we are able to take advantage of this to produce an estimated confidence interval for the risk ratio (as well as for the odds ratio). We briefly encountered the natural log in Chapter 2 when perusing logistic regression. Let us now dig a little deeper.

This requires two steps.

First, an estimated confidence interval is generated for the natural log of the risk ratio, or ln(risk ratio). The equation for this is:

$$\ln(\widehat{\text{RR}}) \pm z\sqrt{\dfrac{\left(n_1 - x_1\right)\big/ x_1}{n_1} + \dfrac{\left(n_2 - x_2\right)\big/ x_2}{n_2}}$$

Recall that n_1 and n_2 refer to the number of persons in group 1 and group 2, while x_1 and x_2 refer to the number of "successes" in group 1 and group 2.

Second, the antilogs of the upper and lower limits of the estimated confidence interval for the ln(risk ratio) are computed to give the upper and lower limits of the estimated confidence interval for the risk ratio. Stick with me now.

The "antilog of the upper and lower limits" is written: exp(Lower limit), exp(Upper limit).

In the spirit that doing is always better than describing, let us proceed with Example A to better illustrate all this somewhat impenetrable verbiage.

Table 6.9 Two-by-two frequency table for gender identity and resting heart rate, n = 80

	Heart rate ≥ 83 bpm	Heart rate < 83 bpm	Total
Cis male	8	32	40
Cis female	12	28	40
Total	20	60	

To begin, we create a familiar table to identify the point estimate for the risk ratio. See Table 6.9.

Our point estimate for the risk ratio is: $\widehat{RR} = \dfrac{\hat{p}_1}{\hat{p}_2}$

$\hat{p}_1 = \dfrac{8}{40} = 0.2$ AND $\hat{p}_2 = \dfrac{12}{40} = 0.3$

Thus, the point estimate for the risk ratio is:

$$\widehat{RR} = \frac{0.2}{0.3} = 0.666$$

The value of 0.666 raises an important concern that we have hit upon before.

As mentioned, if the risk ratio were 1.0 (or 1:1) this would indicate that the proportion of persons in group 1 with a resting heart rate greater than 83 bpm was the same as the proportion of persons in group 2 with a resting heart rate greater than 83 bpm. Therefore, the attribute of interest for persons in group 1 (gender identity) would have had no impact on the outcome of interest (a resting heart rate greater than 83 bpm).

If the risk ratio is greater than 1.0 (or 1:1)—such as 3.0 (or 3:1)—this indicates a higher risk for persons in group 1. More persons in group 1 experience the outcome of interest than persons in group 2.

If the risk ratio is less than 1.0 (or 1:1)—such as 0.666 (or 0.666:1) in our case—this indicates a lower risk for persons in group 1. Fewer persons in group 1 experience the outcome of interest than persons in group 2. The common interpretation of this situation is that the attribute of interest is a "protective" factor. In this case that would be the attribute of cis-male gender identity.

Importantly, risk ratios (and odds ratios) are initially calculated in decimal form. For ease of interpretation we prefer to convert the decimal form to a ratio. For instance, interpreting a risk ratio in decimal form that is less than 1.0 (such as 0.666) can be fairly counterintuitive. See Table 6.10 for the ratio form of select decimal forms of risk ratios.

Thus, the ratio form for a risk ratio of 4.0 indicates that for every four persons exposed to some risk factor who become ill, there is one person *not exposed* to that risk factor who becomes ill.

The ratio form for a risk ratio of 0.25 indicates that for every one person exposed to some risk factor who becomes ill, there are four persons *not exposed* to that risk factor who become ill.

As mentioned, the trick to convert a risk ratio in decimal form (0.666) to a ratio form (1:1.5) is relatively simple. First we write 0.666 in ratio form. This is 0.666:1. Second, we divide each side of the ratio by 0.666. The result is 1:1.5.

The ratio form for our risk ratio of 0.666 thus indicates that for every one person exposed to some risk factor who experiences some condition, there are (approximately) 1.5 persons *not exposed* to that risk factor who experience that condition.

Table 6.10 Risk ratios in decimal form and in ratio form

Decimal form	4.0	3.0	2.0	1.0	0.25	0.333	0.5	0.666	0.75
Ratio form	4:1	3:1	2:1	1:1	1:4	1:3	1:2	1:1.5	1:1.333

In the case of a risk ratio (or odds ratio), it is helpful to remember to read results in decimal form that are less than 1.0 in this fashion.

We thus prefer to report risk ratios (and odds ratios) in ratio form (1:2) rather than as decimals (0.5) for reasons of simplicity. We need the decimal form initially for purposes of calculation. We need the ratio form to more easily make sense of the results of our calculation.

Let us continue with Example A based on a point estimate of 0.666. Our confidence level is a steady 95%, resulting in a z-value of ± 1.96. Now we have a most bodacious two-step maneuver.

$$\ln(\widehat{RR}) \pm z\sqrt{\frac{\left(n_1 - x_1\right)\Big/x_1}{n_1} + \frac{\left(n_2 - x_2\right)\Big/x_2}{n_2}} \rightarrow$$

$$\ln(0.666) \pm 1.96\sqrt{\frac{32\big/8}{40} + \frac{28\big/12}{40}} = -0.406 \pm 0.779\,(-1.185, 0.373)$$

Note that to generate $[\ln(0.666) = -0.406]$ we use the "ln" button on a scientific calculator.

Thus, at a 95% confidence level, the estimated confidence interval for $\ln(\widehat{RR})$ is (−1.185, 0.373).

To now convert this to an estimated confidence interval for $\widehat{RR}$ (the risk ratio between groups) from an estimated confidence interval for $\ln(\widehat{RR})$ (the natural log of the risk ratio between groups), we take the antilog (exp) of the lower and upper limits:

[exp(−1.185), exp(0.373)] result in (0.306, 1.452)

Note that we generate the antilog via Excel.

Simply type: [=exp(−1.185) AND =exp(0.373)] into the formula bar.

Thus, we estimate—at a 95% confidence level—that the true risk ratio between group 1 and group 2 for a resting heart rate above 83 bpm is between 0.306 and 1.452.

Because the estimated confidence interval includes the null value of 1.0 (or 1:1), we cannot rule out no difference between group 1 and group 2 with regard to the proportion of persons with a resting heart rate above 83 bpm or greater. This is consistent with our previous findings for the risk difference with the same values.

Example B

There are 200 high-school long-distance runners in Mandela County. We are concerned that caffeine consumption may be elevating the resting heart rate of our runners. We recruit a random sample of 80 high-school long-distance runners and randomly assign 40 to group 1 and 40 to group 2.

Over six weeks, group 1 consumes three caffeine beverages per day and group 2 consumes no caffeine beverages. We record the resting heart rate for all persons in both groups after

Table 6.11 Two-by-two frequency table for caffeine consumption and resting heart rate, *n* = 80

	Heart rate ≥ 83 bpm	Heart rate < 83 bpm	Total
Caffeine	16	24	40
No caffeine	10	30	40
Total	26	54	

the six weeks and find that 16 of those in group 1 (or 40%) and 10 of those in group 2 (or 25%) have resting heart rates of 83 bpm or greater.

Given these findings, we must estimate—at a certain confidence level—a range of values that aims to capture the true risk ratio between group 1 and group 2 regarding the proportion of persons with a resting heart rate of 83 bpm or greater.

Technical steps

For this we will follow the previous model from Example A. Thus, we begin by creating a table to help identify the point estimate for the risk ratio for Example B. See Table 6.11.

Our point estimate for the risk ratio is: $\widehat{RR} = \dfrac{\hat{p}_1}{\hat{p}_2}$

$$\hat{p}_1 = \frac{16}{40} = 0.4 \quad \text{AND} \quad \hat{p}_2 = \frac{10}{40} = 0.25$$

Thus, the point estimate for the risk ratio is:

$$\widehat{RR} = \frac{0.4}{0.25} = 1.6$$

With a value greater than 1.0, this indicates that group 1 (with the exposure to caffeine) has a greater risk for the outcome (a resting heart rate of 83 bpm or greater) than group 2 (with no exposure to caffeine).

Specifically, this indicates that persons who consume three caffeine beverages per day have 1.6 times the risk of a resting heart rate of 83 bpm or greater than persons who consume no caffeine beverages.

We now have a point estimate of 1.6 and a 95% confidence level. Thus, our *z*-value is once again ±1.96. We proceed with our two-step maneuver.

$$\ln(\widehat{RR}) \pm z\sqrt{\frac{(n_1 - x_1)/x_1}{n_1} + \frac{(n_2 - x_2)/x_2}{n_2}} =$$

$$\ln(1.6) \pm 1.96\sqrt{\frac{24/16}{40} + \frac{30/10}{40}} = 0.470 \pm 0.657 \, (-0.187, 1.127)$$

Note that we generate [ln(1.6) = 0.470] via the "ln" button on a scientific calculator.

Thus, at a 95% confidence level, the estimated confidence interval for ln($\widehat{RR}$) is (−0.187, 1.127).

To now convert this to an estimated confidence interval for $\widehat{RR}$ (the risk ratio between groups) from an estimated confidence interval for $\ln(\widehat{RR})$ (the natural log of the risk ratio between groups), we take the antilog (exp) of the lower and upper limits:

[exp(–0.187), exp(1.127)] result in (0.829, 3.086)

Note that we generate the antilog via Excel.

Simply type: [=exp(–0.189) AND =exp(1.129)] into the formula bar.

Thus, we estimate—at a 95% confidence level—that the true risk ratio between group 1 and group 2 for a resting heart rate above 83 bpm is between 0.829 and 3.086.

Because the confidence interval includes the null value of 1.0 (or 1:1), we cannot rule out no difference between group 1 and group 2 with regard to the proportion of persons with a resting heart rate of 83 bpm or greater. This is consistent with our previous findings for the risk difference with similar values.

Notice again, however, what happens when we increase the sample sizes from 40 to 4,000. Suddenly our new estimated confidence interval is (1.49, 1.71). Thus, we estimate—at a 95% confidence level and with sample sizes of 4,000—that the true risk ratio between group 1 and group 2 for a resting heart rate above 83 bpm is between 1.49 and 1.71. This is a nice, precise interval between a risk ratio of 1.49:1 and a risk ratio of 1.71:1.

Hypothesis testing and operation 7.2 and risk ratio

Example A

There are 200 high-school long-distance runners in Mandela County. Of these, 110 identify as cis males and 90 as cis females. We want to know if there is any difference between the proportion of cis-male runners and the proportion of cis-female runners with a resting heart rate of 83 bpm or greater. We recruit a random sample of 40 cis-male and 40 cis-female high-school long-distance runners. We find that eight cis males (or 20%) and 12 cis females (or 30%) have a resting heart rate of 83 bpm or greater.

Given these results, we calculate the risk ratio. We then determine the probability of finding a risk ratio of this size between the proportion of cis-male runners and the proportion of cis-female runners with a resting heart rate greater than 83 bpm.

Technical steps

To begin, we return to our two-by-two frequency table to generate our risk ratio. See Table 6.12.

Let us then proceed with our five steps for hypothesis testing.

Table 6.12 Two-by-two frequency table for gender identity and resting heart rate, $n = 80$

	Heart rate ≥ 83 bpm	Heart rate < 83 bpm	Total
Cis male	8	32	40
Cis female	12	28	40
Total	20	60	

The null hypothesis is that the risk ratio between group 1 and group 2 is 1.0 (or 1:1). The alternative hypothesis is that the risk ratio between group 1 and group 2 is not 1.0 (or 1:1).

We choose a 5% significance level, or $\alpha = 0.05$.

STATISTICAL TEST

We replace our previous z-test for hypothesis testing in the case of risk difference. This time we adopt a chi-square test of independence. This is also commonly written as a χ^2 test of independence. The symbol χ^2 is pronounced "kai" square.

$$\chi^2 = \Sigma_{(r*c)} \frac{(O - E)^2}{E}$$

CRITERIA FOR DECISION RULE

We must find the critical value of chi-square to determine if we reject the null hypothesis. (Note that the chi-square test of independence is an upper-tailed test.) We first find the degrees of freedom. This pertains to the notation $(r*c)$, wherein r = rows and c = columns. The degrees of freedom for the chi-square test of independence are: (rows − 1) × (columns − 1).

For us, this is: $(2 - 1) \times (2 - 1) = 1$. We then refer to Table A.3 and find that the critical value of chi-square associated with 1 degree of freedom is 3.841. This will result in a p-value smaller than 0.05 that satisfies our 5% significance level.

Importantly, while a chi-square value greater than 3.841 does indicate a difference, it does not indicate the direction—greater than or less than—of that difference. For this, we must examine the data.

Thus, the decision rule is to reject the null hypothesis if our chi-square value is ≥ 3.841.

CALCULATE STATISTICAL TEST

We return to our two-by-two table (Table 6.12). Based on these data we generate two additional tables. The first table (Table 6.13) is the expected proportions that we would find if there was no difference between group 1 and group 2. The second table (Table 6.14) transforms the values in the first table for our chi-square analysis.

To create Table 6.13 there are four steps. First, in the upper left box, we multiply the total number of persons with a resting heart rate of 83 bpm or more (20) by the total number of cis males (40) and divide this by the total number of persons in both groups (80). The expected value is 10.

Table 6.13 Expected values based on Table 6.12

Heart rate ≥ 83 bpm	Heart rate < 83 bpm
$\frac{20 \times 40}{80} = 10$	$\frac{60 \times 40}{80} = 30$
$\frac{20 \times 40}{80} = 10$	$\frac{60 \times 40}{80} = 30$

Table 6.14 Transformed expected values

Heart rate ≥ 83 bpm	Heart rate < 83 bpm
$\dfrac{(8-10)^2}{10} = 0.4$	$\dfrac{(32-30)^2}{30} = 0.133$
$\dfrac{(12-10)^2}{10} = 0.4$	$\dfrac{(28-30)^2}{30} = 0.133$

Second, in the lower left box, we multiply the total number of persons with a resting heart rate of 83 bpm or greater (20) by the total number of cis females (40) and divide this by the total number of persons in both groups (80). The expected value is 10.

Third, in the upper right box, we multiply the total number of persons with a resting heart rate less than 83 bpm (60) by the total number of cis males (40) and divide this by the total number of persons in both groups (80). The expected value is 30.

Fourth, in the lower right box, we multiply the total number of persons with a resting heart rate less than 83 bpm (60) by the total number of cis females (40) and divide this by the total number of persons in both groups (80). The expected value is 30.

To create Table 6.14, there are also four steps. First, in the upper left box, we square the difference between the actual number of cis males with a resting heart rate of 83 bpm or more (eight) and the expected value for this (10). We then divide this by the expected value (10). The transformed expected value is 0.4.

Second, in the lower left box, we square the difference between the actual number of cis females with a resting heart rate of 83 bpm or less (12) and the expected value for this (10). We then divide this by the expected value (10). The transformed expected value is 0.4.

Third, in the upper right box, we square the difference between the actual number of cis males with a resting heart rate less than 83 bpm (32) and the expected value for this (30). We then divide this by the expected value (30). The transformed expected value is 0.133.

Fourth, in the lower right box, we square the difference between the actual number of cis females with a resting heart rate less than 83 bpm (28) and the expected value for this (30). We then divide this by the expected value (30). The transformed expected value is 0.133.

We add these four transformed expected values to find our chi-square value:

$$0.4 + 0.4 + 0.133 + 0.133 = 1.066$$

ASSESSMENT OF FINDINGS

We do not reject the null hypothesis because 1.066 is not larger than 3.841. We do not have statistically significant evidence, at $\alpha = 0.05$, that the risk ratio between group 1 and group 2 is not 1.0 (or 1:1) with regard to the proportion of persons with a resting heart rate of 83 bpm or greater.

This is consistent with findings for similar data in Example A for confidence interval estimation and risk ratios.

Example B

There are 200 high-school long-distance runners in Mandela County. We are concerned that caffeine consumption may be elevating the resting heart rate of our runners. We recruit a random sample of 80 high-school long-distance runners and randomly assign 40 to group 1 and 40 to group 2.

Over six weeks, group 1 consumes three caffeine beverages per day and group 2 consumes no caffeine beverages. We record the resting heart rate for all persons in both groups after the six weeks and find that 16 of those in group 1 (or 40%) and 10 of those in group 2 (or 25%) have resting heart rates of 83 bpm or greater.

Given these results, we calculate the risk ratio. We then determine the probability of finding a risk ratio of this size between the proportion of group 1 and the proportion of group 2 with a resting heart rate greater than 83 bpm.

Technical steps

Again, we return to our two-by-two frequency table to generate our risk ratio (Table 6.15).
Let us proceed with our five steps for hypothesis testing.

Hypotheses and significance level

The null hypothesis is that the risk ratio between group 1 and group 2 is 1.0 (or 1:1). The alternative hypothesis is that the risk ratio between group 1 and group 2 is not 1.0 (or 1:1).
We choose a 5% significance level, or $\alpha = 0.05$.

Statistical test

We adopt the chi-square test of independence.

$$\chi^2 = \Sigma_{(r*c)} \frac{(O - E)^2}{E}$$

Criteria for decision rule

We must find the critical value of chi-square to determine if we reject the null hypothesis. We first find the degrees of freedom. As with Example A, we have a two-by-two table and so our degree of freedom is one. We refer to Table A.3 and find that the critical value of chi-square associated with one degree of freedom and a 5% significance level. This is 3.841.

Thus, the decision rule is to reject the null hypothesis if our chi-square value is ≥ 3.841.

Calculate statistical test

We return to our two-by-two table (Table 6.15). Based on these data we generate two additional tables. The first table (Table 6.16) is the expected proportions that we would find

Table 6.15 Two-by-two frequency table for caffeine consumption and resting heart rate, n = 80

	Heart rate ≥ 83 bpm	Heart rate < 83 bpm	Total
Caffeine	16	24	40
No caffeine	10	30	40
Total	26	54	

Table 6.16 Expected values based on Table 6.15

Heart rate ≥ 83 bpm	Heart rate < 83 bpm
$\dfrac{26 \times 40}{80} = 13$	$\dfrac{54 \times 40}{80} = 27$
$\dfrac{26 \times 40}{80} = 13$	$\dfrac{54 \times 40}{80} = 27$

Table 6.17 Transformed expected values

Heart rate ≥ 83 bpm	Heart rate < 83 bpm
$\dfrac{(16-13)^2}{13} = 0.692$	$\dfrac{(24-27)^2}{27} = 0.333$
$\dfrac{(10-13)^2}{13} = 0.692$	$\dfrac{(30-27)^2}{27} = 0.333$

if there was no difference between group 1 and group 2. The second table (Table 6.17) transforms the values in the first table for our chi-square analysis.

To create Table 6.16 there are four steps. First, in the upper left box, we multiply the total number of persons with a resting heart rate of 83 bpm or greater (26) by the total number of caffeine consumers (40) and divide this by the total number of persons in both groups (80). The expected value is 13.

Second, in the lower left box, we multiply the total number of persons with a resting heart rate of 83 bpm or greater (26) by the total number of non-consumers of caffeine (40) and divide this by the total number of persons in both groups (80). The expected value is 13.

Third, in the upper right box, we multiply the total number of persons with a resting heart rate less than 83 bpm (54) by the total number of caffeine consumers (40) and divide this by the total number of persons in both groups (80). The expected value is 27.

Fourth, in the lower right box, we multiply the total number of persons with a resting heart rate less than 83 bpm (54) by the total number of non-consumers of caffeine (40) and divide this by the total number of persons in both groups (80). The expected value is 27.

To create Table 6.17 there are four steps. First, in the upper left box, we square the difference between the actual number of caffeine consumers with a resting heart rate of 83 bpm or greater (16) and the expected value for this (13). We then divide this by the expected value (13). The transformed expected value is 0.692.

Second, in the lower left box, we square the difference between the actual number of non-consumers of caffeine with a resting heart rate of 83 bpm or greater (10) and the expected value for this (13). We then divide this by the expected value (13). The transformed expected value is 0.692.

Third, in the upper right box, we square the difference between the actual number of caffeine consumers with a resting heart rate less than 83 bpm (24) and the expected value for this (27). We then divide this by the expected value (13). The transformed expected value is 0.333.

Fourth, in the lower right box, we square the difference between the actual number of non-consumers of caffeine with a resting heart rate less than 83 bpm (30) and the expected value for this (27). We then divide this by the expected value (27). The transformed expected value is 0.333.

We add these four transformed expected values to find our chi-square value:

$$0.692 + 0.692 + 0.333 + 0.333 = 2.05$$

ASSESSMENT OF FINDINGS

We do not reject the null hypothesis because 2.05 is not larger than 3.841. We do not have statistically significant evidence, at $\alpha = 0.05$, to reject the null hypothesis that the risk ratio between group 1 and group 2 is 1.0 (or 1:1), with regard to the proportion of persons with a resting heart rate of 83 bpm or greater. This is consistent with Example B for confidence interval estimation and risk ratio.

As before, let us raise the sample sizes from 40 to 4,000 and see what results.

We thus follow the same steps to create our table of expected values and our table of transformed expected values based on our two-by-two table. (See Tables 6.18, 6.19, and 6.20.) We then add these four transformed expected values to find our chi-square value:

$$69.23 + 69.23 + 33.33 + 33.33 = 205.12$$

Remarkably, we experience a veritable quantum leap, with our chi-square value ballooning from 2.05 to 205.12. We saw the very same dramatic swing when considering operation

Table 6.18 Two-by-two frequency table for caffeine consumption and resting heart rate, n = 8,000

	Heart rate ≥ 83 bpm	Heart rate < 83 bpm	Total
Caffeine	1600	2400	4000
No caffeine	1000	3000	4000
Total	2600	5400	

Table 6.19 Expected values based on Table 6.15

Heart rate ≥ 83 bpm	Heart rate < 83 bpm
$\dfrac{2600 \times 4000}{8000} = 1300$	$\dfrac{5400 \times 4000}{8000} = 2700$
$\dfrac{2600 \times 4000}{8000} = 1300$	$\dfrac{5400 \times 4000}{8000} = 2700$

Table 6.20 Transformed expected values

Heart rate ≥ 83 bpm	Heart rate < 83 bpm
$\dfrac{(1600 - 1300)^2}{1300} = 69.23$	$\dfrac{(2400 - 2700)^2}{2700} = 33.33$
$\dfrac{(1000 - 1300)^2}{1300} = 69.23$	$\dfrac{(3000 - 2700)^2}{2700} = 33.33$

7.1 and risk difference. There we increased the sample size to 4,000 for Example B and hypothesis testing and we saw our z-value soar to new heights in a similar manner. Indeed, the details of both examples were (purposely) identical. This only further demonstrates the strong influence of sample size, insofar as the values of no other factors were altered in value.

Configuration #7: operation 7.3 and odds ratio

Confidence interval estimation and operation 7.3 and odds ratio

Example

There are 200 high-school long-distance runners in Mandela County. We are concerned that caffeine consumption may be elevating the resting heart rate of our runners. We recruit a random sample of 80 high-school long-distance runners and randomly assign 40 to group 1 and 40 to group 2.

Over six weeks, group 1 consumes three caffeine beverages per day and group 2 consumes no caffeine beverages. We record the resting heart rate for all persons in both groups after six weeks and find that 14 of those in group 1 (or 35%) and four of those in group 2 (or 10%) have resting heart rates of 95 bpm or greater.

Given these results, we must estimate—at a certain confidence level—a range of values that aims to capture the true odds ratio between group 1 and group 2 regarding the proportion of persons with a resting heart rate of 95 bpm or greater.

Technical steps

An odds ratio is, naturally, a ratio between the odds for two groups regarding some outcome. The odds in each group is itself a ratio between the number of "successful" outcomes (x) and the number of unsuccessful outcomes ($n - x$). We place the odds for group 2 in the denominator, or the second position in the ratio form (group 1: group 2). Our measures of concern are the odds for each group. Each of these provides the point estimate.

Our estimation equation for the odds ratio between two groups is:

$$\widehat{OR} = \frac{\hat{p}_1 / 1.0 - \hat{p}_1}{\hat{p}_2 / 1.0 - \hat{p}_2}$$

Note that the numerator $\left(\dfrac{\hat{p}_1}{1.0 - \hat{p}_1} \right)$ is the odds of a certain outcome for an individual in group 1 and the denominator $\left(\dfrac{\hat{p}_2}{1.0 - \hat{p}_2} \right)$ is the odds for an individual in group 2. We will revisit the consequences of this in Chapter 9.

As with a risk ratio, an odds ratio does not follow the rules of the standard normal distribution or a binomial distribution. Fortunately, a natural log (ln) does follow the standard normal distribution and we make use of this to produce an estimated confidence interval for an odds ratio. This requires two steps.

First, we estimate a confidence interval for the natural log of the odds ratio, or ln(odds ratio).

Table 6.21 Two-by-two frequency table for caffeine consumption and resting heart rate, n = 80

	heart rate ≥ 95 bpm	Heart rate < 95 bpm	Total
Caffeine	14	26	40
No caffeine	4	36	40
Total	18	62	

$$\ln(\widehat{OR}) \pm z \sqrt{\frac{1}{x_1} + \frac{1}{(n_1 - x_1)} + \frac{1}{x_2} + \frac{1}{(n_2 - x_2)}}$$

Recall that n_1 and n_2 refer to the number of persons in group 1 and group 2, while x_1 and x_2 refer to the number of "successes" in group 1 and group 2.

Second, the antilogs of the upper and lower limits of the estimated confidence interval for $\ln(\widehat{OR})$ are computed to give the upper and lower limits of the estimated confidence interval for the odds ratio.

The antilogs of the upper and lower limits are written: exp(Lower limit), exp(Upper limit).

Let us proceed with our example to better illustrate such things. To begin, we create another two-by-two table to help identify the point estimate for the odds ratio. See Table 6.21.

The point estimate for the odds ratio between group 1 and group 2 is:

$$\widehat{OR} = \frac{\hat{p}_1 / 1.0 - \hat{p}_1}{\hat{p}_2 / 1.0 - \hat{p}_2} \rightarrow \widehat{OR} = \frac{0.35 / 1.0 - 0.35}{0.1 / 1.0 - 0.1} = 4.846$$

This indicates that—for our two groups—caffeine consumers have 4.85 times the odds of non-consumers to have a resting heart rate greater than 95 bpm. We now estimate a confidence interval for this point estimate at a 95% confidence level.

$$\ln(\widehat{OR}) \pm z \sqrt{\frac{1}{x_1} + \frac{1}{(n_1 - x_1)} + \frac{1}{x_2} + \frac{1}{(n_2 - x_2)}}$$

$$\ln(4.846) \pm 1.96 \sqrt{\frac{1}{14} + \frac{1}{(26)} + \frac{1}{4} + \frac{1}{(36)}} = 1.578 \pm 1.219 (0.359, 2.797)$$

To now estimate a confidence interval for the odds ratio, we take the antilog (exp) of the lower and upper limits: exp(0.359), exp(2.797)—resulting in (1.432, 16.395).

Thus, we estimate—at a 95% confidence level—that the true odds ratio between group 1 and group 2 for a resting heart rate above 95 bpm is between 1.43 and 16.39. This is a fairly large interval. However, as you can probably guess by now, were we to increase our sample size of each group from 40 to 4,000 we could shrink this interval dramatically from between 1.43 and 16.39 to between 4.81 and 4.88.

Hypothesis testing and operation 7.3 and odds ratios

Hypothesis testing and the odds ratio adopts the chi-square test of independence.

$$\chi^2 = \Sigma_{(r*c)} \frac{(O-E)^2}{E}$$

This is the same statistical test as we applied for hypothesis testing and the risk ratio. The technical steps match those of hypothesis testing and the risk ratio and we thus forgo repeating these steps here.

Configuration #8

Goal: To compare the proportions of two independent groups for a dichotomous outcome variable based on differences in multiple attributes and/or exposures.

See Chapter 7 for these technical steps.

Configuration #9

Goal: To compare two or more independent groups regarding the distribution of cases across multiple response options for an ordinal or categorical outcome variable. Groups differ based on an attribute or exposure.

Confidence interval estimation and configuration #9

Given more than two groups and the inclusion of categorical and/or ordinal outcome variables, we cannot apply confidence interval estimation to configuration #9.

Hypothesis testing and configuration #9

Example A

There are 300 high-school long-distance runners in Machel County. We suspect that an attribute (blood type) may be linked to a runner's resting heart rate. We create four ordinal categories for resting heart rates. These are: low (50 bpm or lower), moderate (51–82 bpm), elevated (83–99 bpm), and very high (100 bpm or higher). We create three groups of runners based on the three most common blood groups in the population (A, B, and O).

Our groups are thus group A, group B, and group O. (We combine the positive and negative subgroups for each of these that—along with AB positive and negative—form the eight blood types.) We then recruit 50 high-school long-distance runners for each blood group, record each participant's resting heart rate, and catalogue her or him according to our ordinal categories. Table 6.22 provides the distribution of runners across ordinal categories for each group.

Table 6.22 Distribution of blood types across levels of resting heart rates, $n = 150$

	Low rate	Moderate rate	Elevated rate	Very high rate	Totals
Group A	9	26	8	7	50
Group B	14	21	7	8	50
Group O	10	22	12	6	50
Total	33	69	27	21	150

Given these results, we must determine the probability of finding differences of this size in the distribution of responses across ordinal categories for the three groups that differ by blood type.

Technical steps

Similar to configuration #7, operation 7.2 for risk ratio and operation 7.3 for odds ratio, Examples A and B for configuration #9 rely on the chi-square test of independence

$$\chi^2 = \Sigma_{(r*c)} \frac{(O - E)^2}{E}$$

The chi-square test of independence allows us to compare the distribution of responses linked to the ordinal or categorical outcome variable (with multiple response options) among two or more independent comparison groups. The null hypothesis is that there is no difference in the distribution of responses among the comparison groups. The alternative hypothesis is that there is some difference in the distribution of responses among comparison groups.

For this purpose, we organize our data in a modified two-way table. See Table 6.23.

Group r is the final independent group. Response option c is the final response option. N refers to the total number of people in all samples. (This equals the total number of responses.) Each intersection of a row and column is a cell of the table.

The table is identical to the two-by-two table that we used for configuration #7, operations 7.2 and 7.3. However, Table 6.23 is also known as an "r by c" table ($r \times c$), depending upon the number of rows and columns. For example, if we have three groups and five responses, it is a "3 by 5" table (or 3×5).

We are almost set to roll out the five steps of hypothesis testing. But first we have a brief but vital detour to review the concept of "independence" between variables. This will help to better set things up for applying the chi-square test of independence to configuration #9. First, the basic logic:

Two events are independent if: $P(A \mid B) = P(A)$ or $P(A \mid B) = P(B)$.

OR, equivalently, two events are independent if $P(A \text{ and } B) = P(A) \times P(B)$.

Formal complexity aside, the basic underlying logic here is simple. Imagine there is a 20% probability that a person who competes in 5k races will have lung cancer and there is a 20% chance that any person from the population will have lung cancer. This indicates that a person who competes in 5k races and any random person from the population have equal probabilities of having lung cancer. Therefore, there is no connection between lung cancer and competing in 5k races—they are independent.

Table 6.23 Two-way table for data lay-out for chi-square test of independence

Grouping Variable	Response Option 1	Response Option 2	—	Response Option C	Row totals
Group 1					
Group 2					

Group r					
Column totals					N

Second, the *implication* of this basic logic:

> Mathematically, this suggests that if A and B are independent, then the probability of their intersection can be computed by multiplying the probability of each.
>
> However, to conduct the chi-square test of independence, we need expected *frequencies* and *not expected probabilities*. So ...
>
> *To convert a probability to a frequency, we multiply that probability by the total sample size (N).*

Third, an *application* of this basic logic:

> Imagine we conduct a chi-square test of independence and generate the following observed frequency data in Table 6.24.
>
> The frequencies in the cells are the observed frequencies and $N = 150$. This is the total number of responses.
>
> If the groups are independent (meaning the null hypothesis is not rejected), we will find that:
>
> P(Group 1 and Response 1) = P(Group 1) × P(Response 1)
>
> This reads: The probability that someone in group 1 chooses response 1 is equal to the probability that someone in the sample is a member of group 1 *multiplied by* the probability that anyone in the sample chooses response 1.
>
> Thus, we have: P(Group 1) × P(Response 1) = $\dfrac{25}{150} \times \dfrac{62}{150} = 0.069$.
>
> The probability that a person in the sample is a member of group 1 and chose response 1 is 0.069.
>
> Thus, for example, the expected frequency for the cell corresponding with group 1, response 1 in Table 6.24 is: $150 \times 0.069 = 10.4$.

Fortunately, given this, we have a simpler equation to determine the expected cell frequency (E) for the chi-square test of independence. This is:

$$E = \frac{(\text{row total})(\text{column total})}{N}$$

Thus, the expected frequency for the cell corresponding with group 3, response 3 in Table 6.24 is:

$$E = \frac{(75) \times (37)}{150} = 18.5$$

Now on to those five familiar steps. To refresh, here again see Table 6.22 with data for Example A.

Table 6.24 Observed frequency data for chi-square test of independence, $N = 150$

Grouping variable	Response 1	Response 2	Response 3	Row totals
Group 1	10	8	7	25
Group 2	22	15	13	50
Group 3	30	28	17	75
Total	62	51	37	150

The null hypothesis is that there are no differences in the distribution of resting heart rate levels among the three groups that differ by blood type. The alternative hypothesis is that there are differences in the distribution of resting heart rate levels among the three groups that differ by blood type.

We choose a 5% significance level, or $\alpha = 0.05$.

STATISTICAL TEST

We have identified the statistical test as the chi-square test of independence.

$$\chi^2 = \Sigma_{(r*c)} \frac{(O-E)^2}{E}$$

We know that to apply this statistical test, the *expected* frequency for each cell of the $r \times c$ table of data for the chi-square test of independence must be at least five. (We assess this below.)

CRITERIA FOR DECISION RULE

The decision rule for the chi-square test of independence depends on the significance level (5%) and the degrees of freedom. Our degrees of freedom are determined by:

$$df = (r-1)(c-1) = (3-1)(4-1) = 6$$

From Table A.3, we find that, with six degrees of freedom and a 5% significance level, the critical value of chi-square is 12.59.

Thus, the decision rule is to reject the null hypothesis if our chi-square statistic ≥ 12.59.

CALCULATE STATISTICAL TEST

There are two steps for the statistical test. First, we find the expected frequencies to confirm that the expected frequency is at least five for all cells. The equation for this is:

$$E = \frac{\left(\text{row total}\right)\left(\text{column total}\right)}{N}$$

Tables 6.25 and 6.26 apply this equation to our data and we find:
Four cells are highlighted to illustrate how the expected frequency for each cell was calculated.

Cell for low rate, group A $\rightarrow \dfrac{50 \times 33}{150} = 11$

Cell for moderate rate, group B $\rightarrow \dfrac{50 \times 69}{150} = 23$

Cell for elevated rate, group A $\rightarrow \dfrac{50 \times 27}{150} = 9$

Cell for very high rate, group O $\rightarrow \dfrac{50 \times 21}{150} = 7$

Table 6.25 Observed frequency data for chi-square test of independence, N = 150

	Low rate	Moderate rate	Elevated rate	Very high rate	Totals
Group A	9	26	8	7	50
Group B	14	21	7	8	50
Group O	10	22	12	6	50
Total	33	69	27	21	150

Table 6.26 Expected frequency data for chi-square test of independence, N = 150

	Low rate	Moderate rate	Elevated rate	Very high rate	Totals
Group A	11	23	9	7	50
Group B	11	23	9	7	50
Group O	11	23	9	7	50
Total	33	69	27	21	150

We thus see that all "expected" cell values are five or greater and we are free to use the chi-square test of independence.

Our next step is to apply the chi-square test of independence to our data.

We begin with this gargantuan equation:

$$\chi^2 = \Sigma_{(r*c)} \frac{(O-E)^2}{E} \rightarrow$$
$$\left\{ \frac{(9-11)^2}{11} + \frac{(14-11)^2}{11} + \frac{(10-11)^2}{11} \right\} + \left\{ \frac{(26-23)^2}{23} + \frac{(21-23)^2}{23} + \frac{(22-23)^2}{23} \right\} +$$
$$\left\{ \frac{(8-9)^2}{9} + \frac{(7-9)^2}{9} + \frac{(12-9)^2}{9} \right\} + \left\{ \frac{(7-7)^2}{7} + \frac{(8-7)^2}{7} + \frac{6-7)^2}{7} \right\}$$

This yields

χ^2 = {0.364 + 0.818 + 0.091} + {0.391 + 0.174 + 0.043} + {0.111 + 0.444 + 1.0} + {0.0 + 0.143 + 0.143} = 3.722

ASSESSMENT OF FINDINGS

We do not reject the null hypothesis because 3.722 < 12.59. We do not have statistically significant evidence, at α = 0.05, that there are differences in the distribution of resting heart rate levels among the three groups that differ by blood type.

Thus, a runner's blood type and the ordinal level of her or his resting heart rate are "independent." Each has no bearing upon the other.

Example B

There are 300 high-school long-distance runners in Machel County. We are concerned that an exposure (caffeine consumption) may be impacting the resting heart rate of our runners.

Table 6.27 Distribution of levels of caffeine consumption across levels of resting heart rates, N = 150

	Low rate	Moderate rate	Elevated rate	Very high rate	Totals
Group 1	0	9	29	12	50
Group 2	8	28	12	2	50
Group 3	12	33	4	1	50
Total	20	70	45	15	150

We create four ordinal categories for resting heart rates. These are: low (50 bpm or lower), moderate (51–82 bpm), elevated (83–99 bpm), and very high (100 bpm or higher). We recruit 150 high-school long-distance runners and randomly assign 150 runners to three groups.

Group 1 will consume three or more daily caffeine beverages. Group 2 will consume one to two daily caffeine beverages. Group 3 will consume no caffeine beverages. After six weeks, we record each participant's resting heart rate and catalogue her or him according to our ordinal categories for resting heart rates. Table 6.27 provides the distribution of runners across our ordinal categories based on group membership.

Given these results, we must determine the probability of finding differences of this size in the distribution of responses across ordinal categories for the three groups that differ by level of caffeine consumption.

Technical steps

With Example A under our belt, we slide straight into the five steps of hypothesis testing.

HYPOTHESES AND SIGNIFICANCE LEVEL

The null hypothesis is that there are no differences in the distribution of resting heart rate levels among the three groups that differ by level of caffeine consumption. The alternative hypothesis is that there are differences in the distribution of resting heart rate levels among the three groups that differ by level of caffeine consumption.

We choose a 5% significance level, or $\alpha = 0.05$.

STATISTICAL TEST

Our statistical test is the chi-square test of independence.

$$\chi^2 = \Sigma_{(r*c)} \frac{(O - E)^2}{E}$$

We know that to apply this statistical test, the *expected* frequency for each cell of the $r \times c$ table of data for the chi-square test of independence must be at least five. (We assess this below.)

CRITERIA FOR DECISION RULE

The decision rule for the chi-square test of independence depends on the significance level (5%) and the degrees of freedom. Our degrees of freedom are determined by:

$$df = (r - 1)(c - 1) = (3 - 1)(4 - 1) = 6$$

From Table A.3, we find that, with six degrees of freedom and a 5% significance level, the critical value of chi-square is 12.59.

Thus, the decision rule is to reject the null hypothesis if our chi-square statistic ≥ 12.59.

CALCULATE STATISTICAL TEST

There are two steps for the statistical test. First, we find the expected frequencies to confirm that the expected frequency is at least five for all cells. The equation for this is:

$$E = \frac{(\text{row total})(\text{column total})}{N}$$

This equation is applied in Tables 6.28 and 6.29, which illustrate the results.

Four cells are highlighted to illustrate how the expected frequency for each cell was calculated.

Cell for low rate, group 1 $\rightarrow \dfrac{50 \times 20}{150} = 6.67$

Cell for moderate rate, group 2 $\rightarrow \dfrac{50 \times 70}{150} = 23.33$

Cell for elevated rate, group 3 $\rightarrow \dfrac{50 \times 45}{150} = 15$

Cell for very high rate, group 1 $\rightarrow \dfrac{50 \times 15}{150} = 5$

All expected cell values are thus five or greater and we continue with the chi-square test of independence.

We now apply the chi-square test of independence to our data.

Table 6.28 Observed frequency data for chi-square test of independence, $N = 150$

	Low rate	Moderate rate	Elevated rate	Very high rate	Totals
Group 1	0	9	29	12	50
Group 2	8	28	12	2	50
Group 3	12	33	4	1	50
Total	20	70	45	15	150

Table 6.29 Expected frequency data for chi-square test of independence, $N = 150$

	Low rate	Moderate rate	Elevated rate	Very high rate	Totals
Group 1	6.67	23.33	15	5	50
Group 2	6.67	23.33	15	5	50
Group 3	6.67	23.33	15	5	50
Total	20	69.99	45	15	150

$$\chi^2 = \Sigma_{(r*c)} \frac{(O-E)^2}{E} \rightarrow$$

$$\left\{ \frac{(0-6.67)^2}{6.67} + \frac{(8-6.67)^2}{6.67} + \frac{(12-6.67)^2}{6.67} \right\} + \left\{ \frac{(9-23.33)^2}{23.33} + \frac{(28-23.33)^2}{23.33} + \frac{(33-23.33)^2}{23.33} \right\} +$$

$$\left\{ \frac{(29-15)^2}{15} + \frac{(12-15)^2}{15} + \frac{(3-15)^2}{15} \right\} + \left\{ \frac{(12-5)^2}{5} + \frac{(2-5)^2}{5} + \frac{(1-5)^2}{5} \right\}$$

this yields

$$\chi^2 = \{6.67 + 0.265 + 4.259\} + \{8.802 + 0.935 + 4.008\} + \{13.067 + 0.6 + 9.6\} + \{9.8 + 1.8 + 3.2\} = 62.99$$

ASSESSMENT OF FINDINGS

We reject the null hypothesis because 62.99 > 12.59. We have statistically significant evidence, at $\alpha = 0.05$, that there are differences in the distribution of resting heart rate levels among the three groups that differ by level of caffeine consumption.

Thus, a runner's level of caffeine consumption and the ordinal level of her and his resting heart rate are somehow linked, or dependent.

We return to Table A.3 to find a more precise p-value associated with a chi-square value of 62.99 with six degrees of freedom. We first find the row of chi square values associated with six degrees of freedom. This row crosses five columns, from 0.10 to 0.005. The chi-square value in the row for six degrees of freedom and in the column for 0.005 is 18.55. Because the column values do not go below 0.005, we settle for declaring that $p < 0.005$.

There is now one final step. Because we reject the null hypothesis, we must review the sample data to better understand the nature of the relationship.

Given that it is easier to find patterns with percentages rather than frequencies, we create a further table—with percentages—to better illustrate the pattern. See Tables 6.30 and 6.31.

Table 6.30 Observed frequency data for chi-square test of independence

	Low rate	Moderate rate	Elevated rate	Very high rate	Totals
Group 1	0	9	29	12	50
Group 2	8	28	12	2	50
Group 3	12	33	4	1	50
Total	20	70	45	15	150

Table 6.31 Observed percentages for data for chi-square test of independence

	Low rate	Moderate rate	Elevated rate	Very high rate	Totals
Group 1	0%	18%	58%	24%	50
Group 2	16%	56%	24%	4%	50
Group 3	24%	66%	8%	2%	50
Total	–	–	–	–	150

Tables 6.30 and 6.31 further clarify that those in group 1 in the first row—high consumers of caffeine—have higher resting heart rates and those in group 3 in the third row—non-consumers of caffeine—have lower resting heart rates. Hence, as expected, it appears that higher levels of caffeine consumption result in higher resting heart rates.

Example C

There are 200 high-school long-distance runners in Lumumba County. We want to know how many runners have resting heart rates that are low (50 bpm or lower), moderate (51–82 bpm), or high (83 bpm or greater). Statewide data from two years earlier indicate that the distribution among all high-school long-distance runners was 20% low, 40% moderate, and 40% high.

We hypothesize that the distribution for all current high-school long-distance runners in Lumumba County is similarly 20% low, 40% moderate, and 40% high. We then recruit a random sample of 40 high-school long-distance runners and find that the distribution for this sample is 4 (10%) low, 18 (45%) moderate, and 18 (45%) high.

Thus, we have data for two populations. Population 1 has a distribution of resting heart rates of 20% low, 40% moderate, and 40% high. Population 2, based on sample data, has a distribution of resting heart rates of 10% low, 45% moderate, and 45% high.

Given these results, we must determine the probability of finding differences of this size between population 1 and population 2 regarding the distribution of responses across ordinal categories.

Technical steps

Here we are comparing two populations based on data for population 1 and data for a sample from population 2. Recall that this example resembles Example C for configuration #2 and hypothesis testing as well as configuration #7, operation 7.0.

In this case, we find an outcome variable (resting heart rate) with three ordinal categories—low, moderate, or high. We need to compare the distribution of responses from a sample of 40 high-school long-distance runners across these three levels with the known distribution for a population of high-school long-distance runners from two years earlier. This is treated as an ordinal variable, in that the three categories are akin to first, second, and third place. Each level represents greater consumption when moving from low to moderate to high.

The distribution of responses is the percentage of participants in each ordinal category. In our case, this is three ordinal levels of caffeine consumption—20% low, 40% moderate, and 40% high for our population.

Note that whereas the two previous examples for configuration #9 had data for three independent groups across four ordinal categories (levels of resting heart rates), Example C has data for one sample and one population across three ordinal categories (levels of caffeine consumption). We must shift, therefore, from the chi-square test of independence to the chi-square goodness-of-fit test.

$$\chi^2 = \Sigma_k \frac{(O-E)^2}{E}$$

The chi-square goodness-of-fit test allows us to compare the observed frequencies in our sample for each ordinal category and the expected frequencies we would find if our sample from population 2 matched the data for population 1. For this, we must first confirm that the expected frequency for each ordinal category is at least five.

Let us now proceed with the five steps for hypothesis testing.

HYPOTHESES AND SIGNIFICANCE LEVEL

The null hypothesis is that the population distribution of responses across ordinal categories is 20% low, 40% moderate, and 40% high for both population 1 and population 2. The alternative hypothesis is that the distribution of responses across ordinal categories is NOT 20% low, 40% moderate, and 40% for population 2.

We choose a 5% significance level, or $\alpha = 0.05$.

STATISTICAL TEST

Our statistical test is the chi-square goodness-of-fit test. (Again, this is pronounced "kai" squared.) This is an upper-tailed test when determining whether or not to reject the null hypothesis. The equation for the chi-square goodness-of-fit test is:

$$\chi^2 = \Sigma_k \frac{(O-E)^2}{E}$$

We first confirm that there are at least five expected responses for each response option. We calculate:

$$\min[n(p_1) \dots n(p_k)] \geq 5 \rightarrow \min[40(0.20), 40(0.40), 40(0.40)] = \min[18, 18, 8] = 8$$

Eight is greater than five, thus we are free to use the chi-square goodness-of-fit test in this case.

Note that the statistical test for the chi-square goodness-of-fit test is *nearly* identical to the chi-square test of independence that we applied to configuration #9, Examples A and B, as well as, configuration #7, operations 7.2 and 7.3.

chi-square goodness-of-fit test: $\chi^2 = \Sigma_k \frac{(O-E)^2}{E}$

chi-square test of independence: $\chi^2 = \Sigma_{(r*c)} \frac{(O-E)^2}{E}$

The tiny-yet-impressive difference between these two statistical tests is the notation beside the *summa* symbol Σ.

The notation beside the *summa* symbol Σ for the chi-square goodness-of-fit test is "k." This is the number of response categories. This determines the degrees of freedom. For example, here we have three response categories. Thus, the degrees of freedom are: $(3 - 1) = 2$. This determines the critical value of chi-square in Table A.3.

For the chi-square test of independence, the notation beside the *summa* symbol Σ is $(r*c)$. This is the number of rows multiplied by the number of columns in a chi-square contingency table. These values determine the degrees of freedom. For example, if we have three rows and four columns, the degrees of freedom are: $(3 - 1)*(4 - 1) = 6$. This determines the critical value of chi-square in Table A.3.

CRITERIA FOR DECISION RULE

We must now find the critical value of chi-square to determine if we reject the null hypothesis. Note that we use the same table (Table A.3) to find the critical value of chi-square, whether we are using the chi-square goodness-of-fit test or the chi-square test of independence. This requires the degrees of freedom and the significance level.

As noted, our degrees of freedom are defined as $df = k - 1$, where k is the number of response categories. In our example, $k = 3$. Thus, our degrees of freedom is $3 - 1 = 2$. We chose a 5% significance level, naturally.

Given a 5% significance level—or $\alpha = 0.05$—and two degrees of freedom, the critical value of chi-square is 5.99. This we know from Table A.3.

Thus, our decision rule is to reject the null hypothesis if our chi-square statistic ≥ 5.99.

CALCULATE STATISTICAL TEST

We begin by creating a table of expected frequencies. See Table 6.32.

Table 6.32 combines observed and expected frequencies. We see that among the 40 runners observed in our sample, 18 had a moderate resting heart rate. Assuming that the sample and population distribution are similar, we would expect 40% of the sample (16 persons) to have a moderate resting heart rate.

This is the meaning of [40(0.4) = 16] in the "moderate" column.

Let us now apply the numbers from Table 6.32 to our chi-square goodness-of-fit test.

$$\chi^2 = \Sigma_k \frac{(O - E)^2}{E}$$

$$\chi^2 = \frac{(4-8)^2}{8} + \frac{(18-16)^2}{16} + \frac{(18-16)^2}{16} = 2.0 + 0.25 + 0.25 = 2.5$$

ASSESSMENT OF FINDINGS

We do not reject the null hypothesis because 2.5 < 5.99. We do not have statistically significant evidence, at $\alpha = 0.05$, that the distribution of responses across ordinal categories for population 2 is NOT 20% low, 40% moderate, and 40%.

Again, however, we cannot help but to wonder what might happen if we bump the sample size from 40 to 4,000, while retaining our 5% significance level and the original distribution of responses from for population 1. See Table 6.33.

$$\chi^2 = \Sigma_k \frac{(O - E)^2}{E}$$

$$\chi^2 = \frac{(400-800)^2}{800} + \frac{(1800-1600)^2}{1600} + \frac{(1800-1600)^2}{1600} = 200.0 + 25.0 + 25.00 = 250.0$$

Table 6.32 Table of expected frequencies, n = 40

	Low	Moderate	High	Total
Observed frequencies	4	18	18	40
Expected frequencies	40(0.2) = 8	40(0.4) = 16	40(0.4) = 16	40

Table 6.33 Table of expected frequencies, $n = 4,000$

	Low	Moderate	High	Total
Observed frequencies	400	1,800	1,800	4,000
Expected frequencies	$4,000(0.2) = 800$	$4,000(0.4) = 1,600$	$4,000(0.4) = 1,600$	4,000

Thus, we reach an astoundingly (and statistically) significant chi square value of 250.0 after raising the size of our sample from 40 to 4,000. Indeed, it is evident from this and a prior example that for chi square tests increasing a sample size (or group size) from 40 to 4,000 simply moves the decimal point two spaces to the right. With two groups of 40 persons our chi square value was 2.5. With two groups of 4,000, this value becomes 250.

Previously, we saw our chi square value grow in similar fashion from 2.05 to 250.12 for Example B for configuration #7 and operation 7.2 for hypothesis testing. Hence, sample size alone possesses a great capacity for determining the significance of a given scenario.

Our pace now quickens as we hasten along to multiple regression analysis. The shoreline soon will be visible ahead of us. For now, however, we still remain in quite choppy waters.

Chapter 7

Configurations for Biostatistical Analysis
Technical Steps (3)

We turn now to the technical steps for configurations #5 and #8. Some may view this chapter as oddly placed. If so, they would be wrong ... but also slightly correct. In a narrow sense, this chapter is the natural follow-up to the material presented so many pages back in Chapter 2. That chapter addressed the conceptual understanding of regression analysis and its nest of assumptions and presuppositions. The present chapter details the technical steps for carrying out regression analysis—hence, the link between the two.

However, there is a further context for the present chapter. We began Chapter 2 exhorting the purported virtues of regression analysis. Namely, within biostatistical analysis, it is contended that regression analysis—and multiple regression specifically—allows us one of the better opportunities to include a fuller context for (and relationships among) phenomena within health and medicine. This would appear to better approximate a holistic model contra a reductive model.

Investigating this claim remains a principal objective for Chapter 2 and Chapter 7. We, therefore, return to this notion of a fuller context at the close of this chapter. First, however, we must pour our energies into the technical minutiae and analytical pathways that comprise linear and logistic regression. To begin, we consider linear regression.

Linear regression

To unwrap the techniques (and interpretations) of linear and logistic regression, we begin with certain conceptual tools that allow each to unfold. Here we begin with a discussion of two such tools—correlation and least squares estimates. In fact, with these tools conquered, we are a good 90% of the way home with regard to linear regression.

Correlation

Correlation is what you think it is. It is the nature of the linear relationships—or correlations—between two continuous variables. The first variable in this relationship is the causal (or independent) variable. This we designate "x." The second variable is the outcome (or dependent) variable. This we designate "y." To begin, we wish to know two basic things—the strength and direction of this linear relationship between "x" and "y."

To gauge this we generate something called a correlation coefficient. In fact, there are many to choose from. To illustrate the general principles of correlation, we will adopt the ever-popular Pearson product-moment correlation coefficient. This is abbreviated as Pearson's r. (The letter "r" is pronounced "row.") For the Pearson's r correlation coefficient, the strength (or magnitude) of a linear relationship ranges in value between -1.0 and $+1.0$. Thus,

DOI: 10.4324/9781003316985-7

$r = +0.9$ indicates a strong and positive correlation between x and y
$r = -0.2$ indicates a weak and negative correlation between x and y
$r = 0.0$ indicates no correlation between x and y

The direction of a correlation is either positive or negative. The terminology here is slightly confusing. If positive, then as we increase the value of x, we increase the value of y. However, for this same "positive" correlation, it also true that as we decrease the value of x, we decrease the value of y. At the same time, for a negative correlation, as we increase the value of x, we decrease the value of y—and as we decrease the value of x, we increase the value of y. Scatterplot diagrams help depict such correlations and Pearson's r values (see Figures 7.1 and 7.2).

As we move from left to right, the values of x increase. As we move from bottom to top along the y axis, the values of y increase. In Figure 7.1, as x increases in value for the data points, the values on the y axis increase as well. In Figure 7.2, as x increases for the data points, the values on the y axis decrease.

Ok then. Let's set this in motion. To demonstrate the calculation of Pearson's r, we will estimate the correlation between caffeine consumption (x) and the resting heart rate (y) for 10 high-school long-distance runners. For this purpose, we work with some hypothetical data. See Table 7.1. Again, note that "$n = 10$" indicates that our sample includes 10 runners. The aim of this example is three-fold.

First, we identify the six steps (and calculations) to determine the correlation between two continuous variables (x and y).

Second, we examine the nature of this correlation with the data from Table 7.1. For example, what are the consequences for the value of y when we increase (or decrease) the value of x?

Third, we reinforce the exceptionally minimal math skills that are required—addition, subtraction, division, multiplication, exponents, and the big "square root" button on a calculator.

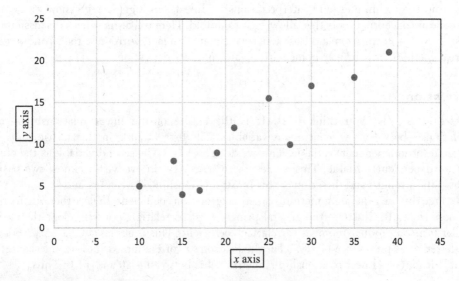

Figure 7.1 Scatterplot diagram for a positive correlation, $r = 0.6$

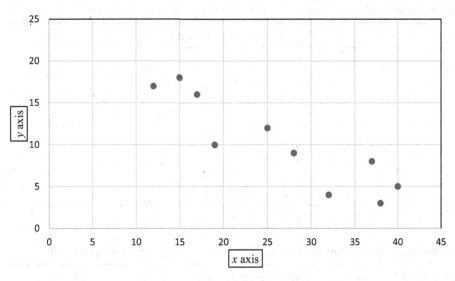

Figure 7.2 Scatterplot diagram for an inverse correlation, $r = -0.6$

Table 7.1 Caffeine consumption and resting heart rates for high-school long-distance runners, $n = 10$

Runner	Caffeine beverages (daily)	Resting heart rate (beats per minute)
1	1	62
2	0	55
3	3	81
4	2	76
5	2	72
6	4	93
7	0	51
8	4	99
9	1	65
10	3	85

Our first step in calculating the correlation between caffeine consumption and the resting heart rate is to find the mean level of caffeine consumption for our 10 runners. Table 7.2 indicates a mean of 2.0 daily caffeine beverages.

Second, we calculate the variance for our data. Table 7.3 indicates a variance of 2.22 caffeine beverages per day.

Symbolic notations in Tables 7.2 through 7.6:

- X is an independent variable.
- Y is a dependent variable.
- $\bar{X}$ is pronounced "x-bar" and is the mean of the independent variables for all persons in the sample.
- $\bar{Y}$ is pronounced "y-bar" and is the mean of the values for all persons in the sample.
- s_x^2 and s_y^2 are the variance for "x" and for "y"; they are a measure of the variability of the sample data.

Table 7.2 Mean daily caffeine consumption for high-school long-distance runners, $n = 10$

Runner	Caffeine beverages (daily)
1	1
2	0
3	3
4	2
5	2
6	4
7	0
8	4
9	1
10	3
	$\bar{X} = 20 / 10 = 2.0$

Table 7.3 Variance of daily caffeine consumption for high-school long-distance runners, $n = 10$

High-school long-distance runner	Caffeine beverages (daily)	$X - \bar{X}$	$(X - \bar{X})^2$
1	1	$1 - 2 = -1$	1
2	0	$0 - 2 = -2$	4
3	3	$3 - 2 = 1$	1
4	2	$2 - 2 = 0$	0
5	2	$2 - 2 = 0$	0
6	4	$4 - 2 = 2$	4
7	0	$0 - 2 = -2$	4
8	4	$4 - 2 = 2$	4
9	1	$1 - 2 = -1$	1
10	3	$3 - 2 = 1$	1
	$\bar{X} = 2.0$		$s_x^2 = \Sigma(X - \bar{X})^2$
	$s = 1.49$		$\Sigma(X - \bar{X})^2 = 20$
			$20 / 9 = 2.22$

- s_x and s_y are the standard deviation for "x" or for "y"; they are a measure of the variability of the sample data based on the variance.
- Σ is pronounced "summa" and indicates that we must add those values following this symbol.
- $\text{cov}(x, y)$ is the covariance of "x" and "y" and is a measure of the degree by which these increase or decrease in relation to one another.

Third, we calculate the mean resting heart rate for our high-school long-distance runners. Table 7.4 finds a mean resting heart rate of 73.9 bpm.

Fourth, we calculate the variance of the data for the resting heart rate. Table 7.5 finds a variance of 253.21.

Fifth, we calculate the covariance for caffeine consumption (x) and resting heart rates (y). This is written: $\text{cov}(x, y)$. This is a measure of the degree by which these increase or decrease in relation to one another. Table 7.6 finds a covariance of 23.44.

We now have all the values that we need to calculate Pearson's r for these data. Again, there are six steps for this—most of which we have just completed.

Table 7.4 Mean resting heart rate for high-school long-distance runners, $n = 10$

Runner	Resting heart rate (bpm)
1	62
2	55
3	81
4	76
5	72
6	93
7	51
8	99
9	65
10	85
	$\bar{Y} = 739 / 10 = 73.9$

Table 7.5 Variance of resting heart rates for high-school long-distance runners, $n = 10$

High-school long-distance runner	Resting heart rate (bpm)	$Y - \bar{Y}$	$(Y - \bar{Y})^2$
1	62	$62 - 73.9 = -11.9$	141.61
2	55	$55 - 73.9 = -18.9$	357.21
3	81	$81 - 73.9 = 7.1$	50.41
4	76	$76 - 73.9 = 2.1$	4.41
5	72	$72 - 73.9 = -1.9$	3.61
6	93	$93 - 73.9 = 19.1$	364.81
7	51	$51 - 73.9 = -22.9$	524.41
8	99	$99 - 73.9 = 25.1$	630.01
9	65	$65 - 73.9 = -8.9$	79.21
10	85	$85 - 73.9 = 11.1$	123.21
	$\bar{Y} = 73.9$		$s_y^2 = \Sigma(Y - \bar{Y})^2$
	$s = 15.91$		$\Sigma(Y - \bar{Y})^2 = 2{,}278.9$
			$2{,}278.9 / 9 = 253.21$

Table 7.6 Covariance of caffeine consumption and resting heart rates for high-school long-distance runners, $n = 10$

Runner	$X - \bar{X}$	$Y - \bar{Y}$	$(X - \bar{X})(Y - \bar{Y})$
1	−1	−11.9	11.9
2	−2	−18.9	37.8
3	1	7.1	7.1
4	0	2.1	0
5	0	−1.9	0
6	2	19.1	38.2
7	−2	−22.9	45.8
8	2	25.1	50.2
9	−1	−8.9	8.9
10	1	11.1	11.1
			$\text{cov}(x, y) = \Sigma(X - \bar{X})(Y - \bar{Y})$
			$\Sigma(X - \bar{X})(Y - \bar{Y}) = 211$
			$211 / 9 = 23.44$

1. Find mean caffeine consumption:

$$\bar{X} \to \frac{\sum X}{n} \to \frac{20}{10} = 2.0 \text{ beverages}$$

2. Find variance of caffeine consumption:

$$s_x^2 \to \frac{\sum(X - \bar{X})^2}{n - 1.0} \to \frac{20}{9} = 2.22 \text{ beverages}$$

3. Find mean resting heart rate:

$$\bar{Y} \to \frac{\sum Y}{n} \to \frac{739}{10} = 73.9 \text{ bpm}$$

4. Find variance of resting heart rate:

$$s_y^2 \to \frac{\sum(Y - \bar{Y})^2}{n - 1.0} \to \frac{2{,}278.9}{9} = 253.21 \text{ bpm}$$

5. Find covariance of caffeine consumption and heart rate:

$$\text{cov}(x, y) \to \frac{\sum(X - \bar{X})(Y - \bar{Y})}{n - 1.0} \to \frac{211}{9} = 23.44$$

6. Find correlation coefficient:

$$r \to \frac{\text{cov}(x, y)}{\sqrt{(s_x^2)(s_y^2)}} \to \frac{23.44}{\sqrt{(2.22)(253.21)}} = \frac{23.44}{23.71} = 0.989$$

Our Pearson's r is 0.989. This indicates a positive and extremely strong degree of correlation. Thus, there is a nearly perfect positive correlation between a change in caffeine consumption and a change in the resting heart rate. Keep in mind, of course, that we deliberately chose these hypothetical data to better illustrate the steps for deriving a correlation coefficient.

Least squares estimates (and simple linear regression)

Alongside correlation, the least squares estimate is an essential mathematical tool for linear regression. Here, we will initially consider simple linear regression, with a single, causal (or independent) variable and a single, continuous outcome (or dependent) variable. Note that "linear" specifies the type of relationship between the independent and dependent variables. Other types of regression analysis are based on other kinds of relationships, such as curvilinear or exponential relationships. These operate with different mathematical logics and different types of dependent variables.

Simple linear regression employs least squares estimates to estimate the equation for a line that best describes the association between the independent and dependent variables. Pound-for-pound, the previous sentence may be the hardest-hitting sentence in all of biostatistical analysis and it will require great effort on our part for its full unwinding.

Again, with attitude:

> Simple linear regression employs least squares estimates *to estimate the equation for a line that best describes the association between the independent and dependent variables.*

For the moment, we note only that the equation generating this line *that best describes the association between the independent and dependent variables* is labeled the "simple linear regression equation."

This equation is written:

$$\hat{y} = b_0 + b_1 x_1$$

Table 7.7 identifies the elements of the simple linear regression equation.

Let us proceed with a simple, if slightly off kilter, example to develop each of these elements of the simple linear regression equation in greater detail.

Bill the monkey performs backflips for bananas. For each banana (x) that we give Bill, he will perform one backflip (y). Note that y is the actual number of observed backflips and $\hat{y}$ is the number of backflips that we predict he will perform after Bill the monkey is given a certain number of bananas. The banana is the causal (or independent) variable. The backflip is the outcome (or dependent) variable.

Note also that if we had wanted to include more independent variables—such as Bill the monkey's educational level, marital status, or employment history—to more fully explain how many backflips he will perform, we would write these as:

$$b_1 x_1, b_2 x_2, b_3 x_3, b_4 x_4 \ldots$$

In this case, $b_1 x_1$ represents number of bananas, $b_2 x_2$ represents educational level, $b_3 x_3$ represents marital status, and $b_4 x_4$ represents employment history. Including these additional independent variables would elevate *simple* linear regression to *multiple* linear regression, as we shall see shortly.

We begin with the equation that we are currently deciphering: $\hat{y} = b_0 + b_1 x_1$. The purpose of this equation is to produce a line that best fits our data. But what does it mean to say that a line "best fits" our data? The answer to this question, you will see, provides a key that opens a great many doors. It is, therefore, very much worth the trouble of decoding what

Table 7.7 Elements of the simple linear regression equation

Elements of equation	Examples of elements
$\hat{y}$ is the predicted value of the dependent variable; pronounced y-hat	Number of backflips by Bill the monkey
x_1 is the independent variable	Number of bananas given to Bill the monkey
b_0 is the predicted y-intercept when the independent variable (x_1) equals zero	0.0
b_1 is the estimated regression coefficient that forms the estimated slope of the least squares regression line	1.0

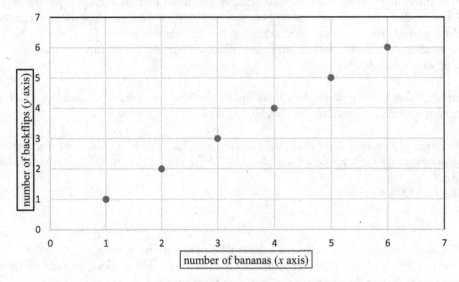

Figure 7.3 Plot points for number of backflips for bananas for Bill the monkey

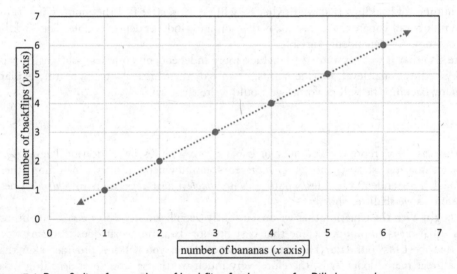

Figure 7.4 Best fit line for number of backflips for bananas for Bill the monkey

many mathematically inclined statisticians too often make utterly obscure. Let us see what Bill the monkey can teach us in this regard.

When we give Bill the monkey one banana he performs one backflip. When we give him three bananas he performs three backflips, and so on. It is a perfectly positive relationship. For each banana, we get the same number of backflips. In this case, there is little need to calculate the line that best fits our data. Figure 7.3 provides the plot points for this. Figure 7.4 produces the "best fit line" that traces through each plot point. With this linear relationship we see that the data points all line up impeccably.

Enter Bill's cousin, Murray the monkey. Give Murray a banana and he performs three backflips. Give Murray two bananas and you will get six backflips. You get the idea. Our

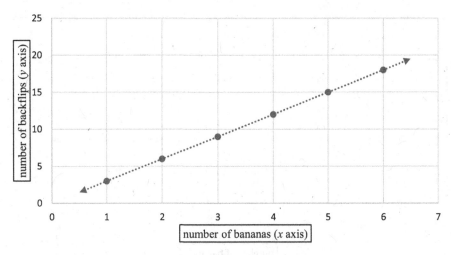

Figure 7.5 Best fit line for number of backflips for bananas for Murray the monkey

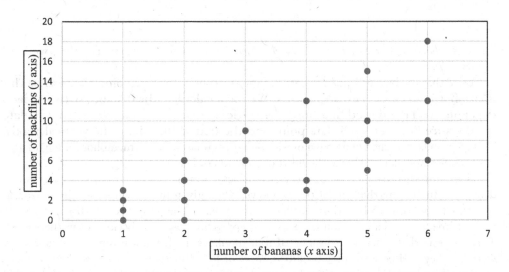

Figure 7.6 Plot points number of backflips for bananas for Bill the monkey and his three relatives

graph of the line that best fits Murray the monkey's data produces a predictable line with all the data points again lining up impeccably—though crossing different plot points along the y axis than was the case for Bill the monkey. Compare Figure 7.4 and Figure 7.5 in this regard.

Charting each individual's "best fit line," of course, serves little purpose. We want to know what the best fit line looks like for a number of individuals. For this, we gather Bill the monkey, Murray the monkey, and two other relatives, and we plot the data linking bananas and backflips for all four monkeys. We begin with Figure 7.6, where we plot the data points for all four monkeys based on the number of backflips each will perform for a certain number of bananas.

The picture now appears more muddled when trying to draw a dotted line that best fits the data. Obviously, no *one* line will intersect all 24 data points. What we want to

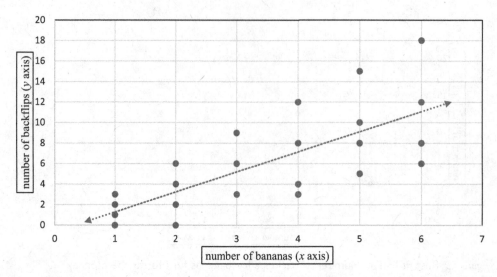

Figure 7.7 Best fit line for number of backflips for bananas for Bill the monkey and his three relatives

know is *what single line best fits the 24 data points for all four monkeys*. For this, we have Figure 7.7.

Notice that the best fit line in Figure 7.7 intersects only one data point (and barely). This is fine. But it makes our next step critical. **We must calculate the distance between each data point and the dotted line along the vertical *y* axis.** We repeat. **We must calculate the distance between each data point and the dotted line along the vertical *y* axis.** This step, in fact, is the whole bowl of wax—that peculiar Western metaphor for any matter of supreme importance. This is the heart of least squares estimates.

Calculating this distance is not especially difficult in this case. For example, there is one data point indicating that one of the monkeys, when given five bananas (on the horizontal *x* axis), will perform 15 backflips (on the vertical *y* axis). The dotted best fit line crosses the vertical line for five bananas (on the *x* axis) at approximately nine backflips (on the *y* axis). This suggests that when we consider all four monkeys, if they are given five bananas—*on average*—they will perform nine backflips, more or less. But there is *no monkey* who actually performs nine backflips when given five bananas. Two perform more than nine backflips and two perform fewer than nine.

Let us continue examining these four data points along the vertical *y* axis where it intersects with five bananas along the horizontal *x* axis. Again, no two are plotted in the same place along the *y* axis. (Note that when two or more monkeys share an identical data point—for example, there are two monkeys who perform three backflips when given three bananas—this will appear as a single data point on the chart. For purposes of creating the best fit line, however, these are calculated as two distinct data points.) The average of the four data points along the *y* axis is 9.5 backflips. This, in fact, is roughly where the dotted best fit line intersects the *y* axis when a monkey is given five bananas.

However, this will not always be the case. After all, the best fit line must account for the average of each set of four data points along the horizontal *x* axis representing the number of bananas we gave each monkey—in this case, one through seven. Ordinarily, we do not try to figure out the exact placement of the best fit line on our own. This is better left to statistical programs. (The best fit line here was generated with Excel.) For us, it is the underlying rationale guiding the calculations of these programs that interests us—that is to say, least squares estimates.

Least squares estimates are premised upon the fact that almost all observed data points will lie somewhere above or below the estimated best fit line. Very simply, the statistical program yearns to generate the best fit line that—*for all data points*—creates the shortest possible distance between each actual (observed) data point and the best fit line at any point along the horizontal x axis. The best fit line thus represents the predicted value ($\hat{y}$) at different points along the horizontal x axis. In this sense, regression analysis is essentially a measure of data variability—or the dispersal of data points around their mean.

Again, an actual observation is designated y and a predicted data point (along the best fit line) is designated $\hat{y}$. Thus, when we subtract $\hat{y}$ from y (written, $y - \hat{y}$) this allows us to find the distance between (a) an observed data point (y) and (b) the predicted point on the best fit line ($\hat{y}$).

An example of this from Figure 7.7 is the difference between our monkey who performs 15 backflips (y) when given five bananas and the predicted point on the best fit line ($\hat{y}$) at that same point along the x axis (five bananas)—indicating that our four monkeys on "average" perform nine backflips when given five bananas. Thus, for this monkey who performs 15 backflips:

$$[y - \hat{y}] \rightarrow 15 - 9 = 6$$

Importantly, we only need the absolute value of the distance between y and $\hat{y}$. So below, when the result is a negative number, we report this as an absolute value for illustration. (When statistical programs actually perform this drudgery, the results of $y - \hat{y}$ are squared to eradicate all negative values from our sight.)

One way to confirm your rock solid grasp of this principle is to return to Figure 7.7 and consider the following.

> If you give a monkey six bananas and she or he performs 15 backflips this results in
> $18 - 11 = 7$.
> If you give a monkey six bananas and she or he performs six backflips this results in
> $6 - 11 \doteq 5$.
> If you give a monkey two bananas and she or he performs six backflips, this results in
> $6 - 3 = 3$.
> If you give a monkey two bananas and she or he performs zero backflips, this results in
> $0 - 3 = 3$.

To proceed, it is essential to be clear eyed about the origin for all of the numbers in these four equations. Indeed, we are about to encounter some very rough going.

Now, given this reasonably simple notion—explaining $y - \hat{y}$—let us borrow an obscure and complicated language from mathematics to thoroughly confuse and mystify this entire situation before applying all of this to an example involving our high-school long-distance runners. We begin by restating the simple linear equation and again identifying each of its parts.

$$\hat{y} = b_0 + b_1 x_1$$

$\hat{y}$ is the predicted value of the dependent variable; **these values sit along the best fit line!!!**
x_1 is the independent variable.

b_0 is the predicted y-intercept when the independent variable (x_1) equals zero.

b_1 is the estimated regression coefficient that forms the estimated slope of the least squares regression line.

See how we snuck that one in; do not worry about the "estimated slope" reference just yet.

We offer one further comment before continuing. If you are able to grasp the next few pages in your first read through that makes you a complete freak of nature. For mere mortals, this will require *at least* three read throughs. There are a lot of moving pieces. Keep that in mind as we trudge along.

We will work with two formulations of the general rule for the simple linear equation. The first formulation, gifted to us by some of our more loquacious friends in mathematics, reads as follows:

> Formulation 1: The estimates of the y-intercept (b_0) and the slope (b_1) *minimize the sum* of the squared differences between the observed (y) and the predicted ($\hat{y}$) values—thus, our estimates minimize $\Sigma(\hat{y} - y)^2$.

However, after a brief technical side journey, we can render this quite confusing, formal description of the simple linear equation—and of least squares estimates—into a wholly indecipherable tribute to heroic mathematical rigor.

This second, abbreviated reformulation of the very same rule reads:

> Formulation 2: The least squares estimates of the regression coefficients (b_0 and b_1) minimize the sum of the squared residuals—$\Sigma(\hat{y} - y)^2$.

Tracing how this reformulation takes place, in fact, provides a window into the parts and rationale that propel this rule. What follows is a *non-mathematical* explanation of this mathematical rule via a rendering of the shared logic behind the opaque language of these two formulations of the exact same rule.

We begin with the wording from the first formulation of the rule. **Bold font** indicates language taken directly from the rule. Okay, hold on to your fairy dust.

> First, if we know the **estimates of the y-intercept (b_0) and the slope (b_1)**, then we can determine the best fit line because we will know (a) where the best fit line intersects the y axis when the value of an independent variable (x_1) is zero and (b) the slope of the best fit line. The slope of the best fit line is the expected change in the dependent variable (y), given a one-unit change in the independent variable (x). Put differently, as we move from left to right on the x axis we want to know what happens along the y axis.
>
> For example, Bill the monkey increases his number of backflips (y) by one for each additional banana (x) he is given. (This is a move from left to right along the x axis.) Therefore, the slope of the line (b_1) is 1.0 and the y-intercept (b_0) is 0.0 when x is 0.0. This is because if you give Bill the monkey zero bananas, he will perform zero backflips. So we know that the best fit line will intersect with the zero point along the y axis when x is 0.0.
>
> Second, estimates of the y-intercept (b_0) and of the slope (b_1) **minimize the *sum of the squared differences* between the observed data point (y) and the predicted data point ($\hat{y}$)**. This summons three steps.

> Step 1: We take each observed data point (y) and subtract the predicted data point ($\hat{y}$) that lies at the same spot along the best fit line where the observed data

point (y) intersects the horizontal x axis. This yields $y - \hat{y}$. (This is what we explored above with Figure 7.7.)

Step 2: As noted above, all results of $y - \hat{y}$ will be either a positive number, a negative number, or zero. When we add these numbers, the sum will always equal zero. To avoid a sum equal to zero, we square all the results of $y - \hat{y}$. This eliminates negative numbers. We refer to the result of this as *the squared differences* between the observed data points (y) and the predicted data points ($\hat{y}$). (It may prove helpful to shout this last sentence several times out loud for emphasis.)

Step 3: We now sum *the squared differences* between the observed data points (y) and the predicted data points ($\hat{y}$).

Steps 2 and 3 can be combined and rewritten: $\Sigma(\hat{y} - y)^2$.

In this way, **our estimates minimize $\Sigma(\hat{y} - y)^2$**. Again, the symbol summa (Σ) requires that we add all that immediately follows Σ in an equation. Notice that most of steps 1–3 simply repeat what we did with Figure 7.7. The only additional maneuvers are (a) to square the results of $y - \hat{y}$ to eliminate negative values and (b) to sum all of the squared differences that are produced from this to set up the next steps.

So far, so good.

Third, there are four technical terms introduced from the world of mathematics, but the weary need not despair.

Residuals: We refer to the **differences** between the observed data points (y) and the predicted data points ($\hat{y}$) as **residuals**. Thus, in the second formulation of the rule, "**the sum of the squared differences**" simply becomes **the *sum of the squared residuals***. (Again, this is worth shouting.)

Least squares regression line: To class it up a bit, the line that we have been calling "the best fit line" is more formally known as the **least squares regression line**.

Least squares estimates: Here we go. The "estimates of the y-intercept (b_0) and the slope (b_1)" that form the **least squares regression line** by minimizing **the *sum of the squared residuals*** are referred to as **least squares estimates**.

The term "estimates" indicates that these are the "predicted" values of y (meaning $\hat{y}$), not the actual observations of y. Therefore, **least squares estimates** are values along the best fit line—which we now call the **least squares regression line**.

Examples of **least squares estimates** from Figure 7.7 are: "1" when a monkey is given two bananas; "3" when a monkey is given two bananas; "5" when a monkey is given three bananas, and so on.

Regression coefficients: We refer to "the y-intercept (b_0) and the slope (b_1)" as **regression coefficients**. Therefore, "estimates of the y-intercept (b_0) and the slope (b_1)" in formulation one is rewritten in formulation two as **the least squares estimates of the regression coefficients (b_0 and b_1)**.

Fourth, our task is to find the values for the **regression coefficients (b_0 and b_1)** that make the *sum of the squared residuals* as small as possible. As a technical matter, this we leave to statistical software programs. The fifth consideration, however, details the basics of this.

Fifth, the **least squares estimates of the regression coefficients (b_0 and b_1)**—that is, the y-intercept (b_0) and the slope (b_1)—are calculated as follows:

$$b_0 = \bar{Y} - b_1 \bar{X}$$

b_0 is the estimate of the y-intercept; the number of backflips when the number of bananas (x) = 0.

$\bar{Y}$ and $\bar{X}$ are the mean values for the dependent variable (y) and independent variable (x_1).

$$b_1 = (r)\frac{s_x}{s_y}$$

r refers to the correlation coefficient, or Pearson's r—the steps to calculate this were outlined above.

s_x and s_y are the standard deviations for the dependent variable (y) and independent variable (x_1).

Returning to our data above for caffeine consumption (x) and the resting heart rate (y) among high-school long-distance runners, we calculate the least squares estimates of the regression coefficients (b_0 and b_1). For reference, Table 7.8 provides raw and summary data from our earlier example for correlation.

In this case, b_0 (the estimate of the y-intercept) is the estimated resting heart rate when $x = 0.0$ and b_1 (the estimate of the slope of the least squares regression line) is the change in resting heart rate relative to a one-unit change in daily caffeine consumption.

Given the data in Table 7.8, these are:

$$b_0 = \bar{Y} - b_1(\bar{X}) = 73.9 - 10.57(2.0) = 52.76$$

$$b_1 = (r)\frac{s_x}{s_y} = (0.99)\frac{15.91}{1.49} = 10.57$$

The equation of the regression line ($\hat{y} = b_0 + b_1 x_1$) thus yields: $\hat{y}$ = 52.76 + 10.57 (number of caffeine beverages).

Table 7.8 Caffeine consumption and resting heart rates for high-school long-distance runners, $n = 10$

Runner	Caffeine beverages (daily)	Resting heart rate (beats per minute)
1	1	62
2	0	55
3	3	81
4	2	76
5	2	72
6	4	93
7	0	51
8	4	99
9	1	65
10	3	85
	$\bar{X}$ = 2.0	$\bar{Y}$ = 73.9
	s_x = 1.49	s_y = 15.91
		r = 0.99

These data allow us to then estimate the resting heart rate of a high-school long-distance runner given her or his level of daily caffeine consumption. If a runner's daily caffeine consumption is one beverage, her or his estimated resting heart rate will be:

52.76 + 10.57(1) = 63.33 bpm

If a runner's daily caffeine consumption is four beverages, her or his estimated resting heart rate will be:

52.76 + 10.57(4) = 95.04 bpm

We conclude this overview of least squared estimates (and simple linear regression) with some qualifying remarks. First, estimating a runner's resting heart rate in this manner is only valid when her or his daily caffeine consumption falls within the range of consumption levels for those in the sample—in this case, zero to four beverages.

Second, given consistent differences in resting heart rates based on gender identity within the general population, we would not ordinarily combine a sample of cis-male and cis-female long-distance runners without adjusting for gender identity. However, that would make this an example of multiple linear regression, rather than simple linear regression. And it is this that we turn to next.

Multiple linear regression

We are now able to bring in multiple linear regression. But first let us remember how we got here. Of all the tools and techniques unveiled in an introductory biostatistics course, multiple regression analysis provides the most ambitious claims regarding the contextual and holistic nature of health and medicine. Both a combination of factors (and their interactions) are considered when explaining certain outcomes via multiple linear regression. This much is so. Let us now see what this looks like.

As will hopefully be evident, mastering the basic conceptual tools of simple linear regression—especially correlation and least squares estimates—go quite far in preparing one to take on multiple regression. We will thus build on many lessons already learned.

Multiple linear regression assesses the association between two or more causal (or independent) variables and a single, continuous outcome (or dependent) variable. Again, the *simple* linear regression equation is:

$$\hat{y} = b_0 + b_1 x_1$$

The *multiple* linear regression equation is thus an extension of this:

$$\hat{y} = b_0 + b_1 x_1 + b_2 x_2 + \ldots b_p x_p$$

$\hat{y}$ is the predicted value of the dependent variable.
x_1 through x_p are our independent variables.
b_0 is the predicted y-intercept when all independent variables are equal to zero.
b_1 through b_p are the estimated regression coefficients that form the estimated slope of the least squares regression line.

Note that each of the estimated regression coefficients ($b_1 \ldots b_p$) is the expected change in the value of y relative to a one-unit change in the respective independent variable, *while holding all other independent variables constant.* For example, we might want to know if new shoes for our runners will decrease ankle injuries, while keeping all other conditions the same.

Incidentally, recall that within mathematics when we see the notation $(b_1 \dots b_p)$ this refers to a list of items that number from one through some unknown number. In this case, this tells us that theoretically we can add any number of independent variables to the equation.

Confounding variables

Multiple linear regression is commonly brought in to assess possible confounding variables. In Chapter 2, we walked through the underlying concepts and principles behind the use of this tool for this purpose. Now, we consider the technical steps. Again, we turn to our high-school long-distance runners to help illustrate.

We thus begin with a single independent variable (long-distance running) which we denote x_1 and a single, continuous dependent variable (the resting heart rate) that we denote $\hat{y}$. With simple linear regression, we wrote the equation:

$$\hat{y} = b_0 + b_1 x_1$$

The estimated regression coefficient (b_1) gives us a value that determines the slope of a line that best fits the relationship between long-distance running (x_1) and the resting heart rate $(\hat{y})$.

$\hat{y} = b_0 + b_1 x_1$ becomes:
[the resting heart rate] = [the resting heart rate of a high school student who is not a long-distance runner] + [$(b_1) \times 1$ (if a person is a runner) or 0 (if a person is not a runner)]

Thus the goal is to find the value of b_1.

Now imagine we want to determine if a second causal variable (daily meditation) acts as a confounder. We designate this potential confounder as x_2. Our multiple linear regression equation is then:

$$\hat{y} = b_0 + b_1 x_1 + b_2 x_2$$

In this case, the estimated regression coefficient (b_2) quantifies the correlation between meditation (x_2) and the resting heart rate $(\hat{y})$. Now we compare the value of our first regression coefficient (b_1) from our simple linear regression equation with the value of b_1 in the new multiple linear regression equation that now includes $b_2 x_2$. Convention holds that, if this regression coefficient (b_1) changes by 10% or more—after adding x_2 (meditation)—then meditation is considered confounding.

Thus, once a variable is identified as a potential confounder, we can use multiple linear regression to estimate the correlation between the original exposure (long-distance running) and the outcome (the resting heart rate), after adjusting for that confounder (meditation).

We organize this task into two steps. In the first step, we analyze the correlation between long-distance running and the resting heart rate. This requires simple linear regression. In the second step, we add the correlation between meditation and the resting heart rate. This requires multiple linear regression.

Let's begin with the first step. We have data for 50 high-school students, of whom, 15 (or 32%) are long-distance runners. The mean resting heart rate for all 50 students is 68.3

Table 7.9 Simple linear regression analysis, *n* = 50

R Square	0.77645		
Independent variable	Regression (or beta) coefficient	t Statistic	p-Value
Intercept	76.62857	65.06932	1.78E-48
Long-distance runner	– 27.7619	– 12.9121	3.14E-17

bpm, with a standard deviation of 2.06. This time, rather than working this out by hand as in Chapters 5 and 6, we rely on Excel. Table 7.9 has our results.

The simple linear regression equation yields:

$$\hat{y} = b_0 + b_1 x_1 \rightarrow 76.63 - 27.76(1) = 48.87\,\text{bpm}$$

Thus, it is estimated that the resting heart rate for students who are long-distance runners will be 48.87 bpm. This reflects a regression coefficient of –27.76 bpm for students who are long-distance runners. Note that (b_0), **the regression coefficient for the intercept** (76.63), is the value on the *y* axis when the value on the *x* axis is zero. (In this case, the value on the *x* axis is zero when someone is not a long-distance runner.)

In addition, note that the *p*-value for the intercept (1.78E-48) does not actually provide useful information regarding the relationship between variables.

Reviewing the values and symbols in Table 7.9:

48.87 bpm is $\hat{y}$, the estimated resting heart rate for a student who is a long-distance runner.
76.63 bpm is the *y*-intercept (b_0) when the independent variable (long-distance runner) is no, or (zero).
27.76 bpm is the regression coefficient associated with long-distance running.
(1) indicates the person is a long-distance runner; (0) would indicate that the person is not.
t statistic refers to the "test statistic" that is run by a statistical software program.
R square is an estimate of the proportion of the value of $\hat{y}$ that is attributable to the independent variables.

The *R* square value indicates that long-distance running accounts for 77.6% of the factors explaining a person's resting heart rate. (This is generated by statistical software programs, as is the *t* statistic.) The magnitude of the *t* statistic identifies the relative importance of each of the independent variables. This relative importance is better illustrated below, when we consider multiple independent variables.

Lastly, the *p*-value for "long-distance runner" is written "3.14E-17." This indicates an exceptionally tiny value. For example, 3.14E-5 is 0.0000314. In general, any *p*-value below 0.05 is considered statistically significant. This tells us that the correlation between long-distance running and a resting heart rate is statistically significant in this case. The *p*-value is also generated by a statistical software program.

Before moving to the second step, there is one more consideration. You may have noticed that to proceed with the first step we needed three pieces of information. These included the sample size (50), the mean resting heart rate (68.3), and the standard deviation for the resting heart rates (2.06). We chose the sample size ourselves for this hypothetical case and the mean is simply an average that you have known how to calculate since 4th grade. But what about the standard deviation, which we have encountered a few times already? We will have more to say about this in Chapter 10.

For now, we merely treat the standard deviation as a measure of variability within the sample data for resting heart rates. Whether 2.06 is "low" or "high" is not relevant for now. The relevance of 2.06 is how it affects the other values in our results. Our highly significant p-value here suggests the variability in our sample data was not too great.

Now the second step. We add the relationship between meditation and the resting heart rate to determine if meditation may be playing a confounding role. In doing so, it is helpful to remind ourselves that a confounding variable must have the potential to interact with both the independent variable (long-distance running) and the outcome variable (resting heart rate). From Chapter 2, we recall that meditation interacts with long-distance running via a mandate that all runners must meditate as part of their training. The link between meditation and a person's resting heart rate has been established by prior research.

We then resume our analysis with the same sample of 50 high-school students. Among these students, 15 (or 32%) are long-distance runners and 28 (or 58%) regularly meditate. A most mellow high school, indeed.

Because all long-distance runners must meditate as part of their training, we know that of the 28 students in our sample who meditate, 15 are long-distance runners and 13 are not. The mean resting heart rate and standard deviation for all students remain unchanged.

The results of the multiple linear regression analysis are displayed in Table 7.10.

The multiple linear regression equation yields:

$$\hat{y} = b_0 + b_1 x_1 + b_2 x_2 \;\rightarrow\; 80.67 - 21.704(1) - 10.09(1) = 48.88 \, \text{bpm}$$

Thus, it is estimated that a student who is a long-distance runner that meditates will have a resting heart rate of 48.88 bpm. This reflects regression coefficients of –21.704 bpm and –10.095 bpm for long-distance running and meditation, respectively. Notice that the regression coefficient for long-distance running has "increased" by 22.6%—from –27.76 to –21.48 bpm from Table 7.9. Given that this change is greater than 10%, this suggests that, indeed, meditation is a confounding variable, when considering the correlation between long-distance running and the resting heart rate.

The R square value indicates that the combination of long-distance running and meditation accounts for 85.9% of the factors explaining a person's resting heart rate. Note further that the p-value for the association between long-distance running and the resting heart rate (8.08E-14) is statistically significant, as is the p-value for the association between meditation and the resting heart rate (3.92E-06). (Again, 3.92E-06 = 0.00000392.)

We also find that the t statistic indicates a greater relative importance for long-distance running (–10.43) over meditation (–5.22). Both values are negative because we are interested in *reducing* the resting heart rate. Thus, the value of the t statistic for long-distance running (–10.43) can be said to be "greater" than that for meditation (–5.22).

Now is a good time to repeat that there is nothing especially complicated about what we are doing. The only complicatedness—were that a word—concerns the substitution of written concepts, such as "the percentage of the explanation of some outcome that can be

Table 7.10 Multiple linear regression analysis, $n = 50$

R Square	0.85859		
Independent variable	Regression (or beta) coefficient	t Statistic	p-Value
Intercept	80.66667	66.01296	5.35E-48
Long-distance runner	–21.7048	–10.4302	8.08E-14
Meditation	–10.0952	–5.22494	3.92E-06

attributed to the factors (or variables) we are considering," for its symbolic shorthand, "R square." For whatever reason, this use of symbolic shorthand is more intuitive for some people than it is for others.

However, as described in Chapter 2, everyone has the experience of explaining which movie or international badminton champion is better than another movie or international badminton champion. Remember, when we line up the reasons for our preference, we are demonstrating the basics of multiple regression analysis—whether or not we use any symbolic shorthand.

Effect modification

Now we consider the role of multiple linear regression for detecting effect modification. This time we want to understand the impact of caffeine consumption on the resting heart rate of high-school students who are long-distance runners. Again, we face two steps. In the first step, we assess the impact of caffeine consumption, at any level, for the resting heart rates of long-distance runners. In the second step, we assess the impact of caffeine consumption, at different levels, on the resting heart rates of long-distance runners.

First then, we assess caffeine consumption without attention to level. (Again, we do this via Excel.) We simply add "caffeine consumption" as a third independent variable, alongside "long-distance runner" and "meditation."

Table 7.11 provides the results of our multiple linear regression analysis.

The multiple linear regression equation yields:

$$\hat{y} = b_0 + b_1 x_1 + b_2 x_2 + b_3 x_3 \rightarrow 71.82 - 16.89(1) - 11.57(1) + 10.32(1) = 53.68 \, \text{bpm}$$

Thus, it is estimated that a student who is a long-distance runner that meditates and consumes caffeine will have a resting heart rate of 53.68 bpm. This includes regression coefficients of −16.89 bpm and −11.57 bpm for long-distance running and meditation, respectively, along with a regression coefficient of 10.32 bpm for caffeine consumption.

The p-values for all three independent variables, including caffeine consumption (1.43E-07), are again statistically significant. So to consume caffeine—without distinguishing between consumption levels—appears to have a significant impact on the resting heart rate.

The R square value indicates that long-distance running, meditation, and caffeine consumption combine to now account for a whopping 92.3% of the variation in a student's resting heart rate.

The t-statistic is slightly counterintuitive here, requiring a brief discussion. There are two considerations, the direction and the magnitude. A positive or negative value indicates the direction—that is, whether the resting heart rate is rising or falling. The magnitude indicates the absolute value of any rise or fall. Here, the t-statistic for both long-distance

Table 7.11 Multiple linear regression analysis, $n = 50$

R Square	0.92302		
Independent variable	Regression (or beta) coefficient	t Statistic	p-Value
Intercept	71.82075	42.44578	1.53E-38
Long-distance runner	−16.8886	−9.73266	9.57E-13
Meditation	−11.5696	−7.922	3.85E-10
Caffeine consumption	10.32024	6.204803	1.43E-07

running and meditation are negative, indicating a fall in the resting heart rate. The *t*-statistic for caffeine consumption is positive, indicating a rise in the resting heart rate.

However, it is the magnitude of the absolute value of each *t* statistic, *regardless of direction*, that provides the true measure of the impact of each independent variable. By this measure, the largest *impact* is long-distance running (9.73 bpm), followed by meditation (7.92 bpm) and then caffeine consumption (6.204 bpm). Again, these are the absolute values for each *t*-statistic linked to each independent variable in Table 7.11.

In the second step, we put aside these results and assess the impact of caffeine consumption at five different levels—0, 1, 2, 3, or 4 daily caffeinated beverages. This maneuver, however, will require a minor, unscheduled digression. This concerns how we organize ordinal (or categorical) data for multiple regression analysis.

We have five ordinal categories of data with defined levels. These are: zero daily caffeinated beverages; one daily caffeinated beverage; two daily caffeinated beverages; three daily caffeinated beverages; and four daily caffeinated beverages. These "levels" are thus the functional equivalent of five categorical variables from "low" to "high."

Accordingly, there are several steps to prepare our ordinal categories for this analysis. First, we set aside one level of caffeine consumption to serve as a reference group. The four other levels of caffeine consumption will be compared with that level of coffee consumption.

Consider the following example in which those who consume **three daily caffeine beverages** serve as the reference group.

> Imagine there is a push-up competition. The mean number of push-ups for those consuming two daily caffeine beverages is five below the mean for those consuming **three daily caffeine beverages**. However, the mean number of push-ups for those consuming four daily caffeine beverages is five above the mean of those consuming **three daily caffeine beverages**.

This makes a bit more sense visually. See Table 7.12.

> Described this way, those consuming **three daily caffeine beverages** are the reference group that provides the basis for a comparison across the four other levels of caffeine consumption. The mean number of push-ups for those consuming zero daily caffeine beverages can then be compared with the mean of those consuming two daily caffeine beverages *based on the distance of each from the common reference mean* of those consuming **three daily caffeine beverages**.

Thus we know that the mean number of push-ups for those consuming zero daily caffeine beverages is five below the mean number of push-ups by those consuming two daily caffeine beverages.

This example introduces two features. First we identify a "reference" variable. In this case, the reference variable is those consuming three **daily caffeine beverages**. Second,

Table 7.12 Mean push-ups and daily caffeine beverages

Daily caffeine beverages	Mean number of push-ups
0	−10
1	−7
2	−5
3	−
4	+5

we create "indicator" variables. (These are also known as "dummy" variables.) Indicator variables are ordinal or nominal categories (in this case, consumption levels) that stand in relation (a) to the reference variable and (b) to other indicator variables *vis-à-vis* the reference variable.

This is like the time you and your friends all settled the matter that Lin Dan was clearly the greatest cis-male badminton player of all time. If 10 is absolute perfection, you and your friends agreed that Lin Dan would be rated a 9.5. You then went on to rate Taufik Hidayat, Lee Chong Wei, Peter Gade, and Rudy Hartono based on how close each was to the talent of Lin Dan. In this way, Lin Dan set the standard for the others. However, it also allowed you to say that Peter Gade may not have been as good as Lee Chong Wei but he was certainly better than Rudy Hartono—in relation to Lin Dan.

"But wait a minute!" you are no doubt asking yourself. "Why in tarnation can't I just draw up a list of groups by most push-ups to fewest push-ups." Indeed, this you can do. However, sorting out if 25 push-ups is more than 18 push-ups is not our concern here. Our concern is the challenge of clearly distinguishing between these five groups purely based on the ordinal level of caffeine consumption.

The reason that we need to identify a reference group and create indicator variables concerns the dreaded scourge of collinearity, or worse yet multicollinearity. This occurs when two or more independent variables are so similar (or redundant) that both essentially vary in unison *vis-à-vis* the dependent variable. An example might be the age of a student and her class year. We would expect a strong correlation between a student's age and her class year in high school. To include both age and class year among our independent variables would thus likely create a redundancy.

Given such collinearity, efforts within regression analysis to tease out differences among our independent variables can cause significant distortions across our final results. These distortions include inaccuracies among regression coefficients and p-values—even when we still have a large R square.

In the case of ordinal or categorical data, the source of collinearity is a redundancy built into the nature of how the data are organized. Imagine we want to know the relation between a runner's family life and the time it takes a runner to complete a race. We place each runner in one of three categories: (1) single parent, (2) two parents, or (3) orphan. If we know a runner's answer to the first two options then we know the answer to the third option. Hence, to ask the third option is not necessary and is logically redundant. Thus, the redundancy is a function of how the data are organized.

In this case, identifying a reference group (such as orphans) and creating indicator variables for each of the other two independent variables can correct the design flaw that is creating redundancy and is the source of collinearity. This same principle holds in the case of five ordinal categories—zero, one, two, three, or four daily caffeinated beverages. If we know whether or not a person consumes zero, one, two, or three daily caffeinated beverages, then logically we know whether or not s/he consumes four daily caffeinated beverages. Thus, redundancy is similarly built into the organization of our data and for this reason we must assign a reference group.

Any group can serve as the reference group. Indicator variables are then created for the remaining groups and each is coded 1 (for those who belong to that group) or 0 (for those who do not belong to that group).

In multiple linear regression, the regression coefficient associated with each indicator variable—in this case varying levels of caffeine consumption—is the estimated difference between (a) the mean of the outcome variable (the resting heart rate) for a particular level

Table 7.13a Multiple linear regression analysis, $n = 50$

R Square	0.99762		
Independent variable	Regression (or beta) coefficient	t Statistic	p-Value
Intercept	75.90099	286.5095	3.47E-72
Long-distance runner	−14.7544	−45.3329	6.13E-38
Meditation	−11.9002	−44.6838	1.13E-37
Caffeine (0 daily beverages)	−5.34276	−14.5337	3.37E-18
Caffeine (2 daily beverages)	3.930924	11.41773	1.33E-14
Caffeine (3 daily beverages)	7.990022	23.46724	3.85E-26
Caffeine (4 daily beverages)	12.0591	35.06356	2.88E-33

of caffeine consumption and (b) the mean resting heart rate for the reference group, *holding all other independent variables constant.* In any event, the choice of reference group is arbitrary. Here we choose those consuming one daily caffeinated beverage.

The results from our multiple regression analysis (Table 7.13a) are as follows:

The multiple linear regression equation yields:

$$\hat{y} = b_0 + b_1 x_1 + b_2 x_2 + b_3 x_3 + b_4 x_4 + b_5 x_5 + b_6 x_6 \rightarrow$$
$$75.9 - 14.75(1) - 11.9(1) - 5.34(0) + 3.93(0) + 7.99(1) + 12.05(0) = 57.24 \text{ bpm}$$

The linear regression equation represents a person who consumes three daily caffeine beverages. These results indicate two things. First, the regression coefficient for caffeine consumption in the second column does vary based on level of consumption. Thus, there is evidence of some effect modification in the case of caffeine consumption.

Second, the results *seem to indicate* that for the specific case of a high-school student who is a long-distance runner that meditates and consumes three daily caffeine beverages, she or he will have a resting heart rate of 57.24 bpm. But this is not precisely the case.

Technically, the regression coefficients for zero, two, three, or four daily caffeine beverages are *in relation to a person who consumes one daily caffeinated beverage.* For instance, Table 7.13a indicates that the heart rate of a person consuming three daily beverages will be 7.99 bpm higher than a person who consumes one daily caffeine beverage. But what if we alter things and make those who consume two daily caffeine beverages the reference group? See Table 7.13b.

(Keep in mind, of course, that we can always perform multiple linear regression analysis with "two daily beverages" as the sole independent variable for caffeine consumption to find a more precise estimate. But our interest here is whether or not a difference in the magnitude of coffee consumption results in a difference *of any kind* in resting heart rate.)

The multiple linear regression equation yields:

$$\hat{y} = b_0 + b_1 x_1 + b_2 x_2 + b_3 x_3 + b_4 x_4 + b_5 x_5 + b_6 x_6 \rightarrow$$
$$75.9 - 14.75(1) - 11.9(1) - 9.27(0) - 3.93(0) + 4.06(1) + 8.13(0) = 53.31 \text{ bpm}$$

Our reference group is now those who consume two daily caffeine beverages. Again, the linear regression equation is for a person who consumes three daily caffeine beverages. Notice what has happened. Most strangely, the estimated resting heart rate for a high-school student who is a long-distance runner that meditates and consumes three daily caffeine beverages has *fallen* from 57.24 to 53.31 bpm.

Indeed, when we compare Tables 7.13a and 7.13b, the regression coefficients for three independent variables (zero, three, and four daily beverages) have each fallen. More remarkably, each has fallen by precisely 3.93 bpm. The reason for such results is the following.

Table 7.13b Multiple linear regression analysis, n = 50

R Square	0.99762		
Independent variable	Regression (or beta) coefficient	t Statistic	p-Value
Intercept	79.83192	277.0963	1.46E-71
Long-distance runner	−14.7544	−45.3329	6.13E-38
Meditation	−11.9002	−44.6838	1.13E-37
Caffeine (0 daily beverages)	−9.27368	−26.2564	4.19E-28
Caffeine (1 daily beverage)	−3.93092	−11.4177	1.33E-14
Caffeine (3 daily beverages)	4.059098	11.80241	4.48E-15
Caffeine (4 daily beverages)	8.128174	22.78383	1.25E-25

Table 7.14 Change in resting heart rates associated with independent variables

Independent variable	Resting heart rate value
Long-distance runner	−15 bpm
Meditation	−12 bpm
Caffeine (1 daily beverage)	6 bpm
Caffeine (2 daily beverages)	10 bpm
Caffeine (3 daily beverages)	14 bpm
Caffeine (4 daily beverages)	18 bpm

First, and most importantly, the absolute impact of an independent variable cannot alter just because we change the reference group from one daily beverage to two daily beverages. *This drop for the three independent variables is only possible precisely because the regression coefficients, in this case, are not measures of absolute value.* Rather, they are measures of values that are relative to the values between and among five (ordinal-categorical) independent variables—zero, one, two, three, and four daily caffeine beverages.

For example, in both Table 7.13a and Table 7.13b, it is estimated that the absolute difference between the resting heart rate of those consuming three daily caffeine beverages and those consuming zero daily caffeine beverages is *exactly* 13.33278 bpm. This is no mere happy coincidence. This reflects the fact that no matter which level of caffeine consumption serves as our reference group, the relative differences between and among the regression coefficients for each of the five levels of consumption remain unaltered.

Lastly, notice two startling items. First, our R square value remains unchanged—a most impressive 99.8%—for both Table 7.13a and Table 7.13b. Second, in these same two tables, our regression coefficients for both runner and meditation also remain unchanged, −14.7544 and −11.9002, respectively. This clearly indicates that when we alter the reference group the only values that vary are those associated with different levels of caffeine consumption in relation to the alternating reference groups in Table 7.13a and Table 7.13b. This all but closes the case in favor of effect modification.

Importantly, there is a further reason why we find fairly exacting results in Tables 7.13a and 7.13b. The data for this sample of 50 students have been contrived to better demonstrate certain features of multiple linear regression. A student who did not participate in long-distance running, who did not meditate, and who did not consume caffeine was assigned a resting heart rate of 70 bpm. Each independent variable was given a specific resting heart rate value in bpm. The independent variables were then distributed among the 50 students and the presence of each added (or subtracted) to a student's common baseline of 70 bpm. (See Table 7.14.)

Simultaneous assessment of independent variables

A third common application of multiple linear regression is to assess (and compare) the impact of multiple independent variables simultaneously on a single, continuous outcome variable. As noted, for multiple linear regression, these independent variables can be continuous, dichotomous, ordinal, or categorical. Here we use categorical variables and provide a further demonstration of working with reference groups and indicator variables.

Our plan is to throw an assortment of independent variables into the pot, stir, and see what results. For example, we might want to combine caffeine consumption, long-distance running, and years of running experience as our independent variables and assess the impact of this combination on a student's resting heart rate. Depending upon our results, we may then want to distinguish between levels of caffeine consumption or compare cis-female and cis-male outcomes to assess effect modification based on gender identity.

Alternatively, we may have suspected these issues earlier and included differential consumption levels and gender identity among our independent variables from the beginning. In other words, what are essential in carrying out multiple linear regression are the circumstances of confounding and effect modification, along with the simultaneous assessment of independent variables. Less important is the precise order of investigation, which can vary.

For this example, we introduce a new categorical variable, religious identity, for our independent variables. We are again off to a local high school. This time we wander over to Gina Mlakabeni High School, where we meet with coach Christina Okolo who introduces us to her 35 long-distance runners. Perhaps somewhat surprisingly, these runners happen to include seven Methodists, seven Jehovah's Witnesses, seven Shia Muslims, seven Sikhs, and seven atheists.

Among other considerations, we wish to investigate any differences in resting heart rates associated with a runner's religious identity. The other independent variables to be assessed simultaneously for their relative effect on our continuous outcome variable (the resting heart rate) are a student's gender identity, age, and BMI.

To begin, there are again a number of steps to prepare our categorical variables for inclusion in the analysis. First, we designate those students who identify as Sikhs as our reference group. Those identifying with each of the other religions (or atheism) will be our indicator variables. As noted above, the regression coefficients associated with each of the indicator variables—in this case religious identities—are interpreted as: the estimated difference between the mean of the outcome variable for a particular religious identity and the mean of that variable for the reference group, *holding all other independent variables constant.*

We asked each runner to pray to her or his religion's God for calm resolve—or to consciously not pray if atheist—10 minutes prior to a big race. We then measured each runner's resting heart rate to determine whose God is most powerful. For fuller context, coach Okolo wanted to know if there were any differences among our 35 runners' resting heart rates based on gender identity, age, and BMI, along with religious identity. The data for our sample indicate:

- 41.7% are cis female.
- The mean age is 15.5 years, with a standard deviation of 1.20.
- The mean BMI is 21.4, with a standard deviation of 2.23.
- 20% are Methodists, 20% Jehovah's Witnesses, 20% Shia Muslims, 20% Sikhs, and 20% atheists.
- The mean resting heart rate for all 35 runners is 69.71 bpm, with a standard deviation of 6.81.

Table 7.15 Multiple linear regression analysis, $n = 35$

R square	0.893		
Independent variable	Regression (or beta) coefficient	t Statistic	p-Value
Intercept	9.389	1.420	0.167076
Cis female	−3.940	−4.509	0.000114
Age	1.147	1.449	0.15884
BMI	1.802	4.527	0.000108
Methodist	7.418	5.505	0.00000786
Jehovah's Witness	5.819	4.248	0.000229
Shia Muslim	6.302	4.547	0.000103
Atheist	9.354	6.816	0.000000254

The results of our multiple linear regression analysis are displayed in Table 7.15. The multiple linear regression equation yields:

$$\hat{y} = b_0 + b_1 x_1 + b_2 x_2 + b_3 x_3 + b_4 x_4 + b_5 x_5 + b_6 x_6 + b_7 x_7 \rightarrow$$
$$9.4 - 3.9(1) + 1.1(16) + 1.8(20) + 7.4(0) + 5.8(0) + 6.3(1) + 9.4(0) = 65.4 \text{ bpm}$$

Notice first that, with the exception of age, all independent variables proved statistically significant, with p-values well below 0.05. The regression coefficient for cis-female gender identity is −3.94 bpm, *adjusting for the other independent variables*. A one-unit increase in BMI increases a long-distance runner's resting heart rate by 1.802 bpm, *adjusting for the other independent variables*. In addition, the R square value is 89.3%.

Based on the linear regression equation for Table 7.15, it is estimated that a 16-year-old, cis-female high-school student with a BMI of 20, who is a long-distance runner and a practicing Shia Muslim, will have a resting heart rate of 65.4 bpm.

Turning then to our indicator variables, we find clear evidence (a) that, in fact, there is a God and (b) that the Sikh's God is the most powerful. The regression coefficients for Methodists, Jehovah's Witnesses, Shia Muslims, and atheists are between 5.819 to 9.354 bpm, *adjusting for the other independent variables*. No data for students who identify as Sikhs are reported because they are the reference group. This means, for instance, that the estimated resting heart rate of Methodists is 7.418 bpm above that for Sikhs.

In fact, the estimated resting heart rates for students who identify as Methodists, Jehovah's Witnesses, Shia Muslims, or atheists are all above the estimated rate for those who identify as Sikhs, after all runners—except atheists—prayed for calm resolve before a big race, *adjusting for the other independent variables*. This provides irrefutable statistical evidence that the Sikh's God is the most powerful. Furthermore, given that atheists have the largest increase in their resting heart rate (a regression coefficient of 9.354 bpm), we also have clear statistical evidence that there is a God.

Logistic regression

Just as our review of linear regression required a preliminary discussion of correlation and least squares estimates, our consideration of logistic regression requires similar attention to a number of key conceptual tools. It is true that we have already been down this road. These are the odds ratio, the natural logarithm, and the logit.

To understand logistic regression, one must understand (a) that it requires a single, dichotomous outcome variable and that (b), as the bad boy of biostatistics, a dichotomous outcome variable does not follow the same mathematical rules as a continuous outcome variable in the case of linear regression. (The rules for linear regression are based on the standard normal distribution that we further detail in Chapter 9.)

In addition, it must be recalled that biostatisticians really, really, *really* like the mathematical rules of linear regression and the standard normal distribution. Therefore, the first step is to rework things so that our dichotomous outcome variable can be disciplined to align with our independent variables in a manner more in tune with the mathematical rules of linear regression, allowing all biostatisticians to better sleep at night.

We align our variables in this fashion with something called a logit. The simplest description of a logit is that it is the natural logarithm of an odds ratio. Unfortunately, that is also a fairly complicated description of a logit. Allow that description to settle in a bit ... the natural logarithm of an odds ratio. This begs two questions. What is a natural logarithm? What is an odds ratio? We begin with an introduction—or reintroduction—to each of these. First, the odds ratio.

Odds ratio

The odds ratio is a fundamental tool for biostatistical analysis when tangling with a dichotomous outcome variable, as is the case for logistic regression. Regrettably, it can also be a significant source of misinterpretation. It is true that we have been down this road once or twice before. But let's again start with the basics.

To unravel the secrets of the odds ratio it is helpful to build up to this by beginning with the difference between the probability of some event and the odds of some event. When considering the *probability* of an event, our concern is the likelihood of ONE outcome, such as an ankle injury. When considering the *odds* of an event, our concern is the ratio between the likelihood of TWO outcomes— an ankle injury AND no ankle injury.

We know there is a 50% probability for "heads" if we flip a coin. That is, the probability of that ONE outcome. However, the odds for "heads"—as a ratio—is 1:1. This indicates that for every one time that you flip a coin and get "heads" you will flip the coin and NOT get "heads"—a ratio of TWO outcomes. It is very, very, very important and yet very, very, very difficult to understand that NOT heads is *not the equivalent of* "tails." Whether or not you get "heads" is event 1, with two possible outcomes (yes/no). Whether or not you get "tails" is event 2, with two possible outcomes (yes/no). Thus, it can be helpful to think in terms of outcomes rather than events.

Of course, there are many ways that people use odds and many of these appear to include more than two outcomes, such as betting on horse racing. However, for our limited purposes here regarding logistic regression, when we discuss odds (or an odds ratio) it will be in terms of only a single event with two possible outcomes—event A happens AND event A does NOT happen. In fact, as we will see, the odds is simply the ratio between *probabilities* for these two outcomes.

When describing a single event with two possible outcomes, wherein outcome A happens AND outcome A does NOT happen, the work of "AND" plays a critical part. First, this indicates that both must be considered, not one OR the other. Second, the nature of an outcome either happening or not happening makes these two outcomes binary and mutually exclusive. If one is true, the other CANNOT be true.

For this reason, each outcome has a probability that is the inverse of the other. If there is a 90% probability of an ankle injury, there must be a 10% probability of no ankle injury. It is the ratio between these probabilities for each outcome that produces the odds for the members of each group—NOT the odds between two groups.

This points to an important mathematical gimmick, or short cut, that we have already run into a few times. This is the expression: $1.0 - p$. (In this case, p is probability.) If we know the probability for an ankle injury is 90%, then:

$$1.0 - p \rightarrow 1.0 - 0.9 = 0.10 \text{ (or 10%)}$$

This is because, in this expression, 1.0 represents 100%. Indeed, $1.0 - p$ (or $1.0 - x$) is always a short cut to find an inverse value.

Let's walk through an example involving ankle injuries and our long-distance runners to better distinguish between the probability, the odds, and an odds ratio. For this, we create two groups of high-school long-distance runners. Group 1 has 50 runners who wore new track shoes this past season. Group 2 has 50 runners who wore their old track shoes this past season. Group 1 had 20 ankle injuries. Group 2 had five ankle injuries.

We want to compare the probability, the odds, and the odds ratio with respect to ankle injuries among the members of group 1 (with new shoes) and group 2 (with old shoes).

We begin with probability. The formula for probability is:

$$\frac{\text{the number of cases}}{\text{the number of potential cases}} \rightarrow \text{a percentage}$$

The probable proportion of persons with an ankle injury in group 1 is: $\frac{20}{50} = 0.40$ (or 40%). Note that this is NOT the probability for any particular person injuring an ankle. Rather, this tells us that if 100 runners in group 1 competed with new shoes, there is a probability that 40 of them would injure an ankle.

The probable proportion of persons with an ankle injury in group 2 is: $\frac{5}{50} = 0.10$ (or 10%).

Now we move to odds. The formula for odds is: $\frac{\text{the probability of an outcome}}{1.0 - (\text{the probability of an outcome})} \rightarrow \frac{p}{1.0 - p} \rightarrow$ a ratio

This equation for the odds is thus a ratio between the probabilities for two outcomes, such as the probability of an ankle injury (the numerator) and the probability of NO ankle injury (the denominator)—for the members of a specific group.

For our example, ankle injury (the numerator) is the proportion of persons who had an ankle injury. This is 40% for group 1. No ankle injury (the denominator) is the proportion of persons who did NOT have an ankle injury. This is 60% for group 1.

Thus, we find:

The odds of an ankle injury for an individual in group 1 are: $\frac{0.40}{1.0 - 0.40} = 0.666$ (or a ratio of 1:1.5).

We derive the ratio of 1:1.5 by dividing both sides of the ratio 0.666:1 by 0.666.

The odds of an ankle injury for an individual in group 2 are: $\frac{0.10}{1.0 - 0.10} = 0.111$ (or a ratio of 1:9).

We derive the ratio of 1:9 by dividing both sides of the ratio 0.111:1 by 0.111.

In group 1, for every 1.0 person who has an ankle injury, 1.5 persons do NOT have an ankle injury. These are the two outcomes for group 1.

In group 2, for every 1.0 person who has an ankle injury, 9.0 persons do NOT have an ankle injury. These are the two outcomes for group 2.

To further clarify, for group 1, we find **a probability** of 0.40 and **odds** of 0.666 (or 1:1.5) because:

- 0.40 is the probability of ONE outcome (an ankle injury)
- 0.666 (or 1:1.5) is the ratio between the probabilities for TWO outcomes (ankle injury *and* NO ankle injury)

Now the odds ratio. As the term suggests, an odds ratio is a ratio between *two odds*. Because the odds already provide a ratio between two probabilities this can get slightly dicey.

For our example, the odds ratio is a ratio between two ratios. These two ratios are:

the ratio between (a) the probable proportion of persons with an ankle injury *and* (b) the probable proportion of persons with NO ankle injury in group 1

AND

the ratio between (a) the probable proportion of persons with an ankle injury *and* (b) the probable proportion of persons with NO ankle injury in group 2

Based on the probabilities and the odds for our example, we find an odds ratio of 6:1.

$$\frac{p_1 / (1.0 - p_1)}{p_2 / (1.0 - p_2)} \rightarrow \frac{0.40 / (1.0 - 0.40)}{0.10 / (1.0 - 0.10)} \rightarrow \frac{0.40 / 0.60}{0.10 / 0.90} \rightarrow \frac{0.40 \times 0.90}{0.60 \times 0.10} \rightarrow \frac{0.36}{0.06} = 6.0 \ (or \ 6:1)$$

In this case, our odds ratio (6:1) tells us that:

The odds of an ankle injury for a person in group 1 are six times greater than the odds for a person in group 2. Or, for every six persons in group 1 with an ankle injury, there will be 1.0 person with an ankle injury in group 2.

Of course, we already had the odds for these outcomes for the persons in group 1 and group 2. The odds ratio allows us now to make comparisons between these two groups based on the data (the odds) for each group.

Finally, notice the following.

Probability tells us TWO things:

- 40% of runners with new shoes will likely have an ankle injury.
- 10% of runners with their old shoes will likely have an ankle injury.

The odds tell us TWO things:

- For every 1.0 runner with new shoes who has an ankle injury, 1.5 runners with new shoes will NOT have an ankle injury.
- For every 1.0 runner with their old shoes who has an ankle injury, 9.0 runners with their old shoes will NOT have an ankle injury.

The odds ratio tells us ONE thing:

• For every 6.0 runners with new shoes who has an ankle injury, 1.0 runner with their old shoes will have an ankle injury.

There is one further source of confusion that merits mention. This is the difference between the risk ratio and the odds ratio. The risk ratio essentially skips a step and produces a ratio between the probability of an outcome for group 1 and the probability of an outcome for group 2. (Whereas the odds ratio produces a ratio between the odds of an outcome for group 1 and the odds of an outcome for group 2.)

From the data above for ankle injuries, the risk ratio would be: $0.40/0.10 = 4.0$. Thus, for every 4.0 runners with new shoes who has an ankle injury, 1.0 runner with their old shoes will have an ankle injury. Often, there is little difference between the risk ratio and the odds ratio. This points to an important consideration when interpreting an odds ratio.

Indeed, there is one very ESSENTIAL feature of an odds ratio to be aware of. Given a 40% probability of an ankle injury for group 1 and a 10% probability for group 2, the odds ratio between the two groups was 6:1. This seems like a pretty high ratio. However, what if we had the same odds ratio (6:1), and there was only a 2% probability (not 40%) of an ankle injury for those with new shoes—and thus an even far teenier probability for those with old shoes?

In theory, it would be possible to alter the numbers for each group and find a 2% probability of an ankle injury for runners with new shoes and an even smaller probability for runners with old shoes, while retaining an odds ratio of 6:1 between the two groups. Clearly, the altered case—with far, far fewer ankle injuries per runner with new shoes—would be much less of a concern than the original case. (To generate such numbers we would need an exceptionally large sample of runners and ankle injuries would need to be exceptionally rare.)

Thus, the importance we give to the size of the odds ratio between two groups is ALWAYS, ALWAYS determined by the underlying probability for each group.

Be sure to repeat this last sentence several times! This notion is akin to finding a statistically significant difference between two medications but determining that the size of this difference is not clinically meaningful. Yes, given strict rules of statistical significance there is an actual measurable difference between the medications. However, this difference is too small to make a practical difference for treating patients.

A related and perhaps more intuitive example of such distortions is a comparison between a 2% increase in the annual number of US deaths due to lung cancer and a 400% increase in the annual number of US deaths due to deep sea diving. Clearly, 400% sounds like a lot—certainly a lot more than 2%. However, it will surprise few people that there are far more annual US deaths due to lung cancer (approximately 130,000) compared to deaths from deep sea diving (approximately 100). Thus, a tiny 2% increase in lung cancer deaths (an increase of 2,600 deaths) still dwarfs a huge 400% increase in deep sea diving deaths (an increase of 400 deaths).

The natural logarithm

Here we provide a very brief review of the natural logarithm to further set up our discussion of the logit. A logarithm is the power (or exponent) to which a number must be raised to equal some other number.

There are two frequent logarithms.

• The common logarithms with base of 10; this is written $\log(100)$ → $\log_{10}(100)$ → $10^x = 100$
• The natural logarithms with base of "e"; this is written $\ln(50)$ → $\log_e(50)$ → $e^x = 50$

The two final equations ($[10^x = 100]$ and $[e^x = 50]$) can be read as follows:

  $10^x = 100$: how many times do we multiply 10 by itself to equal 100; the answer is 2
  ($10 \times 10 = 100$)
  $e^x = 50$: how many times do we multiply "e" by itself to equal 50; the answer is 3.912;
  continue reading for an explanation

As noted, our interest is the natural logarithm. The letter "e" = 2.71828. This is a naturally occurring value that happens to be very common. Leonhard Euler is the one who found the number somewhere in Switzerland. Thus, "e" stands for Euler's number.

  Consider the following example:

$$\ln(3.5) \rightarrow \log_e(3.5) \rightarrow e^x = 3.5 \rightarrow 2.71828^x = 3.5 \rightarrow x = 1.253$$

"e" = 2.71828.

We need to determine what is the power (x) to which we must raise "e," so that it equals 3.5. To solve for x, we use the "ln" function on a scientific calculator.

Type in 3.5 and then press the "ln" key and we find ... 1.253.

You may recall from junior high this technique of raising a number to the base of another number to equal some value.

  This is written: $2_x(16) \rightarrow 2^x = 16 \rightarrow 2^4 = 16$ (or $2 \times 2 \times 2 \times 2 = 16$)

To illustrate this with the notorious "e," keep in mind that: $2.71828 \times 2.71828 = 7.38904616$.

  Thus: $\ln(7.38904616) \rightarrow \log_e(7.38904616) \rightarrow e^x = 7.38904616 \rightarrow 2.71828^x \approx 2.0$

The natural logarithm—based on Euler's number—is foundational for working with the logit and for logistic regression more generally.

The logit

Let us return to that original, bedazzling sentence. "The logit is the natural logarithm of an odds ratio." We can write this in equally edifying style as:

$$\ln(\text{odds ratio}) \rightarrow \log_e(\text{odds ratio}) \rightarrow e^x = (\text{odds ratio}) \rightarrow 2.71828^x = (\text{odds ratio})$$

The math for deriving the odds ratio—detailed above—is not overly taxing and walking through this math can be helpful for better understanding the odds ratio as a concept. This is less helpful in the case of the logit and an introduction to logistic regression. The math is manageable, but the degree of detail can deter us from our larger goals. Therefore, it is better to reserve this for a later biostatistics course. For now, we will leave the math to a statistical software program.

In our example of ankle injuries we had an odds ratio of 6:1 (or 6.0) between those in group 1 with new shoes and those in group 2 with their old shoes. The natural logarithm of this odds ratio [$\ln(6.0)$] is a logit. In this case, our logit is 1.792.

Very, very, very importantly, "1.792" would be the (beta) regression coefficient for "new shoes" were it an independent variable within logistic regression. As we will see, the (beta) regression coefficient is the odds ratio that is associated with a one-unit increase in some attribute or exposure.

Logistic regression thus requires that we transform the dichotomous outcome variable into a logit. The logit can thus be understood as the natural logarithm of the odds ratio between two groups regarding some dichotomous outcome. Logistic regression, in this sense, is designed to predict the logit of a dichotomous outcome variable based on the independent variables. This amounts to the probability of an outcome.

Let us now put all this in motion, beginning with simple logistic regression. The equation for this is:

$$\text{logit}(Y) = \ln\left(\frac{\hat{p}}{1.0 - \hat{p}}\right) \rightarrow \ln\left(\frac{\hat{p}}{1.0 - \hat{p}}\right) = \alpha + b_x \rightarrow \text{logit}(Y) = \alpha + b_x$$

Our goal here is to find the value of $\text{logit}(Y)$. This is equal to $\ln\left(\frac{\hat{p}}{1.0 - \hat{p}}\right)$. AND $\ln\left(\frac{\hat{p}}{1.0 - \hat{p}}\right)$ is equal to $\alpha + b_x$.

So to solve for $\text{logit}(Y)$, we need either the value of $\ln\left(\frac{\hat{p}}{1.0 - \hat{p}}\right)$ OR the value of $\alpha + b_x$.

Keep in mind that $\frac{p}{1.0 - p}$ is the odds between the probability of outcome A and the probability of NOT outcome A. The Greek letter alpha (α) represents some constant value. This value is akin to b_0, the constant value (or intercept) in multiple linear regression.

This equation is then expanded, as follows, for multiple logistic regression:

$$\text{logit}(Y) = \ln\left(\frac{\hat{p}}{1.0 - \hat{p}}\right) \rightarrow \ln\left(\frac{\hat{p}}{1.0 - \hat{p}}\right) = \alpha + b_1 x_1 + b_2 x_2 + b_3 x_3 + b_4 x_4$$

Thus, for multiple logistic regression, to solve for $\text{logit}(Y)$, we need the value of either:

$$\ln\left(\frac{\hat{p}}{1.0 - \hat{p}}\right) \quad \textbf{OR} \quad \alpha + b_1 x_1 + b_2 x_2 + b_3 x_3 + b_4 x_4$$

As with multiple linear regression, solving for these values is the work of statistical software programs.

Thus, we turn now to how we set up our data for a statistical program to analyze things and how we interpret the results of that analysis. We begin with simple logistic regression with one causal (or independent) variable, before turning to multiple logistic regression. As in the case of multiple linear regression, these causal (or independent) variables can be continuous, dichotomous, ordinal, or categorical.

Just a very few further preliminaries

Before diving in, there is just a tiny bit more to pull together. This concerns three basic differences between how we calculate and interpret the results of linear regression and how we calculate and interpret the results of logistic regression. Each of these differences follows from the fundamental difference between working with a continuous outcome variable (linear regression) and working with a dichotomous outcome variable (logistic regression).

Difference #1. Recall that with linear regression we are trying to solve for the continuous value of a dependent variable (y), given the values of our independent variables. The value of y is a number that can be positive or negative as well as infinitesimally small or infinitely large.

For logistic regression, the value of Y (the logit) is not a theoretically infinite value. It is a probability. Therefore, it is finite and its values range between 0.0 and 1.0. (Such that, 0.0 = 0% and 1.0 = 100%.) We are after the probability that a certain outcome actually does occur, given the values of the independent variables. If the outcome does occur we code this as "1.0."

Hence, $p(y = 1.0)$ can be read: the probability that the value of y is "1.0," indicating that the outcome did occur.

Difference #2. What then is the method for generating the values for the regression coefficients (b_1, b_2, b_3, etc.) within the logistic regression equation? (Again, these are also referred to as betas, for the Greek letter β, or "beta.") Recall that for multiple linear regression this requires least squares estimates which we reviewed previously via the esoteric language of formal mathematics. For multiple logistic regression, however, the value of the intercept (b_0) and the values of the betas ($b_1, b_2 \ldots b_p$) are generated by something called the maximum likelihood method.

This is a technique—performed by statistical programs—that maximizes the likelihood of reproducing the data that we are working from, given the parameter estimates of that data. Parameter estimates are those measures of central tendency and variability for that data—such as a mean, median, variance, or standard deviation.

The maximum likelihood method then leads us to measures of the probability of finding the observed results, given these parameter estimates. There are two types of tests for this. The first type is a goodness-of-fit test for the logistic regression model. The hope is that the test will NOT prove to be statistically significant. The goal is thus a p-value GREATER than 0.05. The reason for this is slightly counterintuitive.

The idea is that the larger the p-value the more likely it is to generate our results, given the parameter estimates of our data. This indicates that our model—the logistic regression equation—fits our data. The Hosmer-Lemeshow test is an example of a goodness-of-fit test for this purpose.

The second type of test to assess the probability of finding the observed results is designed to replicate the R squared value found in multiple linear regression, with a range in values from 0.0 to 1.0. The interpretation of these tests is, therefore, comparable to that in multiple linear regression. Examples of these tests include the Cox and Snell R squared and Nagelkerke R squared. Statistical programs generally choose which tests are used.

The use of the maximum likelihood method also means that the statistical software programs will need to run chi-square statistics rather than the t statistics that we saw above with linear regression.

Difference #3. There is one final complication before turning to simple logistic regression. This concerns how to interpret the regression coefficients (or beta values) that we find. Again, these are: ($b_0 + b_1x_1 + b_2x_2 \ldots + b_px_p$).

While the regression coefficient (b_1x_1) holds considerable interest when we are engaged in linear regression, this is less the case for logistic regression. For logistic regression, the regression coefficient represents a value yet to be further transformed into an odds ratio. Our true interest is the antilog of a regression coefficient, more specifically antilog$_e$. Not to confuse matters too much, however, we will commonly see three terms. Each refers to the same thing and each produces an odds ratio.

$\text{antilog}_e \rightarrow e^{b_1} \rightarrow \exp(b_1)$

What we need to know is this. The odds ratio for b_1—and *any beta regression coefficient*—is e^{b_1}. You will recall, that e^{b_1} is equivalent to 2.71828^{b_1}. Thus, we must determine to what power must we raise 2.71828 to equal b_1. For this, we calculate $\exp(b_1)$. This "power" can be calculated with either a scientific calculator or Excel.

The antilog reverses, or undoes, a logarithm. When we calculate the logarithm of a number, we raise the original number to the power of some value. Thus, we are after that *original number*.

For instance, e^2 is equivalent to $2.71828^2 = 7.38905$.
Therefore, the antilog$_e$ of 7.38905 is 2.718282.

This is thus a super important maneuver for transforming a regression coefficient (or beta) into an odds ratio in logistic regression. Let us see some examples of all this below to bring about crystal clarity.

Simple logistic regression

For this presentation of simple and multiple logistic regression, we will work with the same examples from multiple linear regression. Importantly, however, this does NOT include the same data. First, we must replace the previous continuous outcome variable (the resting heart rate) with a dichotomous variable—whether or not the resting heart rate is below 69 bpm. This is the fundamental difference between linear and logistic regression. If a student's resting heart rate is below 69 bpm, her or his outcome value will be coded as "1." If not, this will be coded as "0."

Second, the sample size requirements differ for linear and logistic regression. With one exception, the examples for linear regression had a sample size of 50 students, 23 of whom were runners. For logistic regression we have a sample size of 100, 50 of whom are runners. In fact, an even larger sample size would produce stronger results.

The problems for smaller samples emerge when there are too few cases distributed across all the possible outcomes for our dichotomous independent variables. (This is essentially a problem of multicollinearity.) This creates high degrees of uncertainty that result in all sorts of mayhem, including elevated odds ratios and large estimated confidence intervals. The data for logistic regression here have, therefore, been tailored to better illustrate the key features of logistic regression.

To set the stage, we begin with simple logistic regression. We want to know if there is a relationship between a single independent variable (long-distance running) and a single dichotomous dependent variable (a resting heart rate below 69 bpm). See Table 7.16.

Table 7.16 Simple logistic regression, $n = 100$

Independent variable	(Beta) regression coefficient	Standard error	Wald test	p-Value	Odds ratio	Odds ratio 95% confidence intervals
Constant	– 1.15268	0.331133	12.11747	0.0005	0.315789	1.147561
Runner	0.992337	0.436078	5.178321	0.02287	2.697531	1.147561– 6.34099

Our simple logistic regression equation is:

$$\ln\left(\frac{\hat{p}}{1.0-\hat{p}}\right) \rightarrow -1.15268 + 0.992337 \text{(runner)}$$

Thus, the odds ratio between runners and non-runners indicates that a runner is 2.69 times more likely to have a resting heart rate below 69 bpm than a non-runner. For a more detailed understanding, let us review the categories of this logistic regression table across the seven columns. We begin with the (beta) regression coefficient for the independent variable, the odds ratio, and the estimated confidence interval for the odds ratio based on a 95% confidence level.

The "constant" (beta) regression coefficient is –1.153. Recall that this is NOT a value for the number of "bpm" as it is with linear regression. For logistic regression, this is a measure of the odds that a person will have a resting heart rate below 69 bpm, if all other independent variables have a regression coefficient equivalent to 0.0. Thus we turn our focus to the other independent variables. Here we have one other independent variable—whether or not a student is a long-distance runner.

Remember that to find the odds ratio between two groups for an independent variable we must find the antilog of the (beta) regression coefficient associated with that variable. This is referred to as "exponentiating" the (beta) regression coefficient. This is written: e^b (again, e = 2.71828).

Thus, e^b asks to what power must we raise "e" (or 2.71828) to equal the (beta) regression coefficient?

Assume that our (beta) regression coefficient is 1.2345. The easiest way to "exponentiate" this value is to open Excel, select any cell, and type "=exp(1.2345)" in the function box. This returns an odds ratio.

In this case, the odds ratio is 3.43666.

The (beta) regression coefficient for "runner" is 0.9923. After exponentiating 0.9923—exp(0.9923)—we generate an odds ratio of 2.69 between runners and non-runners. Thus, if a student is a runner, her or his estimated likelihood of a resting heart rate below 69 bpm is 2.69 times greater than that for a student who is not a runner. This is an odds ratio of 2.69:1. Thus, for every 2.69 runners with a resting heart rate below 69 bpm, there will be 1.0 non-runner with a heart rate below 69 bpm.

As Table 7.16 indicates, this odds ratio between runners and non-runners has an estimated confidence interval between 1.15 and 6.34, at a 95% confidence level. Again, this indicates that if we repeat these calculations with 100 different samples from the same population, the true population odds ratio between runners and non-runners would fall somewhere within the resulting estimated confidence intervals 95 times out of 100.

The final three columns provide the standard error, the Wald test result, and the p-value for each (beta) regression coefficient. The standard error is a measure of variability among the values for each student pertaining to a particular (beta) regression coefficient. The smaller the standard error, the less volatility we will have across all our results. The standard error is also necessary for the Wald test.

The Wald test evaluates the relationship between the dependent and independent variables by assessing the null hypothesis as it pertains to each independent variable. The null hypothesis for multiple logistic regression is that ALL (beta) regression coefficients are equal to 0.0. Rejection of the null hypothesis implies that AT LEAST one (beta) regression coefficient does NOT equal 0.0. The Wald test divides the value of each (beta) regression coefficient by the standard error. Thus, the smaller the standard error, the larger the value of the Wald test.

The p-value indicates if the value of the Wald test result is significantly different from 0.0, allowing us to reject the null hypothesis. We reject the null hypothesis if the p-value is below 0.05. In our case, the p-value is below 0.05 for our one independent variable (runner) and we reject the null hypothesis for its (beta) regression coefficient. Happily, this validates the statistical significance of our findings regarding the link between this independent variable and our dependent variable—a resting heart rate below 69 bpm.

Multiple logistic regression

As we move on from simple logistic regression, it is important to clarify a further important distinction between multiple linear regression and multiple logistic regression. Multiple linear regression produces a single, cumulative value for some continuous outcome variable based on a combination of independent variables. Each time we add a new independent variable to the mix, all the other independent variables are recalibrated. This results in a new single cumulative value for the dependent variable, *as well as*, new values for the regression coefficient for each independent variable. Each new calibration is an adjustment to account for some new variable. In this way, we are able to assess any confounding variables as we add new independent variables.

Multiple logistic regression does NOT produce a single, cumulative value (or odds ratio). Odds ratios cannot be combined in this fashion. Rather, multiple logistic regression produces a series of odds ratios associated with each specific independent variable. This indicates the magnitude of the impact of each independent variable (via its odds ratio) on the likelihood of some dichotomous outcome.

Each time we add a new independent variable to the mix, the odds ratio for all the other independent variables is recalibrated resulting in a new odds ratio for each. Thus, each new calibration is an adjustment to account for some new variable in a manner analogous to multiple linear regression. This means that a major purpose of multiple logistic regression is to assess the impact of *individual* independent variables on the probability of the dichotomous outcome variable.

We now want to know if there is a relationship between multiple independent variables (long-distance runners and meditation) and a single, dichotomous dependent variable (a resting heart rate below 69 bpm). Our results are displayed in Table 7.17.

Our multiple logistic regression equation is:

$$\ln\left(\frac{\hat{p}}{1.0 - \hat{p}}\right) \rightarrow -3.12547 + 1.171989(\text{runner}) + 0.035989(\text{weekly meditation minutes})$$

Table 7.17 Multiple logistic regression, $n = 100$

Independent variable	Regression coefficient	Standard error	Wald test	p-Value	Odds ratio	Odds ratio 95% confidence intervals
Constant	−3.12547	0.69514	20.21564	6.92E-06	0.043916	–
Runner	1.171989	0.481777	5.917715	0.014989	3.228406	1.255737 – 8.299994
Meditation	0.035989	0.009955	13.06975	0.0003	1.036645	1.016614 – 1.05707

Our new (beta) regression coefficient for "runner" is 1.1719. After exponentiating 1.1719—exp(1.1719)—we generate an odds ratio of 3.23 between runners and non-runners. If a student is a long-distance runner, her or his estimated likelihood of a resting heart rate below 69 bpm is 3.23 times greater than for a student who is not a runner, after controlling for meditation.

When we compare these data with the data from Table 7.16, we notice that the (beta) regression coefficient for "runner" has increased from 0.9923 (with an odds ratio of 2.69) to a (beta) regression coefficient of 1.1719 (with an odds ratio of 3.23), after adjusting for meditation. Note that this adjustment assumes that the average minutes of meditation is the same for the runner and non-runner being compared.

The odds ratio between runners and non-runners is 3.23:1. Thus, for every 3.23 runners with a resting heart rate below 69 bpm, there will be 1.0 non-runner with a heart rate below 69 bpm. (This odds ratio has an estimated confidence interval between 1.26 and 8.29, at a 95% confidence level.)

The (beta) regression coefficient for "meditation" is 0.0359. After exponentiating 0.0359—exp(0.0359)—we generate an odds ratio of 1.04 between those who meditate and those who do not meditate. Thus, for each additional minute of meditation, a student's estimated likelihood of a resting heart rate below 69 bpm increases by 1.04. (This increase in the odds ratio has an estimated confidence interval between 1.02 and 1.06, at a 95% confidence level.) Note that one reason for such a small value is that the increment of change (one minute) is also very small. Remember, as well, that the (beta) regression coefficient of 0.0359 for meditation (with an odds ratio of 1.04) has been adjusted to account for "runner."

Now the final three columns. The standard error is reasonably small for each (beta) regression coefficient. All p-values for the Wald test are below 0.05, allowing us to reject the null hypothesis for each (beta) regression coefficient. This again validates the statistical significance of our findings regarding the link between our independent variables (running and meditation) and our dependent variable (a resting heart rate below 69 bpm).

We are ready now to bring in the coffee buzz. See Table 7.18.

Our multiple logistic regression equation is now:

$$\ln\left(\frac{\hat{p}}{1.0-\hat{p}}\right) \rightarrow -0.90631+1.36679\,(\text{runner})+0.042251\,(\text{weekly meditation minutes})$$
$$-0.01162\,(\text{caffeine consumption})$$

We again begin with the (beta) regression coefficient for each independent variable, the odds ratio, and the estimated confidence interval for the odds ratio, at a 95% confidence level. The (beta) regression coefficient for "runner" is 1.3668. After exponentiating 1.3668—exp(1.3668)—we generate an odds ratio between runners and non-runners of 3.92. (This

Table 7.18 Multiple logistic regression, n = 100

Independent variable	Regression coefficient	Standard error	Wald test	p-Value	Odds ratio	Odds ratio 95% confidence intervals
Constant	−0.90631	0.901133	1.011526	0.314538	0.404012	–
Runner	1.36679	0.529347	6.666886	0.009822	3.92274	1.38998 – 11.07058
Meditation	0.042251	0.011283	14.02276	0.000181	1.043156	1.020341 – 1.066482
Caffeine	−0.01162	0.003497	11.04896	0.000887	0.988443	0.981691 – 0.995241

is a slight change from a (beta) regression coefficient of 1.172 and an odds ratio of 3.23 in Table 7.17.)

If a student is a runner, her or his estimated likelihood of a resting heart rate below 69 bpm is 3.92 times greater than for a student who is not a runner, after adjusting for meditation and caffeine consumption. Again, this adjustment assumes that the average minutes of meditation and the level of caffeine consumption are the same for the runner and non-runner being compared. The odds ratio between runners and non-runners is 3.92:1. Thus, for every 3.92 runners with a resting heart rate below 69 bpm, there will be 1.0 non-runner with a heart rate below 69 bpm. This odds ratio has an estimated confidence interval between 1.39 and 11.07, at a 95% confidence level.

The (beta) regression coefficient for "meditation" is 0.0422. After exponentiating 0.0422—exp(0.0422)—we generate an odds ratio of 1.04 between those who meditate and those who do not meditate. Thus, for each additional minute of meditation, a student's estimated odds of a resting heart rate below 69 bpm increase by 1.04. This again is after adjusting for a person's runner status and caffeine consumption. This increase in the odds ratio has an estimated confidence interval between 1.02 and 1.07, at a 95% confidence level. Again, one reason for such a small value is that the increment of change (one minute) is also very small.

The (beta) regression coefficient for "caffeine" is –0.0116. After exponentiating –0.0116— exp(–0.0116)—we generate an odds ratio of 0.99. Thus, for each additional microgram of caffeine, a student's estimated odds of a resting heart rate below 69 bpm increase by 0.99. This is after adjusting for a person's runner status and meditation practice. This increase in the odds ratio has an estimated confidence interval between 0.98 and 0.99, at a 95% confidence level.

Note that such a small value this time is again due to a very tiny increment of change (one microgram of caffeine). This is essentially an odds ratio of 1:1, meaning an increase of 1.0 microgram of caffeine consumption adds basically nothing to the likelihood that a person will (or will not) have a resting heart rate below 69 bpm.

Now the final three columns. The standard errors are quite small for each (beta) regression coefficient. All p-values for the Wald test are below 0.05, allowing us to reject the null hypothesis for each (beta) regression coefficient. This then validates the statistical significance of our findings regarding the link between our independent variables (running, meditation, and caffeine consumption) and our dependent variable (a resting heart rate below 69 bpm).

Final remarks

In one sense, most or all of Chapters 5, 6, and 7 have been a sustained exercise in one's willful suspension of disbelief. The material is almost exclusively grounded in a reductive perspective in which discrete parts (or variables) operate and interact with one another independently. And yet ... there remains that promise, first raised back in Chapter 2, that—in the right hands—regression analysis could provide the tools and techniques to sneak a holistic perspective in through a back door of biostatistical analysis.

The principal argument was that by including multiple independent variables—and by adjusting each of these in accord with their interactions with the others—a researcher, inclined to do so, could capture the context for each variable and the relationships between these. Let us then consider these two elements—the context and the relationships between these variables—by contrasting a holistic lens with the (reductive) lens of multiple regression analysis.

From a holistic perspective, consideration of a context would detail the ecological environment that myriad variables occupy. Variables would thus be understood via their origins within—and interactions with—that environment. The variables and the ecological environment would be treated as constituent elements of some larger system whose origins, rationale, and reproduction would enter into our description and explanation of the variables, the environment, and the interactions between them. Thus, consideration of the relationships between variables separate from a system-level analysis would be viewed as a reductive distortion. These are the basic features of a holistic perspective regarding a context for, and the relationships among, variables. The ground for this analysis is necessarily the system, as a holistic and interactive whole.

In turn, from a reductive perspective, consideration of a context would detail the variables that occupy a (presupposed) ecological environment. The environment would be understood as a detached arena for the interaction of discrete variables. Insofar as the ecological environment is an inert and non-reflexive vessel, there is no system, *per se*. Moreover, there is no real need for recourse to a system to explain the behavior of the variables because this behavior emerges from their interactions and from their unique, individual propensities, along with underlying discrete laws that we uncover.

Consequently, consideration of the relationships between variables within a system-level analysis would be viewed as a metaphysical delusion. In line with this perspective, the ground for regression analysis is an admixture of discrete, interacting variables, as parts of a reductive and divisible aggregation.

Hence, while regression analysis certainly extends the reductive perspective beyond certain limitations of bivariate analysis, this cannot ultimately lift biostatistical analysis out of its morass of reductive premises. Importantly, this is not necessarily for lack of imagination. Intentional or not—this sacrifice of a holistic viewpoint is justified by researchers based on the phenomenal reductive insights that have been extraordinarily beneficial to research and to health and medicine more generally.

Thus, the fault lies not in motive, not in ideology, nor in slow-wittedness. The fault lies only in the failure to treat this reductive retreat as a (temporary) willful suspension of disbelief and the stubborn refusal to return one's analysis to a holistic realm after reaping these critical reductive insights.

Chapter 8

Optimal Sample Size—or Benign Manipulation, the Good Kind

Sample size has been a topic of both quiet and loud conversation throughout many previous chapters. Yet, the rationale and technical steps for determining an optimal sample size have remained under wraps. The rationale for an optimal sample size, very simply, is efficiency. The researcher who concocts the smallest possible sample size that delivers sufficiently robust results, saving us both time and money, wins praise far and wide. While we have no objections to a science based on thrift and discount beakers, our interest here is not efficiency alone.

In addition, we shall see that the deliberative nature of sample size determination raises troubling concerns for the notions of detached objectivity within biostatistical analysis more generally. Indeed, determining an optimal sample size requires a host of personal choices by the researcher to better "manage" her or his data with certain ends in mind, such as controlling variability. Put bluntly, the name of the game in biostatistical analysis is "certainty"—more precisely, degrees of certainty. Limiting variability increases certainty. Sample size is one tool for limiting variability.

We thus aim in this chapter—via scrutiny of the optimal sample size—to better understand the roles of both subjective judgment and (quantitative) variability within biostatistical analysis (and its results). Indeed, the latter has a role that will soon metastasize exponentially in our discussion of probability in the next chapter. As we shall see, determining an optimal sample size is largely about identifying, measuring, and managing instruments of variability—such as the standard error of the mean or the standard deviation—within the data generated by one's study. Lastly, it also seems conspicuous that choosing one's sample size to accommodate certain results apparently goes hand-in-hand with efforts to bring order to our chaotic world.

Some preliminary (conceptual) considerations for optimal sample size

In Chapters 5, 6, and 7, we saw how the sample size can impact the results of a statistical test in a number of ways. On the one hand, we often encounter minimal cut-off points, indicating that we must choose one type of test or another. For example, with hypothesis testing we must often opt for either a z-test or a t-test, depending upon the sample size. Framed this way, the accuracy of a test result is dependent on the sample size. However, the logic here seems backwards.

We are told that if we have fewer than 30 persons in a sample we must choose a t-test over a z-test. This is obviously absurd. It is the test that determines the appropriate sample size, not the sample size that determines the test. It is only presented in this backward manner because we can more easily manipulate the sample size, than the statistical test. However,

DOI: 10.4324/9781003316985-8

if it is true concerns over sample size arise, in part, from a need to identify, measure, and manage variability, then it seems that what we really manipulate is not only our sample size, but the variability of that sample.

On the other hand, and perhaps even more stupendously, we have seen that merely increasing one's sample size from say 40 to 4,000 can, at times, magically render our results statistically significant. This occurs notwithstanding that all essential measures—mean, proportion, standard deviation, etc.—remain unchanged from those results previously deemed insignificant.

In other words, if a certain proportion of a group of 40 people report a headache after a hit on the head with a hammer, we have an inkling. But if the same proportion of a group of 4,000 people also report a headache after a similar hammer blow, we have a diagnosis. At the same time, when moving from 40 to 4,000, we reach a certain point along the way when further increasing the sample size begins to have a smaller and smaller impact on our results. This accounts for the efficiency of selecting an optimal sample size.

On the third hand, we also find statistical tests that require a minimum number of expected observations before moving forward with our analysis. The chi-square goodness-of-fit test is an example. This dilemma is directly linked to sample size, insofar as one of our surest methods to meet a minimal requirement for expected observations is to increase our sample size. Notice that increasing the sample size by increments until we meet the minimum requirement for expected observations may or may not alter the distribution of responses among our categories of observations. The details regarding the data themselves that are added when increasing the sample size are, therefore, secondary. What matters is sheer volume. This again is what counters variability.

So what is going on? Why does sample size ordinarily influence our results in this way? The simplest answer is that large samples decrease variability. This decrease has two sources. First, mathematically, the greater the number of observations, the less the influence of extreme cases. Accordingly, techniques for setting a sample size are often quite refined. So refined, in fact, that, depending upon the degree of variability within each group, a small difference between the means of two groups can yield far more statistical significance than a large difference between the means of two smaller groups.

Indeed, this is why the researcher must in general determine if the study results—even when statistically significant to a very high degree—are actually *clinically* significant. For instance, a medication that demonstrates the ability to reduce systolic blood pressure from 121.7 to 121.2, with a p-value of 0.00001, would likely be of little practical value.

Second, methodologically, we know, in general, that the greater the number of cases, the fewer the number of variables. This follows from the parsimonious ethos of biostatistical research. We gather a great many cases and examine a modest number of variables for each. Qualitative research, by contrast, typically gathers a modest number of cases and examines a great many variables for each. With quantitative research, we sacrifice idiosyncrasy for precision.

At the start of biostatistical research, this principle is well understood and consciously pursued. However, along the way, the fallacious notion that a larger sample size provides more details and reduces variability creeps back in long after the decisive actions have been taken—that is, after certain slippery and qualitative phenomena comprising health and medicine have been simplified and quantified.

In Chapter 1, we moved from a broad, eclectic, and qualitative notion of health to a narrow, precise, and quantitative notion (a resting heart rate). As we continue to emphasize *ad nauseam*, this movement—and the "willful suspension of belief" that it entails—is not in itself problematic. However, this assumes that one retains the duality of this concept in their head as a conscious, strategic maneuver, before then returning to the fuller concept.

In fact, because the determination of optimal sample size occurs so long after the original transformation of the subject matter into a quantifiable abstraction, it is at the point of wrangling with sample size that the now hidden and forgotten premises of biostatistical analysis should weigh most heavily on our minds. In other words, the determination of sample size is actually a relatively *late-stage* exercise that prolongs and deepens our willful suspension of disbelief.

Thus, reduced quantitative variability is a function of both sample size, as well as the initial necessary methodological distortion of the subject matter that permits its analysis via biostatistical tools and techniques. Commonly, this is attributed to some (presumed) inherent distinction between qualitative and quantitative analysis. However, as further explored in Chapter 10, all quantitative measures begin as qualitative observations. Quantitative analysis then proceeds in stages, first, to whittle away the number and variety of qualitative observations before, second, to transform the few surviving observations into two-dimensional caricatures of their original forms.

Thus, sample size matters not merely due to certain inherent mathematical principles—such as the need to reduce variability by increasing the number of cases—but due to the reduction of singular, complex, and particular cases to bundles of discrete, simple, and universal units of measurements.

As discussed, especially in Chapter 4 and later in Chapter 10, there are two principal types of quantitative measurement that we perform on a daily basis yet rarely think about. For individual objects this includes consideration of certain dimensions, such as length, weight, or volume. However, when we combine the measures of individual objects, such as the weights of five rocks, we have a second type of quantitative measure for these *combined* items. This includes various aggregate measures, such as the mean, median, or standard deviation.

We move sequentially from a singular and distinct thing (an individual rock) to a thing that can be compared to like things via a common measure (the weight of one rock *vis-à-vis* the weights of other rocks) to a thing whose individual qualities dissolve within the qualities of other like things (the mean weight of five rocks).

In this sense, these (aggregate) quantitative measurements—mean, median, standard deviation, etc.—are expressions of a deliberate homogenization. This second type of quantitative measures somehow repackages and reconstitutes an individual thing and the original rock, for instance, then becomes a particular—yet indistinguishable—bearer of certain communal properties. The first type of quantitative measurement is concrete and individual. This belongs to explicit qualitative description. The second type is abstract and collective. This belongs to implicit quantitative construction.

Some preliminary (technical) considerations for optimal sample size

Alongside conceptual considerations, there are a number of technical matters to wrestle with when contemplating an optimal sample size:

- The type of outcome variable.
- The number of groups.
- The type of relationship between groups (dependent or independent).
- The number of causal (or independent) variables.
- The technical frameworks (confidence interval estimation, hypothesis testing, regression analysis).

All of these elements have their role in determining an optimal sample size. However, two of the technical frameworks—confidence interval estimation and hypothesis testing—play especially consequential roles in this process. Therefore, before proceeding with our nine configurations and their optimal sample sizes, we first draw out some important differences between these two frameworks in this regard. Indeed, a different set of measures determines the optimal sample size for each.

For confidence interval estimation, the measures that determine the optimal sample size are:

- The confidence level (chosen by researcher).
- The margin of error (chosen by researcher).
- The variability of the data determining an outcome variable (for us, this outcome variable is either a mean or a proportion).

For hypothesis testing, the measures that determine the optimal sample size are:

- The significance level (chosen by researcher).
- The effect size (chosen by researcher).
- The power of the test (chosen by researcher).
- The variability of the data determining an outcome variable (for us, this outcome variable is either a mean or a proportion).

Importantly, for both confidence interval estimation and hypothesis testing, the researcher chooses the value for most of these measures and it is the variability of the data determining the mean or proportion that alone remains subject to the vicissitudes of the study population.

First, let us consider the three measures of confidence interval estimation. The margin of error is a range of values that the researcher judges to be of practical significance. An optimal sample size thus allows for a margin of error that is sufficiently precise—meaning small—to be informative. Consider a study comparing the resting heart rates of high-school long-distance runners with the resting heart rates of high-school students who are not long-distance runners.

We find a mean of 65 bpm for runners and a mean of 72 bpm for non-runners, with a margin of error of ±20 bpm for each. Thus, the mean resting heart rate for runners is 65 bpm ±20 and we estimate that the true mean resting heart rate for all students who are long-distance runners is between 45 and 85 bpm. The mean resting heart rate for non-runners is 72 bpm ±20 and we estimate that the true mean resting heart rate for all non-runners is between 52 and 92 bpm. The range in this case is clearly too large. We need a more precise margin of error for our estimate of the resting heart rate for each group.

To rectify things, the researchers regroup and stipulate that the margin of error should be no greater than 3 bpm. The researchers now need to determine the sample size that would generate a margin of error no greater than 3 bpm in this scenario. After adjusting the sample size, our modified results indicate a mean resting heart rate for runners of 65 bpm ±3, with an estimated interval range of 62 to 68 bpm. For non-runners, the mean resting heart rate is 72 bpm ±3, with an estimated interval range of 69 to 75 bpm.

Again, the choice of margin of error—that then requires an adjustment to the sample size—is a subjective clinical decision, not a statistical decision. Recall from Chapter 6 that the equation for the margin of error for an estimated interval range is:

$$\bar{X} \pm z \frac{\sigma}{\sqrt{n}}$$

Note that, for this equation, assuming no change for the standard deviation, any increase in the sample size (n) will narrow the margin of error and any decrease in sample size (n) will widen it. See what happens to the margin of error when we increase our sample size from 40 to 4,000.

$$\bar{X} \pm z\frac{\sigma}{\sqrt{n}} \rightarrow \bar{X} \pm 1.96\frac{5}{\sqrt{40}} = 1.55 \quad \bar{X} \pm 1.96\frac{\sigma}{\sqrt{4000}} = 0.15$$

Thus, the equation for the margin of error can be written more generally as:

$$ME = z\frac{\sigma}{\sqrt{n}}$$

Once a margin of error is specified, this equation can then be reworked to find the sample size (n).

$$ME = z\frac{\sigma}{\sqrt{n}} \rightarrow n = \left(\frac{z(\sigma)}{ME}\right)^2$$

This equation allows us to find the minimum sample size that still ensures that the margin of error for our estimated confidence interval—in a study with one sample—will not exceed the margin of error that the researcher has selected.

Note in Table 8.1 that variations on this equation provide the basis for finding the optimal sample size for configurations #1, #2, and #3, with regard to estimated confidence intervals.

Now we turn to the four measures of hypothesis testing. As seen, for confidence interval estimation there is a pretty simple fix for finding a sample size to suit our needs. We essentially set our preferred margin of error and confidence level and plug these into an equation that produces our sample size. For hypothesis testing, a bit more negotiation comes into play.

Recall that confidence interval estimation produces a range of values for a given measure (such as a mean)—at a certain confidence level—that aims to capture the true mean. Alternatively, hypothesis testing produces a single value (a point estimate)—such as a mean—and assesses the probability of finding such a value, at a certain significance level, if the null hypothesis is true.

Hypothesis testing thus introduces a clear and present danger. What, pray tell, if we were to reject the null hypothesis when actually we should not? In such a case, we would declare a treatment to be effective when, in fact, it was not. Alternatively, what if we failed to reject the null hypothesis when actually we should reject it? In that case, we would declare a treatment to be ineffective when, in fact, it was effective. The first misstep is a so-called type 1 error. The second is a type 2 error.

Finding the optimal sample size for hypothesis testing is largely wrapped up in prescriptions for avoiding each of these errors. Again:

- Type 1 error—treatment is good, we say it is bad.
- Type 2 error—treatment is bad, we say it is good.

At this point, the language gets a bit jargonisty. Let's take things one step at a time. The likelihood of a type 1 error is determined, in part, by the significance level that we choose.

Throughout this book, our default significance level has remained a warm and breezy 5%—or, $\alpha = 0.05$. If we decrease this significance level to $\alpha = 0.01$, we further decrease the likelihood of a type 1 error. If we increase the significance level to $\alpha = 0.10$, we increase the likelihood of a type 1 error.

Have you by chance already forgotten what a type 1 error is? Treatment is good, we say it is bad.

The beta level, which we have not yet addressed, is a measure of the likelihood of a type 2 error. Like the confidence level or significance level, the researcher chooses the beta level. For our purposes, we set our default beta level at 0.20. When we decrease this beta level, we further decrease the likelihood of a type 2 error. When we increase this beta level, we increase the likelihood of a type 2 error. You get the idea.

The beta level we choose also happens to determine the power of a test. For hypothesis testing there is a particular focus on "power." This determines the probability that we (correctly) reject the null hypothesis, when, in fact, we *should* reject the null hypothesis. For example, we correctly declare a treatment to be effective when it is, in fact, effective. ***Power is thus the probability that we correctly reject the null hypothesis***. Thus, beta and power work in tandem to protect against a type 2 error, declaring that a treatment is bad when it is good.

The bottom line is this: As the beta decreases, the power of a test increases and this decreases the likelihood of a type 2 error.

The power of a test ranges between the values of 0.0 and 1.0. It is equal to $1.0 - \beta$. (Again, β is the Greek letter "beta.") For our purposes, the default power of a test will thus be: $1.0 - 0.20 = 0.80$. Within biostatistical analysis, 0.80 (and 0.90) are common levels for the power of a test.

The power of a test is further influenced by:

- the significance level;
- the effect size; and
- the sample size.

The effect size is the degree of change in a parameter (or a statistic) of interest that represents a clinically meaningful difference. Let us again march out our research subjects and strike each in the head with a hammer. This time, however, we ask each person to rate her or his headache that follows on a 10-point scale, with 10 being the greatest pain. We set the effect size at a headache with a rating of six or higher. We thus limit the effect size of interest to only those headaches rated six or higher.

The effect size is obviously akin to the margin of error for confidence interval estimation. Note, however, that the effect size is a minimal threshold and it is written "*no less than* 12 centimeters." The margin of error is a maximum threshold and it is written "*no more than* 12 centimeters." Effect size also helps determine the likelihood of both a type 1 and a type 2 error.

Hence, as detailed below, the importance of sample size for hypothesis testing is tied to the interactions of five measures, each of which requires a *subjective* decision by the researcher.

- significance level (chosen by researcher);
- effect size   (chosen by researcher);
- power of the test ($1.0 - \beta$ [beta], chosen by researcher);
- type 1 error   (requires a small α [alpha] to decrease risk; chosen by researcher); and
- type 2 error   (requires a small β [beta] to decrease risk; chosen by researcher).

Importantly, to decrease α (alpha) and β (beta) requires that we reduce—that is, manipulate—the variability within our data and generate a smaller standard deviation. The principal method for this is to increase the sample size.

This then is the set-up. Table 8.1 identifies the specific equations for determining sample sizes—based on either confidence interval estimation or hypothesis testing—for five of the nine configurations. The four remaining configurations fall into one of two camps. The first is camp complexity. Here we find configurations #4, #5, and #8. In these cases, the statistical test associated with each requires a level of technical complexity that is beyond an introductory level, with regard to determining an optimal sample size.

The second camp is home for configuration #9. The rules for configuration #9 do follow certain general principles, but these are not, in a strict sense, dictated by narrow mathematical rationale. This follows from the use of ordinal or categorical outcome variables that rely upon either the chi-square goodness-of-fit test or the chi-square test of independence.

Table 8.1 Equations for determining sample size for five configurations

	Confidence interval estimation	Hypothesis testing
Configuration #1	$n = \left(\dfrac{z(\sigma)}{ME}\right)^2$	$n = \left(\dfrac{z_{1.0-\alpha/2} + z_{1.0-\beta}}{ES}\right)^2$
Configuration #2 (Examples A, B)	$n_i = 2\left(\dfrac{z(\sigma)}{ME}\right)^2$	$n_i = 2\left(\dfrac{z_{1.0-\alpha/2} + z_{1.0-\beta}}{ES}\right)^2$
Configuration #2 (Example C)	N/A	$n = \left(\dfrac{z_{1.0-\alpha/2} + z_{1.0-\beta}}{ES}\right)^2$
Configuration #3	$n = \left(\dfrac{z(\sigma_d)}{ME}\right)^2$ or $n_i = 2\left(\dfrac{z(\sigma_d)}{ME}\right)^2$	$n = \left(\dfrac{z_{1.0-\alpha/2} + z_{1.0-\beta}}{ES}\right)^2$ or $n_i = 2\left(\dfrac{z_{1.0-\alpha/2} + z_{1.0-\beta}}{ES}\right)^2$
Configuration #4	N/A	N/A
Configuration #5	N/A	N/A
Configuration #6	$n = p(1.0 - p)\left(\dfrac{z}{ME}\right)^2$	$n = \left(\dfrac{z_{1.0-\alpha/2} + z_{1.0-\beta}}{ES}\right)^2$
Configuration #7 (operation 7.0)	N/A	$n = \left(\dfrac{z_{1.0-\alpha/2} + z_{1.0-\beta}}{ES}\right)^2$
Configuration #7 (operations 7.1, 7.2, 7.3)	$n_i = \left[p_1(1.0 - p_1) + p_2(1.0 - p_2)\right]\left(\dfrac{z}{ME}\right)^2$	$n_i = 2\left(\dfrac{z_{1.0-\alpha/2} + z_{1.0-\beta}}{ES}\right)^2$
Configuration #8	N/A	N/A
Configuration #9	N/A	N/A

These two tests compare two or more groups based on their distribution of cases across categories. This requires a minimal number of "expected" cases for each category. Thus, with regard to determining the optimal sample size, these tests do not follow the logic of the other configurations that produce either a mathematical mean or proportion based on either a continuous or dichotomous outcome variable.

For an explanation of the symbols and notation in Table 8.1 see the application of these equations for specific examples below.

In proceeding to the technical steps, there is one further caveat. To this point, we have relied heavily on examples with a population size of 200 high-school long-distance runners ($N = 200$) and this has served us well for simplifying our cases. However, such a small population size will cause us some degree of anguish when calculating an optimal sample size. This follows from basic operational differences between examples with continuous outcome variables and those with dichotomous outcome variables. The former rely on the standard normal distribution. The latter rely on a binomial distribution. We explore the differences between these distributions in Chapter 9. For now, we will continue with our examples based on populations of 200, but with the following proviso.

First, notice that none of the equations in Table 8.1 require the population size (N) for determining an optimal sample size. Assuming a large population—1,000 or more—this is no problem. Even with small populations, examples with a continuous outcome variable tend to do fine. This includes configurations #1 through #5. However, for examples with a dichotomous outcome variable, larger populations are advantageous when calculating an optimal sample size. This includes configurations #6, #7, and #8.

A common rule of thumb for an example with a dichotomous outcome variable is that the population should be at least 10 times larger than our sample. For example, if we have a sample size of 40, this should be taken from a population of at least 400 persons. In fact, for configurations #6 and #7 below we find optimal sample sizes as large as 697 for our examples with a population of 200!

Thus, the purpose for working through the technical steps to calculate the optimal sample size for these examples with dichotomous outcome variables is less the particular sample size that results. Rather, our point of focus remains fixed on the subjective factors that we deploy for controlling variability when creating a sample, as they pertain to both confidence interval estimation and hypothesis testing. (For small populations with a dichotomous outcome variable, there are alternative methods that would suggest, in general, a sample size of ±135 for $N = 200$ at a 95% confidence level or 5% significance level.)

Technical steps for determining an optimal sample size

Configuration #1

Confidence interval estimation and configuration #1

EXAMPLE

There are 200 high-school long-distance runners in Lumumba County. We have limited health data for these runners. We want to know the mean resting heart rate for all high-school long-distance runners in Lumumba County. For this, we recruit a random sample of 40 high-school long-distance runners and find a mean resting heart rate of 73 bpm for this sample, with a standard deviation of 8.0.

Given these results, we must estimate—at a certain confidence level—a range of values that aims to capture the true mean resting heart rate for all high-school long-distance runners in Lumumba County.

Technical steps

In this example, we must estimate the mean resting heart rate for all high-school long-distance runners in Lumumba County based on a sample. We want to determine the optimal sample size for doing so.

The sample size equation for this is:

$$n = \left(\frac{z(\sigma)}{ME}\right)^2$$

Notice two things about this equation.

* As we increase the standard deviation (the numerator), we increase the sample size.
* As we increase the margin of error (the denominator), we decrease the sample size.

To begin then, we make some choices.

First, we choose a 95% confidence level. Thus, we know that $z = 1.96$.

Second, we choose a margin of error no greater than 5.0 bpm.

Third, we are aware of two prior studies similar to ours. The first had a standard deviation of 16.5 bpm. The second had a standard deviation of 11.5 bpm. To be conservative, we choose the larger value.

We now plug our values into the sample size equation.

$$n = \left(\frac{z(\sigma)}{ME}\right)^2 \rightarrow \left(\frac{1.96 \times 16.5}{5.0}\right)^2 = 41.84$$

Thus, the optimal sample size for our study is 42.

Again, to be conservative, we chose the larger standard deviation (16.5 bpm) over the smaller (11.5 bpm). The smaller standard deviation (11.5 bpm) would have generated a sample size of:

$$n = \left(\frac{z(\sigma)}{ME}\right)^2 \rightarrow \left(\frac{1.96 \times 11.5}{5.0}\right)^2 = 20.32$$

Finally, we have one further concern. From experience, we know that about 5% of high-school long-distance runners will fail to attend the testing session. We must, therefore, account for an attrition rate of 5% when recruiting for our sample size of 42. Given, this we calculate:

$$n(0.95) = 42 \rightarrow n = \frac{42}{0.95} \rightarrow n = 44.21$$

Thus, we must recruit 45 runners to yield a minimum of 42 runners, given an expected 5% attrition rate.

Configuration #2

Confidence interval estimation and configuration #2

EXAMPLE A

There are 200 high-school long-distance runners in Mandela County. Of these, 110 identify as cis males and 90 as cis females. We want to know if there is any difference between the mean resting heart rates of our cis-male and cis-female runners. We recruit a random sample of 40 cis-male and 40 cis-female high-school long-distance runners. We find a mean resting heart rate of 70 bpm for cis males, with a standard deviation of 9.0, and 76 bpm for cis females, with a standard deviation of 7.0.

Given these results, we must estimate—at a certain confidence level—a range of values that aims to capture any difference in means between these two groups.

Technical steps

In this example, we want to estimate the difference in mean resting heart rates between cis-male and cis-female high-school long-distance runners in Lumumba County. We need the optimal sample size for each group in such a study.

The sample size equation for this is:

$$n_i = 2\left(\frac{z(\sigma)}{ME}\right)^2$$

Once more, we begin with choices.

First, we choose a 95% confidence level. Thus, we know that $z = 1.96$.

Second, we choose a margin of error no greater than 4.0 bpm.

Third, drawing from a prior study, we find a standard deviation of 9.0.

We then plug these values into our sample size equation:

$$n = 2\left(\frac{z(\sigma)}{ME}\right)^2 \rightarrow n = 2\left(\frac{1.96(9.0)}{4.0}\right)^2 = 38.9$$

Thus, the optimal sample sizes for groups 1 and 2 are $n_1 = 39$ and $n_2 = 39$.

Lastly, given an expected 5% attrition rate, we calculate:

$$n(0.95) = 39 \rightarrow n = \frac{39}{0.95} \rightarrow n = 41.1$$

Thus, we adjust our sample size to 42 for group 1 and group 2 to yield a minimum of 39 in each group. This is a total of 84 persons that we will recruit for our study.

EXAMPLE B

Example A for configuration #2 and confidence interval estimation compares the means of two independent groups based on a difference in attribute. Example B compares the means of two independent groups based on a difference in exposure. Therefore, with respect to determining an optimal sample size, the two are procedurally identical and we need not repeat the steps from Example A.

Hypothesis testing and configuration #2

EXAMPLE A

There are 200 high-school long-distance runners in Mandela County. Of these, 110 identify as cis males and 90 as cis females. We want to know if there is any difference between the mean resting heart rates of our cis-male and cis-female runners. We recruit a random sample of 40 cis-male and 40 cis-female high-school long-distance runners. We find a mean resting heart rate of 70 bpm for cis males, with a standard deviation of 9.0, and 76 bpm for cis females, with a standard deviation of 7.0.

Given these results, we must determine the probability of finding a difference of this size between the means of these two groups.

Technical steps

In this example we want to know if there is a significant difference between the mean resting heart rates for cis-male and cis-female high-school long-distance runners in Mandela County. We need the optimal sample size for each group in such a study.

The sample size equation for this is:

$$n_i = 2 \left(\frac{z_{1.0-\alpha/2} + z_{1.0-\beta}}{ES} \right)^2$$

Table 8.2 identifies the symbols and notation for this equation.

To begin, we must make some choices.

First, we choose a two-tailed, hypothesis test with a 5% significance level, or $\alpha = 0.05$. Thus, $z_{1.0-\alpha/2} = 1.96$.

Table 8.2 Explanation of symbols for: $n = \left(\dfrac{z_{1.0-\alpha/2} + z_{1.0-\beta}}{ES} \right)^2$

Symbol	Explanation
n_i	The sample size required for each group
α	Alpha, the significance level
$z_{1.0-\alpha/2}$	The value from the standard normal distribution, holding $1.0 - \alpha/2$ below it; for example, if $\alpha = 0.05$, then $1.0 - \alpha/2 = 0.975$ and $z = 1.96$
$z_{1.0-\beta}$	The value from the standard normal distribution, holding $1.0 - \beta$ below it
$1.0 - \beta$	The selected power of the test; the two most common choices are: - 80% power, where $z_{0.8} = 0.84$ - 90% power, where $z_{0.9} = 1.282$
ES	The effect size, defined as: $ES = \dfrac{\lvert \mu_1 - \mu_0 \rvert}{\sigma}$
μ_0	The mean for the null hypothesis; often based on prior study—in this case, 70 bpm
μ_1	The mean for the alternative hypothesis; determined by choice of effect size—in this case, 76 bpm
σ	Standard deviation for the outcome of interest; often based on prior study—in this case, 8.0 bpm

Second, we choose a power of the test of 80%. Thus, $z_{1.0-\beta} = 0.84$.

Third, for purposes of calculating our effect size, we choose a clinically meaningful difference of at least 5 bpm between the means of group 1 and group 2.

We turn now to our three steps to determine the sample size, after plugging in these values. We combine all persons in group 1 and group 2 and find a standard deviation of 8.0. The numerator for the effect size equation is simply 5.0 because this is the minimal clinically meaningful difference of interest to us.

First, we compute the effect size.

$$ES = \frac{|\mu_1 - \mu_0|}{\sigma} \rightarrow \frac{5.0}{8.0} = 0.63$$

Second, we plug our values into the sample size equation:

$$n_i = 2\left(\frac{z_{1.0-\alpha/2} + z_{1.0-\beta}}{ES}\right)^2 \rightarrow 2\left(\frac{1.96 + 0.84}{0.63}\right)^2 = 39.5$$

Thus, sample sizes of $n_1 = 40$ and $n_2 = 40$ for groups 1 and 2 will ensure that a two-tailed, hypothesis test with a 5% significance level will have 80% power to detect a difference in the mean resting heart rate of at least 5.0 bpm between the two groups.

Lastly, to account for an expected 5% attrition rate, we calculate:

$$n(0.95) = 40 \rightarrow n = \frac{40}{0.95} \rightarrow n = 42.11$$

Thus, we adjust our sample size to 43 for both group 1 and group 2 to yield a minimum of 40 cis-male runners in group 1 and 40 cis-female runners in group 2. This is a total of 86 persons that we recruit for our study.

Example B

Example A for configuration #2 and hypothesis testing compares the means of two groups based on a difference in attribute. Example B compares the means of two groups based on a difference in exposure. Therefore, with respect to determining an optimal sample size, the two are procedurally identical and we need not repeat the steps from Example A.

Example C

There are 200 high-school long-distance runners in Lumumba County. We have limited health data for these runners. It happens that we have statewide data indicating that four years earlier the mean resting heart rate for all high-school long-distance runners was 70 bpm. We want to know if the current mean resting heart rate for all high-school long-distance runners in Lumumba County differs from the earlier statewide data.

Given this, we hypothesize that the current mean resting heart rate for all high-school long-distance runners in Lumumba County is 70 bpm. We then recruit a random sample of 40 high-school long-distance runners and find a mean resting heart rate for this sample of 73 bpm, with a standard deviation of 8.0.

Thus, we have data for two populations. The mean resting heart rate for population 1 is 70 bpm. The mean resting heart rate for a sample from population 2 is 73 bpm, based on sample data.

Given these results, we must determine the probability of finding a difference of this size between the means of these two populations.

Technical steps

In this example we want to know if there is a significant difference between the mean resting heart rate of population 1 and the mean resting heart rate of population 2. This is based on data for population 1 and a sample for population 2. We thus want to determine the optimal size for the sample from population 2 for this purpose.

The sample size equation for this is:

$$n = \left(\frac{z_{1.0-\alpha/2} + z_{1.0-\beta}}{ES} \right)^2$$

Again, we face three choices.

First, we choose a two-tailed, hypothesis test with a 5% significance level, or $\alpha = 0.05$. Thus, $z_{1.0-\alpha/2} = 1.96$.

Second, we choose a power of the test of 80%. Thus, $z_{1.0-\beta} = 0.84$.

Third, for purposes of calculating our effect size, we choose a clinically meaningful difference of at least 5 bpm between population 1 and population 2.

This requires a bit more explanation. As mentioned, there is an equation for the effect size. This is:

$$ES = \frac{|\mu_1 - \mu_0|}{\sigma}$$

But if there is an equation, how can we just "choose" an effect size? We do this by choosing one of the three values in the equation. This is the value for μ_1. The values for μ_0 and for σ are based on population 1. So when we say that we choose an effect size of 5.0 bpm we mean that we choose a minimal threshold for our alternative hypothesis. In this case, that threshold is an effect size of at least 5.0 bpm above the null hypothesis value (70 bpm).

Now there are three remaining steps to determine the sample size.

First, we compute the effect size. $ES = \dfrac{\mu_1 - \mu_0}{\sigma} \rightarrow \dfrac{75 - 70}{11.5} = 0.43$

Second, we plug our values into the sample size equation:

$$n = \left(\frac{z_{1.0-\alpha/2} + z_{1.0-\beta}}{ES} \right)^2 \rightarrow \left(\frac{1.96 + 0.84}{0.43} \right)^2 = 42.39$$

Thus, a sample size of 43 will ensure that a two-tailed, hypothesis test with a 5% significance level will have 80% power to detect a difference of at least 5.0 bpm in the mean resting heart rate between population 1 and population 2.

Third, given an expected 5% attrition rate, we further calculate:

$$n(0.95) = 43 \rightarrow n = \frac{43}{0.95} \rightarrow n = 45.26$$

Thus, we adjust our sample size to 46 current high-school long-distance runners to yield a minimum of 43 runners.

Configuration #3

Confidence interval estimation and configuration #3

EXAMPLE A

(This example illustrates a before-and-after study.) There are reports from Nyerere County of improved cardiovascular health among its student athletes. We recruit 40 high-school long-distance runners from across Nyerere County to detect if long-distance running impacts a student's resting heart rate. First, we measure the resting heart rate for each runner before the track season. Second, each runner receives an exposure. In this case, the exposure is all those activities comprising the track season.

Third, we measure the resting heart rate for each runner after the exposure. Fourth, we calculate the differences between each runner's resting heart rate before and after the track season. Fifth, we calculate the *mean of these differences between the before-and-after* resting heart rates. We find a mean of these differences of –8.3 bpm, with a standard deviation of 18.0. (Note that a negative value suggests that the exposure decreases the resting heart rate.)

Given these results, we must estimate—at a certain confidence level—a range of values that aims to capture the true *mean of these differences* for the resting heart rates before and after the track season.

Technical steps

In this example we are interested in the mean difference between resting heart rates of high-school long-distance runners before and after the track season. This mean difference is written μ_d. We need the optimal sample size for such a study.

The sample size equation is:

$$n = \left(\frac{z(\sigma_d)}{ME} \right)^2$$

z – value of the standard normal distribution reflecting the confidence level; $z = 1.96$ at $\alpha = 95\%$

ME – the desired margin of error.

σ_d – the population standard deviation of the difference scores—such as our before-and-after scores.

Again we face choices.

First, we choose a 95% confidence level. Thus, we know that $z = 1.96$.

Second, we choose a margin of error no greater than 5.0 bpm.

Third, drawing from a prior study, we have a standard deviation of 15.0.

We then plug our values into our sample size equation.

$$N = \left(\frac{z(\sigma_d)}{ME} \right)^2 \rightarrow \left(\frac{1.96 \times 15.0}{5.0} \right)^2 = 34.57$$

Thus, the optimal sample size is 35 for our group.
Lastly, given an expected 5% attrition rate, we further calculate:

$$n(0.95) = 35 \rightarrow n = \frac{35}{0.95} \rightarrow n = 36.8$$

Thus, we adjust our sample size to 37 for our group to yield a minimum of 35 participants.

EXAMPLE B

Example A for configuration #3 and confidence interval estimation assesses a mean difference based on a before-and-after study design. Example B assesses a mean difference based on a matched pairs design. The technical steps for each are similar, with one exception. Therefore, we need not repeat the same steps from Example A. The one exception is the need to multiply the result of the matched pairs design by "2."

Again, recall that the matched pairs design will require twice the number of persons as the before-and-after design *in both groups*. For example, if we recruit 22 persons for the before-and-after design, we will likely recruit at least 88 to fill our two groups in the matched pairs design. Remember, a before-and-after study with 22 persons yields 22 difference scores, while a matched pairs study with 88 persons yields 44 difference scores.

Here are our two sample size equations:

Before-and-after design: $n = \left(\dfrac{z(\sigma_d)}{ME} \right)^2$

Matched pairs design: $n = 2 \left(\dfrac{z(\sigma_d)}{ME} \right)^2$

Hypothesis testing and configuration #3

EXAMPLE A

(This example illustrates a before-and-after study.) There are reports from Nyerere County of improved cardiovascular health among its student athletes. We recruit 40 high-school long-distance runners from across Nyerere County to detect if long-distance running impacts a student's resting heart rate. First, we measure the resting heart rate for each runner before the track season. Second, each runner receives an exposure. In this case, the exposure is all those activities comprising the track season.

Third, we measure the resting heart rate for each runner after the exposure. Fourth, we calculate the differences between each runner's resting heart rate before and after the track season. Fifth, we calculate the *mean of these differences between the before-and-after* resting heart rates. We find a mean of these differences of −8.3 bpm, with a standard deviation of 18.0. (Note that a negative value suggests that the exposure decreases the resting heart rate.)

Given these results, we must determine the probability of finding a *mean of these differences* of this size for the resting heart rates before and after the track season.

Technical steps

In this example we are again interested in the mean difference (μ_d) between the resting heart rates of high-school long-distance runners before and after the track season. Our aim is to determine if we have reason to reject the null hypothesis that the mean differences for the before-and-after resting heart rates are equal to zero. We need the optimal sample size for such a study.

The sample size equation for this is:

$$n = \left(\frac{z_{1.0-\alpha/2} + z_{1.0-\beta}}{ES} \right)^2$$

We begin, per usual, with choices.

First, we choose a two-tailed, hypothesis test with a 5% significance level, or $\alpha = 0.05$. Thus, $z_{1.0-\alpha/2} = 1.96$.

Second, we choose a power of the test of 80%. Thus, $z_{1.0-\beta} = 0.84$.

Third, for purposes of calculating our effect size, we choose a clinically meaningful difference of at least 5 bpm between before-and-after scores or between the scores for matched pairs.

Fourth, drawing from a prior study, we have a standard deviation of 15.0.

Our next step is to determine the effect size: $ES = \dfrac{\mu_d}{\sigma_d}$

μ_d– the (minimal) mean difference expected under the alternative hypothesis (we choose)
σ_d– the population standard deviation of the difference scores—such as our before-and-after scores

Given this, we have: $ES = \dfrac{\mu_d}{\sigma_d} \rightarrow ES = \dfrac{5.0}{15.0} = 0.333$

We now plug these values into our sample size equation:

$$n = \left(\frac{z_{1.0-\alpha/2} + z_{1.0-\beta}}{ES} \right)^2 \rightarrow n = \left(\frac{1.96 + 0.84}{0.333} \right)^2 = 7.63$$

Thus, a sample size of 71 will ensure that a two-tailed, hypothesis test with a 5% significance level will have 80% power to detect a mean difference of at least 5.0 bpm, given a before-and-after study design.

Lastly, given an expected 5% attrition rate, we further calculate:

$$n(0.95) = 71 \rightarrow n = \frac{71}{0.95} \rightarrow n = 74.7$$

Thus, we adjust our sample size to 75 to yield a minimum of 71 runners.

Notice that the same study design for confidence interval estimation—with a similar mean and standard deviation, and a comparable effect size—requires a sample size of only 35 runners.

Example A for configuration #3 and hypothesis testing assesses a mean difference based on a before-and-after study design. Example B assesses a mean difference based on a matched pairs design. The technical steps for each are similar, with one exception. Therefore, and we need not repeat the same steps from Example A. The one exception is the need to multiply the result of the matched pair design by "2."

Here are our two sample size equations:

$$\text{before-and-after design: } n = \left(\frac{z_{1.0 - \alpha/2} + z_{1.0 - \beta}}{ES} \right)^2 \cdot$$

$$\text{matched pairs design: } n = 2\left(\frac{z_{1.0 - \alpha/2} + z_{1.0 - \beta}}{ES} \right)^2$$

Configuration #4

Given the role of multiple groups, configuration #4 does not apply to confidence interval estimation. Hypothesis testing relies on ANOVA to account for multiple groups, as demonstrated in Chapter 5. However, the technical steps for calculating an optimal sample size for ANOVA are more advanced than we address here.

Configuration #5

Configuration #5 requires multiple linear regression. As in the case of ANOVA, the technical steps for calculating an optimal sample size for multiple linear regression are more advanced than we address here.

Configuration #6

Confidence interval estimation and configuration #6

Example

There are 200 high-school long-distance runners in Lumumba County. We have limited general health data for these runners. We want to know the proportion of all high-school long-distance runners in Lumumba County with a resting heart rate of 83 bpm or greater. For this, we recruit a random sample of 40 high-school long-distance runners and find 10 runners with a resting heart rate of 83 bpm or greater. This is a proportion of 0.25.

Given these results, we must estimate—at a certain confidence level—a range of values that aims to capture the true proportion of high-school long-distance runners in Lumumba County with a resting heart rate of 83 bpm or greater.

Technical steps

In this example, we want to estimate the proportion of all high-school long-distance runners with a resting heart rate above 83 bpm in Lumumba County.

The sample size equation for this is:

$$n = p(1.0 - p)\left(\frac{z}{ME}\right)^2$$

z – the value of z from the standard normal distribution at a 95% confidence level is 1.96.
ME – the desired margin of error.
p – the proportion of successes in the population.

To begin, we must approximate the value of p, the population proportion. This gets a bit tricky.

The range of possible values for p is 0.0 to 1.0, or 0% to 100%.

The range of possible values for $p(1.0 - p)$ is 0.0 to 0.25, or 0% to 25%. We know this because …

The value of p that maximizes the value of $p(1.0 - p)$ is 0.5. And … $0.5(1.0 - 0.5) = 0.25$.

Thus, if we have no data to approximate the value of p, then we choose $p = 0.5$. This generates the most conservative (or largest necessary) sample size.

Now we make choices.

First, we choose a 95% confidence level. Thus, we know that $z = 1.96$.

Second, we choose a margin of error no greater than 0.05—or 5%.

Third, as suggested, we choose 0.5 as our value of p.

We now plug our values into our sample size equation:

$$n = p(1.0 - p)\left(\frac{z}{ME}\right)^2 \rightarrow 0.5(1.0 - 0.5)\left(\frac{1.96}{0.05}\right)^2 = 384.16$$

Lastly, given an expected 5% attrition rate, we further calculate:

$$n(0.95) = 385 \rightarrow n = \frac{385}{0.95} \rightarrow n = 405.26$$

Thus, we adjust our sample size to 406 to yield a minimum of 385.

Recall that configuration #6 and configuration #1 are identical but for the fact that configuration #6 seeks a population proportion based on a dichotomous outcome variable and configuration #1 seeks a population mean based on a continuous outcome variable.

However, we require a sample size of 406 runners for configuration #6 and a sample of 45 runners for configuration #1. The reason for this is tied up in distinctions between a binomial distribution (pertaining to dichotomous variables) and the standard normal distribution (pertaining to continuous variables). Note, for instance, the lack of a standard deviation as a measure of variability for configuration #6. This is a topic for Chapter 9.

However, there is a further wrinkle. To be prudent, we chose 0.5 as our presumed value for the proportion of runners with a resting heart rate of 83 bpm or greater. Imagine, however, that we had a prior study of the same population that had found a proportion of 0.1. We would then plug this value into our sample size equation and find:

$$n = p(1.0 - p)\left(\frac{z}{ME}\right)^2 \rightarrow 0.1(1.0 - 0.1)\left(\frac{1.96}{0.05}\right)^2 = 138.29$$

Our sample size shrinks by 64% from 406 to 147, after further adjusting for a 5% attrition rate. Indeed, any value for p below—or *above*—0.5 will yield a smaller sample size.

Therefore, it is almost always preferable to work with a prior study's value for p when determining an optimal sample size for configuration #6.

Configuration #7 (and operations 7.0, 7.1, 7.2, and 7.3)

Hypothesis testing and operation 7.0

EXAMPLE

There are 200 high-school long-distance runners in Lumumba County. We have limited general health data for these runners. It happens that we have statewide data indicating that four years earlier the proportion of all high-school long-distance runners with a resting heart rate of 83 bpm or greater was 0.25. We want to know if the current proportion of all high-school long-distance runners in Lumumba County differs from the earlier statewide data.

Given this, we hypothesize that the proportion of all current high-school long-distance runners in Lumumba County with a resting heart rate of 83 bpm is 0.25. We then recruit a random sample of 40 high-school long-distance runners and find a proportion of 0.22 for those with a resting heart rate of 83 bpm or greater.

Thus, we have data for two populations. The proportion of those with a resting heart rate above 83 bpm for population 1 is 0.25. The proportion of those with a resting heart rate above 83 bpm for population 2 is 0.22.

Given these results, we must determine the probability of finding a difference of this size between the proportions of these two populations.

TECHNICAL STEPS

In this example we want to know if there is a significant difference between the proportion of high-school long-distance runners with a resting heart rate of 83 bpm or greater in population 1 and the proportion in population 2. This is based on data for population 1 and a sample for population 2. We thus want to determine the optimal size for the sample from population 2 for this purpose.

The sample size equation for this is:

$$n = \left(\frac{z_{1.0-\alpha/2} + z_{1.0-\beta}}{ES} \right)^2$$

However, we have a new equation for the effect size. This is now:

$$ES = \frac{|p_1 - p_0|}{\sqrt{p_0 (1.0 - p_0)}}$$

p_0 – the proportion for the null hypothesis; this is 0.25 in this example.
p_1 – the proportion for the alternative hypothesis; this is set at 0.05 (see below).

First, we choose a two-tailed, hypothesis test with a 5% significance level, or $\alpha = 0.05$. Thus, $z_{1.0-\alpha/2} = 1.96$.

Second, we choose a power of the test of 80%. Thus, $z_{1.0-\beta} = 0.84$.

Third, for purposes of calculating the effect size, we choose a clinically meaningful absolute difference of at least 5% above the prior study proportion of 25%. (Thus, $p_1 - p_0 = 0.05$.) The proportion for the null hypothesis is $p_0 = 0.25$.

There are now a few steps more to determine the sample size.

First, we compute the effect size:

$$ES = \frac{|p_1 - p_0|}{\sqrt{p_0(1.0 - p_0)}} \rightarrow ES = \frac{0.05}{\sqrt{0.25(1.0 - 0.25)}} = 0.115$$

We now plug our values into our sample size equation:

$$n = \left(\frac{z_{1.0 - \alpha/2} + z_{1.0 - \beta}}{ES} \right)^2 \rightarrow n = \left(\frac{1.96 + 0.84}{0.115} \right)^2 = 592.87$$

Thus, a sample size of 593 will ensure that a two-tailed, hypothesis test with a 5% significance level will have 80% power to detect an absolute difference of 5% or more in the proportion of runners with a resting heart rate of 83 bpm or greater.

Lastly, given an expected 5% attrition rate, we further calculate:

$$n(0.95) = 593 \rightarrow n = \frac{593}{0.95} \rightarrow n = 624.21$$

Thus, we adjust our sample size to 625 to yield a minimum of 593 runners.

As with confidence interval estimation, for hypothesis testing we again find a considerable difference in the sample size for configuration #1 ($n = 46$) and configuration #6 ($n = 625$), notwithstanding similar values. The only difference between the two is the role of a continuous outcome variable in configuration #1 and a dichotomous outcome variable in configuration #6.

As with confidence interval estimation, this difference is tied up with distinctions between a binomial distribution (pertaining to dichotomous variables) and the standard normal distribution (pertaining to continuous variables). For instance, as mentioned, we are lacking a standard deviation as a measure of variability for configuration #6.

Operations 7.1, 7.2, 7.3

Recall from Chapters 4 and 6 that operation #7.1 is an application of the risk difference, operation #7.2 is an application of the risk ratio, and operation #7.3 is an application of the odds ratio. The common thread across these three is the comparison of two independent groups and the role of a dichotomous outcome variable.

It is our good fortunate that confidence interval estimation and hypothesis testing each has a single sample size equation that suffices for operations 7.1, 7.2, and 7.3.

For confidence interval estimation this equation is:

$$n_i = \left[p_1(1.0 - p_1) + p_2(1.0 - p_2) \right] \left(\frac{z}{ME} \right)^2$$

n_i – sample size required in each group.

z – the value of z from the standard normal distribution; at a 95% confidence level this is 1.96.

ME – margin of error.

p_1 and p_2 – proportions of successes in each group.

Note that we use p rather than $\hat{p}$ when we rely on a known proportion from a previous study for the sample proportion.

As detailed above, when we have no other data, we use $p = 0.5$ to generate the most conservative (or largest necessary) sample size.

For hypothesis testing, this equation is:

$$n_i = 2\left(\frac{z_{1.0-\alpha/2} + z_{1.0-\beta}}{ES}\right)^2$$

The effect size equation for hypothesis testing is:

$$ES = \frac{|p_1 - p_0|}{\sqrt{p_0(1.0 - p_0)}}$$

$|p_1 - p_0|$ – the absolute value of the difference in proportions between the two groups expected under the alternative hypothesis.

p – the overall proportion, based on pooling the data from the two comparison groups.

For purposes of illustration, we will use an example from Chapters 4 and 6 pertaining to operation 7.1 and risk difference for confidence interval estimation and hypothesis testing. Again, we limit our examples to operation 7.1 and risk difference, insofar as operations 7.2 and 7.3 use the same sample size equations.

Confidence interval estimation and operation 7.1

EXAMPLE

There are 200 high-school long-distance runners in Mandela County. Of these, 110 identify as cis males and 90 as cis females. We want to know if there is any difference between the proportion of cis-male runners and the proportion of cis-female runners with a resting heart rate of 83 bpm. We recruit a random sample of 40 cis-male and 40 cis-female high-school long-distance runners. We find that 20% of cis males (group 1) and 30% of cis females (group 2) have a resting heart rate of 83 bpm or greater.

Given these findings, we must estimate—at a certain confidence level—a range of values that aims to capture the true risk difference between group 1 and group 2 regarding the proportion of persons with a resting heart rate of 83 bpm or greater.

TECHNICAL STEPS

In this example we are estimating a range of values to capture the risk difference between these groups regarding the proportion of persons in each with a resting heart rate of 83 bpm or greater. We need the optimal sample size for group 1 and group 2 for this purpose.

Again, our sample size equation for this is:

$$n_i = [p_1(1.0 - p_1) + p_2(1.0 - p_2)]\left(\frac{z}{ME}\right)^2$$

We thus begin with choices.

First, we choose a 95% confidence level. Thus, we know that $z = 1.96$.

Second, we choose a margin of error no greater than 0.05, or 5%.

We know from a previous study that 12% of the population as a whole—all high-school long-distance runners in Mandela County—has a resting heart rate of 83 bpm or greater. Thus, $p = 0.12$.

We now plug these values into our sample size equation:

$$n_i = [p_1(1.0 - p_1 + p_2(1.0 - p_2)]\left(\frac{z}{ME}\right)^2 \rightarrow [0.12(1.0 - 0.12) + 0.12(1.0 - 0.12)]\left(\frac{1.96}{0.05}\right)^2$$
$$= 324.54$$

Thus, we require a sample size of 325 for both group 1 and for group 2.

Lastly, given an expected 5% attrition rate, we further calculate:

$$n(0.95) = 325 \rightarrow n = \frac{325}{0.95} \rightarrow n = 342.11$$

Thus, we adjust our sample size to 343 for group 1 and the same for group 2 to yield a minimum of 325 for each group. We must recruit a total of 686 persons for our study.

Notice incidentally the large impact of even a small change in the margin of error. If we were to increase the margin of error from 0.05 to 0.06, the optimal sample size—after adjustment for attrition—would drop to 238 for each group.

Hypothesis testing and operation 7.1

EXAMPLE

There are 200 high-school long-distance runners in Mandela County. Of these, 110 identify as cis males and 90 as cis females. We want to know if there is any difference between the proportion of cis-male runners and the proportion of cis-female runners with a resting heart rate of 83 bpm or greater. We recruit a random sample of 40 cis-male and 40 cis-female high-school long-distance runners. We find that 20% of cis males (group 1) and 30% of cis females (group 2) have a resting heart rate of 83 bpm or greater.

Given these results, we calculate the risk difference. We then determine the probability of finding a risk difference of this size between group 1 and group 2, regarding the proportion of persons with a resting heart rate of 83 bpm or greater.

TECHNICAL STEPS

In this example we want to determine the optimal sample size—for group 1 and group 2—to test the null hypothesis regarding the risk difference between two independent groups regarding the proportion of runners with a resting heart rate of 83 bpm or greater in each. We need the optimal sample size for group 1 and group 2 for this purpose.

The sample size equation for this is:

$$n_i = 2\left(\frac{z_{1.0 - \alpha/2} + z_{1.0 - \beta}}{ES}\right)^2$$

We begin with choices.

First, we choose a two-tailed, hypothesis test with a 5% significance level, or α = 0.05. Thus, $z_{1.0-\alpha/2}$ = 1.96.

Second, we choose a power of the test of 80% to detect this difference between the proportions of runners in group 1 and group 2 with a resting heart rate of 83 bpm or greater. Thus, $z_{1.0-\beta}$ = 0.84.

Third, for purposes of calculating the effect size, we choose a clinically meaningful difference of at least 5% between the proportion of persons in group 1 and group 2 with a resting heart rate above 83 bpm.

From a previous study, we know that 12% of the population as a whole has a resting heart rate of 83 bpm or greater, hence p = 0.12.

Now we can calculate the effect size.

$$ES = \frac{|p_1 - p_0|}{\sqrt{p_0(1.0 - p_0)}} \rightarrow \frac{0.05}{\sqrt{0.12(1.0 - 0.12)}} = 0.154$$

Next we plug in our values and calculate the sample size:

$$n_i = 2\left(\frac{z_{1.0-\alpha/2} + z_{1.0-\beta}}{ES}\right)^2 \rightarrow 2\left(\frac{1.96 + 0.84}{0.154}\right)^2 = 661.13$$

Thus, a sample size of 662 for group 1 and group 2 will ensure that a two-tailed, hypothesis test at a 5% significance level will have 80% power to detect a difference of at least 5% between groups for the proportion of runners with a resting heart rate of 83 bpm or greater.

Lastly, given an expected 5% attrition rate, we further calculate:

$$n(0.95) = 662 \rightarrow n = \frac{662}{0.95} \rightarrow n = 696.84$$

Thus, we adjust our sample size to 697 for group 1 and group 2 to yield a minimum of 662 in each group. We must recruit a total of 1,394 persons for our study.

Configuration #8

Configuration #8 requires multiple logistic regression. As in the case of ANOVA and multiple linear regression, the technical steps for calculating an optimal sample size for multiple logistic regression are more advanced than we address here.

Configuration #9

Determining an optimal sample size for configuration #9 is complicated by the role of categorical or ordinal outcome variables. Consequently, again, the technical steps for calculating an optimal sample size for configuration #9 are more advanced than we address here.

Closing material

The optimal sample size is ostensibly a tool for efficiency, saving researchers time and money. This is true enough. However, walking through the technical steps that determine the optimal size for each configuration, we glean two further insights. The first concerns the subjective nature of biostatistical analysis. The second concerns the role and consequences of (quantitative) variability within biostatistical analysis.

It is evident that our otherwise objective researchers rely to a startling degree on a range of personal preferences to manipulate the sample size. These choices include the margin of error, confidence level, significance level, effect size, and power of the test. Each of these directly affects the optimal sample size. Yet each is controlled by the researcher. Certainly these choices are taken openly and explicitly. Secret, backroom deals are not a concern.

However, for all of the elaborate obedience to the objective protocols of a randomized, double-blind, placebo-controlled study design—the pinnacle of scientific, experimental research within health and medicine—this slate of researcher choices would appear to at least compromise, if not subvert, a number of core principles.

As with the Tuskegee "experiment," it is the above-board, non-secret activities that often reveal the most about the taken-for-granted pretenses behind those practices. Long before the *Washington Star* revealed the gruesome details of the Tuskegee experiment in a July 1972 exposé, the medical protocols (deliberately) leading to the slow and painful deaths of 128 Black men were well known within the infectious disease medical community. The findings of the study had been published in medical journals and presented at international medical conferences for decades. Medical researchers offered no objections because they could not fathom any reasons to object.

Analogously, those rhetorically upholding the principles of objectivity, control, and parsimony—best exemplified by randomized controlled trials—over the principles of holistic interpretation, context, and contingency within holistic research do so because within their world no alternative viewpoint is thought necessary. This is the world built by biostatistical analysis and its reductive premises. The regularity and certainty of that world is grounded largely in mathematical probability.

This brings our attention to the curious ways in which the optimal sample size intersects with the variability of data *vis-à-vis* probability. We saw this link between sample size and probability in earlier chapters, when choosing between z-tests and t-tests. When a sample is large enough (30 or more), the z-test and its assumptions of the standard normal distribution are fine. Otherwise, we have the t-test that relies upon a t distribution to accommodate different assumptions about the variability of the sample data.

The choice of confidence level (or significance level) plays a major role in determining the optimal sample size. Each of these is a function of either the standard normal distribution or a binomial distribution for most configurations. These distributions, in turn, are integral to applications of mathematical probability. For instance, with continuous outcome variables, the larger the sample size, the more closely the data will approximate the standard normal distribution—though there is a maximum size after which the benefits begin to fall off.

This is why increasing a sample size from 40 to 4,000, while holding other values constant, had such a dramatic impact for a number of configurations in Chapters 5 and 6. Hence, what is true for a group of 40 persons can be really, really true for 4,000 persons. To understand why will require, admittedly, a not altogether fun time. Yet, practically nothing thus far uncovered can be fully made sense of without recourse to mathematical probability.

The Faustian bargain we next enter into is this. On the one hand, the reader's indulgence to muddle through mathematical probability will leave her or him better equipped to understand why we can benefit from the occasional willful suspension of disbelief that allows us to engage with biostatistical analysis. No probability, no biostatistical analysis. On the other hand, it also better equips our reader to more fully understand the great many consequences that follow in Chapter 10, as a bracing indictment of the tendentious assumptions that make biostatistical analysis possible.

Chapter 9

Probability

From Chaos to Nice, Orderly Distributions

In a sense, all preceding chapters have been a slow and steady march toward an inevitable conversation about probability. Throughout these chapters, we have introduced myriad mathematical rationale and conceptual premises, while parading out an array of biostatistical tools and techniques. Most of these tools and techniques are devices for transforming qualitative things into quantitative things more suitable for biostatistical analysis. The justification for all this—especially the operative rationale and premises—largely lie within mathematical probability.

Probability is itself a branch of mathematics. Therefore, its presentation is ordinarily mathematical in form and draws heavily from uncomplicated examples of highly controlled situations—such as tossing a two-sided coin, rolling a six-sided die, or selecting cards from a 52-card deck. Such examples provide clarity and certainty when introducing the mathematical principles of probability and random events. However, care is required when moving from applications within a random (yet stable) world of inanimate objects to applications within a random (and chaotic) world of human beings with outcomes that are far less certain or circumscribed.

Much can be done to account for uncertainty in the world of human beings. However, even the gold standard of a randomized controlled trial—with its randomized, double-blind, placebo-controlled design—faces difficulties accounting for the mountain of inter-subject variation among otherwise identical human research subjects. Just a brief list of such variation includes fluctuating metabolic rates, undetected diseases or genetic differences, subject fidelity to test protocols, the imprecisions of technical instruments, and degrees of accuracy among researcher observations and documentation. From this, we get a strong sense of the challenges when comparing a coin toss with a stool sample.

Biostatistical analysis thus rests upon a precarious dedication to measure and account for human variation via the application of mathematical principles of probability that originate with experimental research in the natural sciences and assume a random and largely stable world of inanimate objects in a controlled environment with a certain (and knowable) range of possible outcomes.

For this reason, discussions of probability and biostatistical analysis can be especially daunting. On the one hand, probability provides the engine that propels and makes biostatistical analysis possible. On the other hand, as a branch of mathematics, probability is grounded in a logic and a set of conceptual premises that greatly differ from how we understand the subject matter of health and medicine. Indeed, probability is arguably the most ill-fitting (and utterly foreign) subject that students encounter in their introduction to biostatistical analysis. The fact that these tendentious conceptual premises then infect the tools, techniques, and tests that we deploy to explain the meaning and significance of our findings in the social world only further complicates matters.

DOI: 10.4324/9781003316985-9

Indeed, now many decades into an era of routine, computer-driven statistical analysis, with little need to carry out specific probability functions by hand—such as a binomial distribution—the study of probability and its conceptual rationale is especially critical. This is often a student's only opportunity to consider the profound level of willful suspension of disbelief that is required of a researcher whenever pressing "enter" on a keyboard after loading her or his data into this or that statistical program.

Our approach, therefore, in presenting the basic principles and models of probability that all introductory students of biostatistical analysis should know, is to allow the student to gauge for her- or himself how well the underlying logic and conceptual assumptions provide a useful grounding for the study of health and medicine. As students will later learn in their studies and in their professional practice, the dubious nature of this fit has long generated debate among researchers regarding the suitability of p-values, confidence interval estimation, hypothesis testing, and other routine measures across health and medicine.

Within the broader discipline of mathematics, probability is a complex and extensive topic that draws upon various subfields from set theory, logarithms, and differential equations, as well as algebra, calculus, dynamical systems, and chaos theory more generally. Thus, it is well to recognize that a full consideration of probability (and its foundational knowledge) would, in fact, require several volumes of textbooks.

Our task here is to carve out a handful of features limited to that which we need for understanding the basic applications of probability within biostatistical analysis. For us, this largely boils down to two conceptual tools—binomial distributions and the standard normal distribution—and those elements that form the building blocks for these, such as the central limit theorem. In addition, attention must be given to certain topics derived from "classical" probability, such as conditional probability, the total probability rule, and Bayes' theorem.

A binomial distribution allows us to work with dichotomous outcome variables and is thus quite essential within biostatistical analysis. This follows from a strong interest in experimental procedures that commonly rely on dichotomous outcomes, such as randomized controlled trials. Examples of such outcomes include disease/no disease, remission/non-remission, or infection/non-infection.

The standard normal distribution allows us to work with continuous outcome variables. These are essential for biostatistical analysis that measures degrees of difference or degrees of change between experimental groups. Examples of degrees of difference include divergences between the means (or proportions) of two groups that differ in attribute or exposure. Examples of degrees of change include degrees of improvement/deterioration, growth/decay, or expansion/reduction for some variable among the members of an experimental group after some exposure.

There is one further cautionary note. The material below makes liberal use of mathematical symbols and terminology for purposes of abbreviation—more so than previous chapters. However, symbols and terminology notwithstanding, as promised, 99% of this material requires nothing more than addition, subtraction, multiplication, division, exponents, and square roots. (The only additional technique here concerns factorials.)

Certain symbols may appear unfamiliar and intimidating at first blush, just as "2 + 2 = 4" seemed like a foreign language the first time you saw it scribbled across a first-grade whiteboard. Indeed, if you fully wrote out the meaning of that equation, it could well require several pages of prose. Yet the idea of the equation now seems second nature. This is the lesson best taken from that first-grade experience. Abbreviation via mathematical symbols does NOT necessarily imply complexity. Indeed, in this chapter it invariably indicates some combination of steps requiring addition, subtraction, multiplication, division, exponents, and square roots.

Probability distributions

Most plainly, a probability distribution is a type of mathematical function that is based on a mathematical rule. It determines the probabilities for different values for an outcome (or dependent) variable that correspond with the value(s) of one or more causal (or independent) variable(s). For example, for our old friend Bill the monkey we know the number of backflips (the outcome variable) will increase by one for each banana (the causal variable) that we give him. This further underlines why we emphasize the type of outcome variable when distinguishing between the nine configurations.

There are, in fact, a great many probability distributions that differ based on the specific mathematical rules linking dependent and independent variables in this way. These include Bernoulli distributions, beta-binominal distributions, exponential-logarithmic distributions, and Poisson distributions. However, some of the most common probability distributions for biostatistical analysis—at least at an introductory level—are:

- Binomial distributions   (for dichotomous outcome variables)
- The standard normal distribution   (for continuous outcome variables)
- t Distributions   (for continuous outcome variables with fewer than 30 in sample)
- F Distributions   (for ANOVA)
- Chi-square distributions   (for ordinal or categorical outcome variables)

To clarify, one source of initial confusion can be references to a "frequency" distribution. This is not a further *type* of probability distribution. Rather, each type of probability distribution produces its own unique frequency distribution. This simply refers to the frequency of the different outcomes that each probability distribution produces. It is this frequency that indicates the probability of finding a certain outcome when applying different biostatistical tests. For example, when we look up a critical value of t in Table A.2, this relies upon the frequency distribution produced by a t distribution.

Binomial distributions

By way of reminder, we rely on binomial distributions for specific types of situations when there can only be one of two possible outcomes, such as configurations #6, #7, and #8. As noted, these binary outcomes are conventionally labeled "success" and "non-success" (aka, failure), however, a success is not necessarily a *good* thing. For example, our outcome of interest may be cancer cases. In that situation, a "success" is a person who develops cancer.

When analyzing successes and non-successes, we have two basic concerns—the number of "trials" and the probability of success for each trial. A trial refers to the specific event you are observing for some success or non-success. Imagine our concern is ankle injuries among high-school long-distance runners competing in 5k races. Thus, if a runner suffers an ankle injury in a 5k race, this is a "success." If there are eight runners in a 5k race, we have eight "trials." We designate the number of trials as "n." Thus, $n = 8$.

The probability of success (an ankle injury) in each 5k race is reported as the proportion of all runners (all trials) who participate. From past data for Machel County, we know that 32% of the runners in a 5k race will injure an ankle. We designate the probability of success as "p." Thus, $p = 0.32$. For now, hold back any concerns for this rather high rate of ankle injuries.

A basic rule for binomial distributions is that the likelihood of a success or a non-success must be equally probable for each trial. This means that each of the eight runners participating in a 5k race constitutes a "trial" *and* each runner has an equal likelihood of an ankle injury. Thus, the fact that one trial (meaning, one runner) experiences success or failure cannot impact whether another trial (another runner) experiences success or failure. Thus, if Farouq has an ankle injury, this can in no way affect whether Joaquin—or any of the other runners—also suffers an ankle injury. In this sense, each trial is *independent* of all the other trials.

Let us look more closely at this example of a 5k race in Machel County, where $n = 8$ and $p = 0.32$. We formally write this scenario as:

$$X \sim b(n, p) \rightarrow X \sim b(8, 0.32)$$

This reads: X is distributed as a binomial random variable with $n = 8$ and $p = 0.32$.

However, we can make this far more complicated. And we do! We introduce the binomial formula:

$$(_nC_x)(p^x)(q^{n-x})$$

Here we find three elements (in parentheses) to multiply and a number of moving parts. Table 9.1 details these moving parts.

Note with regard to "q" that, by now, we have seen some version of $1.0 - p$ on numerous occasions. Again, it is helpful to read "1.0" as 100%. Thus, we are subtracting something from 100%. Therefore, $(1.0 - x)$ gives us the probability that some event will NOT happen.

In this case, $(1.0 - p) = (1.0 - 0.32)$. This is 0.68. Thus, there is a probability that 68% of runners will NOT injure their ankle.

If we take a moment to dissect the binomial coefficient, we soon discover that:

$$_nC_x \frac{n!}{x!(n-x)!}$$

Notice first that you need nothing more than subtraction, multiplication, and division to figure out a binomial coefficient ($_nC_x$). Notice second the use of **factorials**—such as $n!$ These factorials allow us to work with different subsets of a group. Such subsets are referred to as **combinations without repetition** and these are essential for calculating probability for binomials.

Note that **permutations** are close cousins of combinations. The difference is that combinations do not care about the order of the elements that are combined, while this order of elements is held dear by permutations.

Table 9.1 Explanations of symbols for the binomial formula—$(_nC_x)(p^x)(q^{n-x})$

Symbol	Explanation
$_nC_x$	The binomial coefficient
x	Number of successes from n that we wish to consider; in our case, we might want to know the probability that *exactly* two of our eight runners will have an ankle injury; we write this: $_8C_2$
n	Number of trials; in our case, this is 8 runners
p	The probability of success for each trial; in our case, this is 0.32
q	The probability of failure for each trial, ($q = 1.0 - p$); in our case, ($1.0 - 0.32 = 0.68$)

Importantly, this formula for the binomial coefficient $\left[\dfrac{n!}{x!(n-x)!}\right]$—and its use of factorials—allows us to determine how many different combinations of trials we can form. Again, in our case, a trial (n) is a runner participating in a 5k race and a "success" (x) is an ankle injury. To better illustrate all this, let us consider a series of examples that walk us through how factorials make use of such combinations without repetition as components of a binomial coefficient.

Example 1

We have three runners and we want to know the probability that exactly two runners will injure an ankle. Our three runners are Ava, Bob, and Chu. For now, we only want to know how many *unique* subsets of pairs of runners we can form from this group of three.

$$_3C_2 \to \frac{n!}{x!(n-x)!} \to \frac{3!}{2!(3-2)!} = \frac{3*2*1}{2*1(1)} = \frac{6}{2} = 3$$

Thus, we can create three unique pairs from this group of three runners:

(Ava, Bob), (Ava, Chu), (Bob, Chu)

Example 2

Di joins the others and we have four runners. We want to know how many *unique* subsets of pairs of runners we can form from this group of four.

$$_4C_2 \to \frac{n!}{x!(n-x)!} \to \frac{4!}{2!(4-2)!} = \frac{4*3*2*1}{(2*1)(2*1)} = \frac{24}{4} = 6$$

Thus, we can create six unique pairs from this group of four runners:

(Ava, Bob), (Ava, Chu), (Ava, Di), (Bob, Chu), (Bob, Di), (Chu, Di)

Example 3

Ed and Fin join the others and we have six runners. Now we want to know how many *unique* subsets of four runners we can form from this group of six.

$$_6C_4 \to \frac{n!}{x!(n-x)!} \to \frac{6!}{4!(6-4)!} = \frac{6*5*4*3*2*1}{4*3*2*1(2*1)} = \frac{720}{48} = 15$$

Thus, we can create 15 unique groups of four runners from this group of six runners:

(Ava, Bob, Chu, Di), (Ava, Bob, Chu, Ed), (Ava, Bob, Chu, Fin), (Ava, Bob, Di, Ed), (Ava, Bob, Di, Fin), (Ava, Bob, Ed, Fin), (Ava, Chu, Di, Ed), (Ava, Chu, Di, Fin), (Ava, Chu, Ed, Fin), (Ava, Di, Ed, Fin)

(Bob, Chu, Di, Ed), (Bob, Chu, Di, Fin), (Bob, Chu, Ed, Fin), (Bob, Di, Ed, Fin)

(Chu, Di, Ed, Fin)

Example 4

We have the same six runners from Example 3. We want to know how many different subsets of zero runners we can form from this group of six.

$$_6C_0 \rightarrow \frac{n!}{x!(n-x)!} \rightarrow \frac{6!}{0!(6-0)!} = \frac{6*5*4*3*2*1}{1(6*5*4*3*2*1)} = \frac{720}{720} = 1$$

Thus, we can create one subset that includes zero runners from this group of six runners:

(*not* Ava, Bob, Chu, Di, Ed, or Fin)

As mentioned, the role of factorials for binomial distributions is essential. But why is this? This is because factorials—along with combinations without repetition—determine the *maximum number of possible outcomes*.

Let us go back to Example 2 with four runners.

Imagine we want to know the probability that *exactly two* runners will suffer ankle injuries. We find that there are six possible unique pairs of runners. If exactly two runners suffer ankle injuries, this must represent one—and only one!—of these six pairs. Consequently, we want to know the probability that the two persons in any one of these pairs will suffer ankle injuries. This requires a few more steps.

To continue, let us consider a new set of scenarios that involve eight long-distance runners. (These are Examples 5 through 13.) Recall from above that, with regard to an ankle injury, $p = 0.32$. This indicates a probability that 32% of the eight runners in a 5k race will injure their ankle. (Note that we purposely chose an oddly high percentage of ankle injuries to better illustrate key aspects of binomial distributions.) For reference, 32% of eight is 2.56 runners. Now we can plug these numbers into our equation:

$$(_nC_x)(p^x)(q^{n-x})$$

Example 5

What is the probability that zero of our eight runners will injure an ankle in a 5k race?

First, we calculate the binomial coefficient $(_nC_x)$. Then we plug this value into our formula.

$$_8C_0 = \frac{n!}{x!(n-x)!} \rightarrow \frac{8!}{0!(8-0)!} = \frac{8*7*6*5*4*3*2*1}{(1)(8*7*6*5*4*3*2*1)} = \frac{40,320}{40,320} = \mathbf{1.0}$$

$$P(X = 0) = [_nC_x * p^x * q^{n-x}] \rightarrow [_8C_0 * 0.32^0 0.68^{8-0}] = [1.0 * 1.0 * 0.046] = \mathbf{0.046}$$

Thus, there is a 4.6% probability that zero of our eight runners will injure an ankle. (See Figure 9.1 for the results for all nine probabilities.)

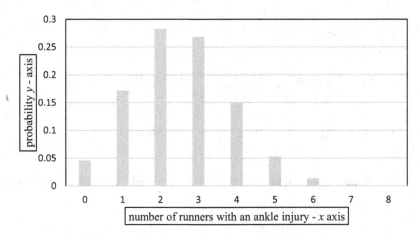

Figure 9.1 Probabilities for a certain number of ankle injuries, *n* = 8

Example 6

What is the probability that exactly one of our eight runners will injure an ankle in a 5k race?

$$_8C_1 = \frac{n!}{x!(n-x)!} \rightarrow \frac{8!}{1!(8-1)!} = \frac{8*7*6*5*4*3*2*1}{7*6*5*4*3*2*1} = \frac{40,320}{5,040} = \textbf{8.0}$$

$$P(X = 1) = [_nC_x * p^x * q^{n-x}] \rightarrow [_8C_1 * 0.32^1 * 0.68^{8-1}] = [8.0 * 0.32 * 0.067] = \textbf{0.172}$$

Thus, there is a 17.2% probability that exactly one of our eight runners will injure an ankle.

Example 7

What is the probability that exactly two of our eight runners will injure an ankle in a 5k race?

$$_8C_2 = \frac{n!}{x!(n-x)!} \rightarrow \frac{8!}{2!(8-2)!} = \frac{8*7*6*5*4*3*2*1}{(2*1)(6*5*4*3*2*1)} = \frac{40,320}{1,440} = \textbf{28.0}$$

$$P(X = 2) = [_nC_x * p^x * q^{n-x}] \rightarrow [_8C_2 * 032^2 * 0.68^{8-2}] = [28.0 * 0.102 * 0.099] = \textbf{0.283}$$

Thus, there is a 28.3% probability that exactly two of our eight runners will injure an ankle.

Example 8

What is the probability that exactly three of our eight runners will injure an ankle in a 5k race?

$$_8C_3 = \frac{n!}{x!(n-x)!} \rightarrow \frac{8!}{3!(8-3)!} = \frac{8*7*6*5*4*3*2*1}{(3*2*1)(5*4*3*2*1)} = \frac{40,320}{720} = \mathbf{56.0}$$

P(X = 3) = $[_nC_x * p^x * q^{n-x}]$ → $[_8C_3 * 0.32^3 * 0.68^{8-3}]$ = [56.0 * 0.033 * 0.145] = **0.268**

Thus, there is a 26.8% probability that exactly three of our eight runners will injure an ankle.

Example 9

What is the probability that exactly four of our eight runners will injure an ankle in a 5k race?

$$_8C_4 = \frac{n!}{x!(n-x)!} \rightarrow \frac{8!}{4!(8-4)!} = \frac{8*7*6*5*4*3*2*1}{(4*3*2*1)*(4*3*2*1)} = \frac{40,320}{576} = \mathbf{70.0}$$

P(X = 4) = $[_nC_x * p^x * q^{n-x}]$ → $[_8C_4 * 0.32^4 * 0.68^{8-4}]$ = [70.0 * 0.010 * 0.214] = **0.150**

Thus, there is a 15.0% probability that exactly four of our eight runners will injure an ankle.

Example 10

What is the probability that exactly five of our eight runners will injure an ankle in a 5k race?

$$_8C_5 = \frac{n!}{x!(n-x)!} \rightarrow \frac{8!}{5!(8-5)!} = \frac{8*7*6*5*4*3*2*1}{(5*4*3*2*1)(3*2*1)} = \frac{40,320}{720} = \mathbf{56.0}$$

P(X = 5) = $[_nC_x * p^x * q^{n-x}]$ → $[_8C_5 * 0.32^5 * 0.68^{8-5}]$ = [56.0 * 0.003 * 0.314] = **0.053**

Thus, there is a 5.3% probability that exactly five of our eight runners will injure an ankle.

Example 11

What is the probability that exactly six of our eight runners will injure an ankle in a 5k race?

$$_8C_6 = \frac{n!}{x!(n-x)!} \rightarrow \frac{8!}{6!(8-6)!} = \frac{8*7*6*5*4*3*2*1}{(6*5*4*3*2*1)(2*1)} = \frac{40,320}{1,440} = \mathbf{28.0}$$

P(X = 6) = $[_nC_x * p^x * q^{n-x}]$ → $[_8C_6 * 0.32^6 * 0.68^{8-6}]$ = [28.0 * 0.001 * 0.462] = **0.013**

Thus, there is a 1.3% probability that exactly six of our eight runners will injure an ankle.

Example 12

What is the probability that exactly seven of our eight runners will injure an ankle in a 5k race?

$$_8C_7 = \frac{n!}{x!(n-x)!} \rightarrow \frac{8!}{7!(8-7)!} = \frac{8*7*6*5*4*3*2*1}{(7*6*5*4*3*2*1)} = \frac{40,320}{5,040} = \mathbf{8.0}$$

P(X = 7) = $[_nC_x * p^x * q^{n-x}]$ → $[_8C_7 * 0.32^7 * 0.68^{8-7}]$ = [8.0 * 0.0003 * 0.68] = **0.002**

Thus, there is a 0.2% probability that exactly seven of our eight runners will injure an ankle.

Example 13

What is the probability that exactly eight of our eight runners will injure an ankle in a 5k race?

$$_8C_8 = \frac{n!}{x!(n-x)!} \rightarrow \frac{8!}{8!(8-8)!} = \frac{8*7*6*5*4*3*2*1}{8*7*6*5*4*3*2*1} = \frac{40,320}{40,320} = \mathbf{1.0}$$

P(X = 8) = $[_nC_x * p^x * q^{n-x}]$ → $[_8C_8 * 0.32^8 * 0.68^{8-8}]$ = [1.0 * 0.0001 * 1.0] = **0.0001**

Thus, there is a 0.01% probability that exactly eight of our eight runners will injure an ankle.

Cumulative probability

If we give this basic idea a slight twist we can generate a **cumulative probability**. This will tell us the probability that there will be x *or more* (or x *or fewer*) trials with a certain outcome. For example, among our eight runners, we may want to know the probability that six or more runners (or five or fewer runners) will have an ankle injury.

The idea is fairly simple. It is just a matter of adding the probability of each possible outcome. Thus:

$$P(X \le 5) = P(X = 0) + P(X = 1) + P(X = 2) + P(X = 3) + P(X = 4) + P(X = 5)$$

Based on data from above for our eight runners in a 5k race, this would be:

$$P(X \le 5) = 0.046 + 0.172 + 0.283 + 0.268 + 0.150 + 0.053 = 0.972$$

Thus, given eight runners and a probability that 32% of all runners will injure an ankle, there is a cumulative probability of 97.2% that five or fewer runners will injure an ankle.

To now determine the cumulative probability that five *or more* runners will injure an ankle, we apply the same strategy by adding those values *above* P(X = 5), instead of below it.

However, if it should happen that there are a large number of cases above P(X = 5) and few below it, we could simply add the numbers below that point and—you guessed it!—subtract this from 1.0. For example, in the case of our eight runners, to determine the cumulative probability that three or more runners will injure an ankle, we follow two steps.

First, we calculate: $P(X = 0) + P(X = 1) + P(X = 2)$ → 0.046 + 0.172 + 0.283 = 0.501.

Second, we calculate: 1.0 − 0.501 = 0.499.

Thus, given eight runners and a probability that 32% of all runners will injure an ankle, there is a cumulative probability of 49.9% that three or more runners will injure an ankle.

Some handy tools

Before turning away from binomial distributions for now, there are a few handy measures that we may want to generate from time to time. These are the mean, variance, and standard deviation. We discuss each of these measures further, as general concepts, in Chapter 10. For now, when working with binomial distributions:

$\mu = n(p)$ the mean (or expected) number of successes

$\sigma^2 = (n)(p)(q)$ the variance for the number of successes

$\sigma = \sqrt{(n)(p)(q)}$ the standard deviation for the number of successes

Applying these equations to our distribution of eight runners and ankle injuries, we find:

$\mu = 8(0.32) = 2.56$

$\sigma^2 = (8)(0.32)(0.68) = 1.741$

$\sigma = \sqrt{(8)(0.32)(0.68)} = 1.319$

Thus, given eight runners and a probability that 32% of all runners in a 5k race will injure an ankle, we project that:

- The mean number of runners who injure an ankle in each 5k race will be 2.4.
- The variance for the number of runners who injure an ankle in each 5k race will be 1.74.
- The standard deviation for the number of runners who injure an ankle in each 5k race will be 1.32.

The standard normal distribution

One of the most familiar uses of the standard normal distribution is to provide summary data for a group of persons based on some continuous measure, such as a person's height. These summaries generally take the form of a frequency distribution. If we collect the individual heights of 100 random students, we have a frequency distribution that almost certainly conforms to the mathematical rules of the standard normal distribution. Within biostatistical analysis, this signals a critical and auspicious moment early in the movement from a qualitative individual to a quantitative aggregation.

A qualitative individual is a concrete thing expressing many qualities, such as 32-year-old María Teresa González, who lives at 29 Chomsky Way in Guymon, Oklahoma, and works at the Kropotkin tire factory. A quantitative aggregation is an abstract concept, such as "all women living in Western Oklahoma." When moving from María Teresa to "all women living in Western Oklahoma" we lose any specificity about María—or any other woman— and imagine that "all women living in Western Oklahoma" is a meaningful and concrete object of study.

María Teresa González, divested of all personal qualities, persists now as a singular data point in a frequency distribution of heights for all women in Western Oklahoma. The frequency distribution thus provides a tool for reframing concrete and qualitative objects as invisible elements within abstract and quantitative concepts. The purpose here is certainly benign—to collect and summarize heights. However, given the complex existential meanings attached to certain concrete objects that are eviscerated when reimagined as an abstract concept, the conceptual implications of this process are potentially catastrophic.

Importantly, nearly all biostatistical analysis makes use of some kind of frequency distribution via mathematical probability. Hence, all biostatisticians warrant some introspection regarding the conceptual premises that guide their work with quantified abstract concepts. Unshockingly, such introspection is rare. However, these premises provide the framework for our consideration of the standard normal distribution.

To begin, a defining feature of the standard normal distribution is its familiar bell-shaped curve. It is happily the case that for many types of continuous data—such as the heights of high-school students—the distribution of their values forms this bell shape in which the largest number of cases (students of average height) gravitate toward the middle and the smaller number of cases (the shortest and the tallest students) accumulate at the outer edges of the curve. In fact, as we will see, even for data that are *not* normally distributed it is possible to generate a similar bell-shaped curve. See Figure 9.2 depicting the standard normal distribution curve.

All, or nearly all, of the important properties of the standard normal distribution—with regard to probability—follow from the so-called **68-95-99.7 rule**. This rule describes the distribution (or dispersal) of the data under the curve and indicates the location of particular data points in relation to the mean for all data points.

Given the mathematical properties of the standard normal distribution, one standard deviation sits one unit above and below the mean. Two standard deviations reside two units

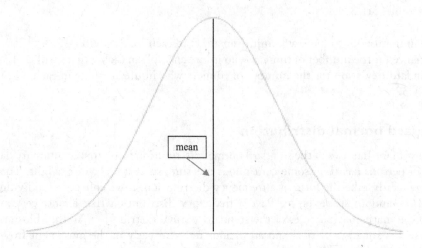

Figure 9.2 Standard normal distribution curve

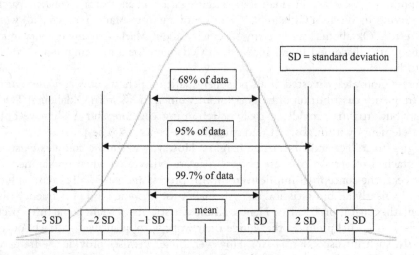

Figure 9.3 The 68-95-99.7 rule

above and below the mean and three standard deviations can be found three units above and below the mean. Our 68-95-99.7 rule indicates that, for the standard normal distribution:

- 68% of all data points will fall within one standard deviation of the mean.
- 95% of all data points fall within two standard deviations of the mean.
- 99.7% of all data points fall within three standard deviations of the mean.

As Figure 9.3 illustrates, the area between the first standard deviation below the mean (–1 SD) and the first standard deviation above the mean (+1 SD) includes 68% of all values under the curve. Thus, there is a 32% probability that we will find some value *above* or *below* the first standard deviation, which is a fairly high likelihood.

The area between the second standard deviation below the mean (–2 SD) and the second standard deviation above the mean (+2 SD) includes 95% of all values under the curve. Thus, there is only a 5% probability that we will find some value above or below the second standard deviation, which is a very low likelihood. It is thus easy to see why a 5% significance level is so popular for hypothesis testing!

The area between the third standard deviation below the mean (–3 SD) and the third standard deviation above the mean (+3 SD) includes 99.7% of all values under the curve. Thus, there is only a 0.3% probability that we will find some value above or below the third standard deviation, which is an exceptionally low likelihood. *In fact, it is the rarity of finding data above or below the second and third standard deviations that generally provides the basis for declaring some result "statistically significant."*

Note further that for the standard normal distribution, the mean, the median, and the mode are identical. Two symbols are important for interpreting the standard normal distribution curve. These are the Greek letter *mu* (*μ*) and the Greek letter *sigma* (*σ*), that designate a population mean and a population standard deviation, respectively. See Figure 9.4 for common uses of these Greek letters.

The standard normal distribution and applications of the 68-95-99.7 rule lead to phenomenal possibilities. However, we must address an obvious sticking point. It is not especially practical to work with ordinal standard deviations (or Greek letters) as our principal units of measure. It makes more sense to adopt the values from whatever item we are measuring.

For example, imagine that the mean weight of all 200 sophomores at Tom, Dick, and Enrique High School in Tweedle Dee County is 77 kilos, with a standard deviation of 10.4 kilos and that the data perfectly fit the standard normal distribution. In this case, a student who weighs 87.4 kilos is one standard deviation above the mean. See Figure 9.5 for a distribution of the weights of all 200 sophomores at Tom, Dick, and Enrique High School.

As it happens, we also have data for the heights of all 200 sophomores at Tom, Dick, and Enrique High School whose motto, "Six of one, or half a dozen of the others! Rah! Rah! Rah!" is affixed to every student's diploma. The mean height for all sophomores at Tom, Dick, and Enrique High school is 165 centimeters, with a standard deviation of 10.51 centimeters. So, in this case, a sophomore 150 centimeters tall would fall somewhere between one standard

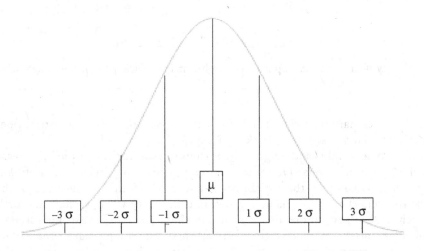

Figure 9.4 Greek letters and the standard normal distribution

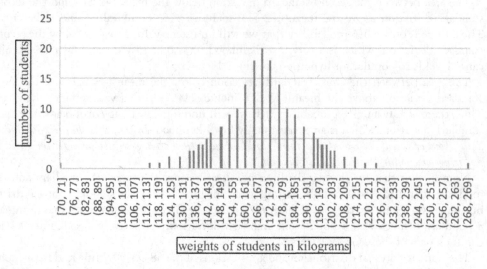

Figure 9.5 Frequency distribution of sophomore weights at Tom, Dick, and Enrique High School, *n* = 200

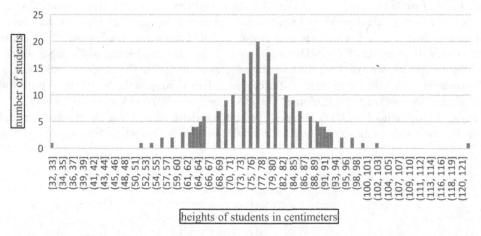

Figure 9.6 Frequency distribution of sophomore heights at Tom, Dick, and Enrique High School, *n* = 200

deviation and two standard deviations above the mean. See Figure 9.6 for a distribution of the heights of all sophomores at Tom, Dick, and Enrique High School.

In comparing these weights and heights, an obvious question arises. Which is "greater" 10.4 kilos or 10.51 centimeters? Or are they roughly equivalent? Indeed, it is often the case that we want to compare the variability of two distinct units of measure, such as kilos and centimeters. This dilemma only grows in complexity when we consider further measures, such as beats per minute for a student's resting heart rate or years for a student's age. We, therefore, need a method to transform all these values—no matter their unit of measure—into one common unit of measure. It is from such a quandary, that z-values were born.

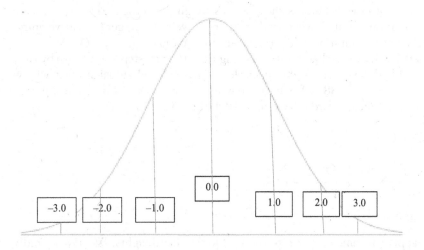

Figure 9.7 z-Values and the standard normal distribution

The development of z-values provided a method for converting all kilos, centimeters, heart beats per minute, years of age, etc. into a single common measure for purposes of comparison. For example, Figure 9.7 provides a basis for comparing the heights and weights of students from a single standard normal distribution that is standardized around the standard deviations from Figure 9.4.

For this, we introduce a method for converting the specific data from Figures 9.5 and 9.6—based on kilos and centimeters—to a common scale on the horizontal axis in Figure 9.7. The numbers along that axis are z-values and, again, 97.5% of all z-values run from –3.0 to 3.0. Thus, any z-value below –3.0 or above 3.0 is exceptionally rare.

At the same time, z-values add a further layer of abstraction to our understanding of the world. We convert concrete and specific measures of students' weights or heights (in kilos or centimeters) into a generic z-value that is then homogenized and aggregated in a mean that is detached from any specific weight or height—or even the concept of a weight or height.

María Teresa González was previously stripped of her entire individual identity, save for her actual height in centimeters. Now her "height" as well disappears. All that remains of María Teresa is the most infinitesimal fragment of data (her re-purposed height), insofar as it contributes to a mean value for the heights of all women living in Western Oklahoma in the form of a z-value. It is this aggregate measure (the mean)—and not any actual, concrete measures of heights—that is retained in the final z-value. It is, in part, the simplicity of calculating a z-value that conceals all of this.

Indeed, converting any measure—such as 77 kilos or 165 centimeters—to a z-value requires a trite equation:

$$z = \frac{(x - \mu)}{\sigma}$$

So what do we have here? This equation has two steps.

First, we have $(x - \mu)$. For this, we subtract the population mean (μ) from a data value for someone in our sample—for example, a student weighing 88.3 kilos. In the example from Tom, Dick, and Enrique High School, this would result in: (88.3 − 77). This determines both the distance of the student's weight from the mean (11.3 kilos) and its relative position—that is, whether that student's weight is larger (a positive number) or smaller (a negative number) than the mean. In this case, it is larger (11.3).

Second, we divide the bare value resulting from the first step (11.3 kilos) by the population standard deviation. In our example, we have an individual student who weighs 88.3 kilos. Thus, x = 88.3. We have a population mean of 77 kilos. Thus, μ = 77. We have a population standard deviation of 10.4 kilos. Thus, σ = 10.4.

Given this, we find:

$$z = \frac{(x - \mu)}{\sigma} \rightarrow \frac{(88.3 - 77)}{10.4} = -1.086$$

Thus, z = 1.09

Now we apply the same equation to the data for student heights. We have an individual student who stands 150 centimeters tall. Thus, x = 150. We have a population mean of 165 centimeters. Thus μ = 165. We have a population standard deviation of 10.51 centimeters. Thus, σ = 10.51.

Given this, we find:

$$z = \frac{(x - \mu)}{\sigma} \rightarrow \frac{(150 - 165)}{10.51} = -1.43$$

Thus, z = −1.43.

The math is simple enough. But what does a z-value of 1.09 or −1.43 mean?

First, it means we have a common unit of measure to compare the distance of two students from the mean, even though one student's weight was measured in kilos and another student's height was measured in centimeters. Our 88.3-kilo student is 1.09 standard deviations from the mean. Our 150-centimeter student is 1.43 standard deviations from the mean. Thus, the 150-centimeter student is 0.43 z-values further from the mean than the 87.4-kilo student.

The z-value thus provides a common method to compare the distance of two students from the mean—regardless of whether they are below or above the mean. To reiterate, the distance from the mean indicates how much a value varies from the average value for the population.

Additionally, we do not technically need the z-value to determine that the 88.3-kilo student is above the mean (a positive value) and the 150-centimeter student is below the mean (a negative value). We know this even before we generate a z-value.

Second, the z-value is based on a ratio in which the numerator is the distance between an individual's score and the mean and the denominator is the standard deviation.

Again, this ratio has the form of: $z = \frac{(x - \mu)}{\sigma}$

As with any ratio:

- If we decrease the numerator, we decrease the ratio.
- If we increase the numerator, we increase the ratio.
- If we decrease the denominator, we increase the ratio.
- If we increase the denominator, we decrease the ratio.

Thus, the larger the ratio—in absolute terms—the greater the variability. Herein lies the link between variability and statistical significance. Remember, for a two-sided hypothesis test at a 95% significance level, a z-value greater than 1.96 or less than –1.96 is considered significant. We achieve this by some combination of increasing the numerator (the distance between a z-value and the population mean) and/or decreasing the denominator (the standard deviation).

Consider the following examples pertaining to the height of our students:

If we decrease the distance between an individual's score and the population mean, we decrease the ratio and lower the z-value:

$$\frac{(150 - 165)}{10.51} = -\mathbf{1.43} \text{ becomes } \frac{(160 - 165)}{10.51} = -\mathbf{0.48}$$

If we increase the distance between an individual's score and the population mean, we increase the ratio and raise the z-value:

$$\frac{(150 - 165)}{10.51} = -\mathbf{1.43} \text{ becomes } \frac{(140 - 165)}{10.51} = -\mathbf{2.38}$$

If we increase the overall variability of the population (the standard deviation), we decrease the ratio and lower the z-value:

$$\frac{(150 - 165)}{10.51} = -\mathbf{1.43} \text{ becomes } \frac{(150 - 165)}{15.25} = -\mathbf{0.98}$$

If we decrease the variability of the population (standard deviation), we increase the ratio and raise the z-value:

$$\frac{(150 - 165)}{10.51} = -\mathbf{1.43} \text{ becomes } \frac{(150 - 165)}{5.25} = -\mathbf{2.86}$$

The equation determining the z-value is, therefore, principally a measure of variability that is based on a ratio between (a) some value's distance from the mean and (b) the standard deviation. The denominator is the standard deviation, which is a cardinal measure of variability and the numerator—the distance between an individual's score and the mean—is a value that *determines* the standard deviation. Thus, denominator and numerator are intrinsically inter-related. This we further explore in Chapter 10.

Controlling for variability can provide significant benefits. At the same time, other than intentionally selecting a population with a large standard deviation, it is difficult to manipulate the standard deviation. Therefore, data points with large values (such as our 88.3-kilo student) are the easiest way to achieve a large z-value. Again, it is the ubiquitous role of z-values throughout biostatistical operations that makes this point so crucial. After all, sometimes the murder weapon is the letter opener sitting in the middle of the room.

It is good to reiterate that whether a value is positive or negative does not impact the size of its distance from the mean. Technically, a score of 50 is a larger number than a score of –100. However, –100 sits further from a mean of zero than does 50. With regard to the z-value equation, our interest is merely a score's absolute distance from the mean.

Let us now consider our example of student weights and heights, along with our z-values, and take our standard normal distribution out for a drive to see what it can actually do for

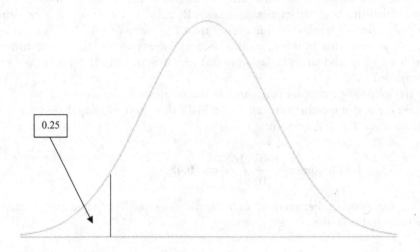

Figure 9.8 Designating 25% of the area under curve

us. Before proceeding, however, there are three important further features of the standard normal distribution that will likely prove helpful.

First, to make use of z-values and derive probabilities from the standard normal distribution, we compute areas under the curve that it creates. The total area under the curve is expressed as 1.0—or 100%. For example, in Figure 9.8, 25% of the area under the curve lies to the left of the line. Therefore, we know that the remaining area is 75%. Understanding this will allow us to infer the total area that is to the left or right of the dividing line.

Second, for the standard normal distribution curve, the probability of any measure being exactly equal to any particular z-value is zero. This is not because a person's BMI cannot equal 25. This is because, in theory, no "area" is represented by a single line, such as the dividing line designating the cut-off point for 25% in Figure 9.8.

So, for the standard normal distribution curve, $P(X = 25)$ is 0. Ordinarily, if we want to know the probability that x is equal to or less than 25, we write this as $P(X \le 25)$. However, when working with the standard normal distribution curve, we write this as $P(X < 25)$. (Note that the probability that $X = 25$ is *not* always zero when working with binomial distributions.)

Third, the standard normal distribution curve is symmetric around the mean. This is the basis for the 68-95-97.5 rule. This symmetry assures that any portion of the area along the horizontal x axis below the mean is equivalent to the same area along the x axis above the mean. Thus, in Figure 9.9, the area beneath the curve that is between the mean (0.0) and −2.0 along the horizontal x axis is equal to the area beneath the curve that is between the mean (0.0) and +2.0.

Let us now walk through some basic operations with the standard normal distribution and z-values. We will work with Table A.1 in the Appendix for this. The basic idea is to demonstrate how we can use the standard normal distribution to determine the probability of finding a person of a given weight or height among the 200 sophomores at Tom, Dick, and Enrique High School in Tweedle Dee County.

To illustrate this, we will make use of data for the weights and heights of students that have been converted to z-values (Figures 9.5 and 9.6). Consequently, the shape of each figure

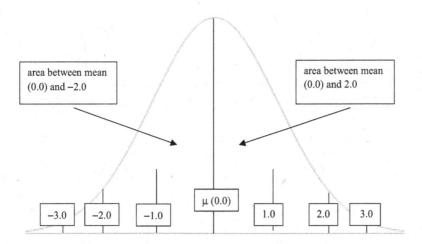

Figure 9.9 Symmetric around the mean

will be identical. The differences between the analyses of each identical figure will turn on the different data and type of problem that we are working with.

To begin, we want to know the probability of finding a student who is less than 185 centimeters tall. To work with Figure 9.6 we first convert 185 centimeters to a z-value.

$$z = \frac{(x - \mu)}{\sigma} \rightarrow \frac{(185 - 165)}{10.51} = 1.9$$

Then we find the value in Table A.1 associated with this z-value. Importantly, the values in this table pertain to the area beneath the curve to the left of our specific value—meaning the area that is less than our specific value. Thus, in this case, this value is the answer to the question of the probability of finding a student who stands less than 185 centimeters tall. Based on Table A.1, that probability is 97.13%. See Figure 9.10.

Shifting from our students' heights to their weights, we consider the probability of finding a student who weighs less than 55 kilos. Again, we first convert 55 kilos to a z-value to find its location along the horizontal axis of Figure 9.5.

$$z = \frac{(x - \mu)}{\sigma} \rightarrow \frac{(55 - 77)}{10.4} = -2.12$$

We next find the value in Table A.1 associated with this z-value. This then reveals the probability of finding a student who weighs less than 55 kilos. That probability is 1.7%. See Figure 9.11.

Now we investigate the probability of finding a student who is taller than 185 centimeters. Again, we begin by converting 185 centimeters to a z-value, which we know from above is 1.9. Then we find the value in Table A.1 associated with this z-value, which again we know is 0.9713. At this point, our path deviates.

The value 0.9713 from Figure 9.10 is that area to the left of our z-value. It is the portion beneath the curve that is *less than* 185 centimeters. Therefore, to determine that portion that is *greater than* 185 centimeters—lying to the right of our z-value—we bring in our old friend 1.0 − x. (Again, this can be understood as 100% − x%.)

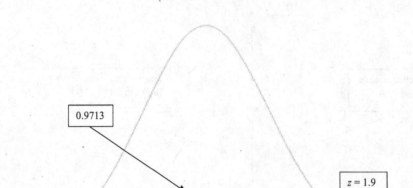

Figure 9.10 Probability of student less than 185 centimeters tall

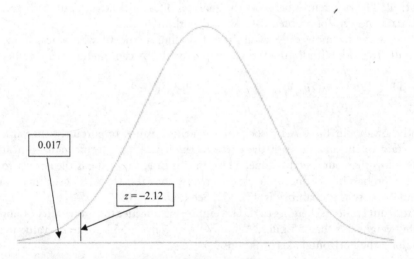

Figure 9.11 Probability of student less than 55 kilograms

Because $1.0 - 0.9713 = 0.0287$, we know that the probability of finding a student who is taller than 185 centimeters is 2.87%. See Figure 9.12.

Finally, we consider the probability of finding a student weighing more than 55 kilos. It follows that we convert 55 kilos to a z-value and find the value associated with this in Table A.1. From above, we know that the z-value is -2.12 and that the value associated with this in Table A.1 is 0.017.

Thus, we move directly to calculate $1.0 - 0.17 = 0.9868$, indicating that the probability of finding a student who weighs greater than 55 kilos is 98.68%. See Figure 9.13.

Now we complicate matters slightly and consider the probability of finding a student who is between 160 and 185 centimeters tall. This requires that we combine the previous steps taken to find the probability of a student standing less than (or greater than) a certain

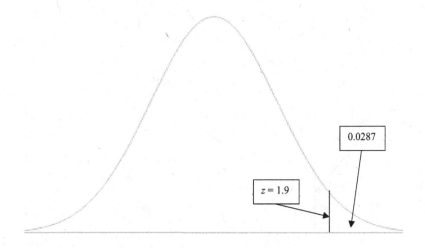

Figure 9.12 Probability of student more than 185 centimeters tall

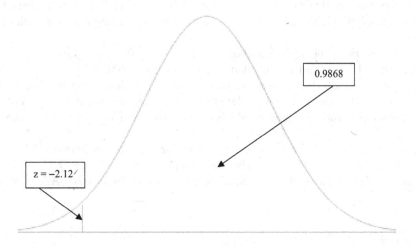

Figure 9.13 Probability of student more than 55 kilograms

height. See Figure 9.14. We first convert each height to a z-value. Next we go to Table A.1 and find the probability associated with each of these z-values.

$$z = \frac{(x - \mu)}{\sigma} \rightarrow \frac{(160 - 165)}{10.51} = -0.48 \ (p = 0.3156)$$

$$z = \frac{(x - \mu)}{\sigma} \rightarrow \frac{(185 - 165)}{10.51} = 1.9 \ (p = 0.9713)$$

The probability associated with the smaller z-value (-0.48) is 0.3156. This is the probability of finding a student less than 160 centimeters tall.

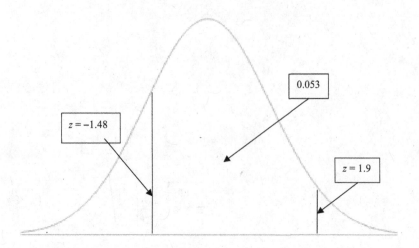

Figure 9.14 Probability student is 160 to 185 centimeters tall

The probability associated with the larger z-value (1.9) is 0.9713. We then further calculate: $1.0 - 0.9713 = 0.0287$. Thus, 0.0287 is the probability of finding a student taller than 180 centimeters.

We then add these two probabilities and derive: $0.3156 + 0.0287 = 0.3443$.

Again, we turn to $1.0 - x$, and we find that: $1.0 - 0.3443 = 0.656$.

This represents the area beneath the curve that *excludes* all students who are shorter than 160 centimeters and all students who are taller than 185 centimeters. Thus, there is a 65.6% probability of finding a student whose height is between 160 and 185 centimeters tall. See Figure 9.14.

Lastly, we examine the probability of finding a student who weighs between 50 and 55 kilos. This follows the same procedure as the previous problem. See Figure 9.15. To begin, we convert each weight to a z-value and find the probabilities from Table A.1 associated with each of these.

$$z = \frac{(x - \mu)}{\sigma} \rightarrow \frac{(50 - 77)}{10.4} = -2.6 \ (p = 0.0047)$$

$$z = \frac{(x - \mu)}{\sigma} \rightarrow \frac{(55 - 77)}{10.4} = -2.12 \ (p = 0.017)$$

The value associated with the smaller z-value (-2.6) is 0.0047. Thus, 0.0047 is the probability of finding a student weighing less than 50 kilos.

The probability associated with the larger z-value (-2.12) is 0.017. We then calculate: $1.0 - 0.017 = 0.983$. Thus, the probability of finding a student weighing more than 55 kilos is 0.983.

We then add these two probabilities and derive: $0.0047 + 0.983 = 0.9877$.

Lastly, we calculate: $1.0 - 0.9877 = 0.0123$.

This represents the area beneath the curve that *excludes* all students who weigh less than 50 kilos and all students who weigh more than 55 kilos. Thus, there is a 1.23% probability of finding a student who weighs between 50 and 55 kilos. See Figure 9.15.

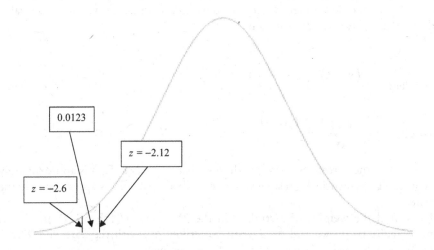

Figure 9.15 Probability student weighs 50 to 55 kilograms

Percentiles and the standard normal distribution

To refresh everyone's memory from past math experiences, a percentile is a value in a distribution that sits above a certain percentage of the population and below the remaining percentage of the population. For example, if a student weighs 88 kilos and is in the 92nd percentile, this indicates that 8% of students weigh more than that student and 92% weigh less. If another student weighs 41 kilos and is in the 8th percentile, this indicates that 92% of students weigh more than that student and 8% weigh less.

Percentiles thus help us to determine where an individual fits—based on height, weight, or some other measure—within a particular population. In addition, percentiles are useful for charting changes over time within a population. For example, perhaps 20 years ago the 50th percentile for weight among all adolescents was 63 kilos and now it is 68 kilos.

With this in mind, we turn to the z-value conversion equation to address two common questions:

1. Based on our data for 200 students, what is an individual student's percentile ranking for her weight or height?
2. Based on our data for 200 students, what is the 90th percentile for student weights or heights? What is the 10th percentile?

For the first question, we generate a z-value based on our data. We then convert that z-value to a percentile based on—you guessed it—a table of values of percentiles based on z-values. This is Table A.5 in the Appendix.

For the second question, we generate a value—such as, a specific weight or height—based on our data and the z-value corresponding to the percentile that we choose. This corresponding z-value is again found in Table A.5. Our equation for this is:

$$x = \mu + (z)\sigma$$

First, let us find the percentiles for both a student weighing 63 kilos and a student weighing 90 kilos. For this, we draw on our data for the heights and weights of sophomores at Tom, Dick, and Enrique High School. Thus, we know that the mean is 77 kilos and the standard deviation is 10.4. So we merely need to convert each student's weight to a z-value and plug all these numbers into the equation.

Thus, we find:

$$63\text{-kilo student: } z = \frac{(x-\mu)}{\sigma} \rightarrow \frac{(63-77)}{10.4} = -1.35$$

$$90\text{-kilo student: } z = \frac{(x-\mu)}{\sigma} \rightarrow \frac{(90-77)}{10.4} = 1.25$$

Based on Table A.5, the percentile corresponding with a z-value of -1.35 is approximately the 8th percentile. The percentile corresponding with a z-value of 1.25 is approximately the 93rd percentile.

Second, let us find the weight for a student in the 25th and 97.5th percentiles based on these same data. To begin we find the z-value corresponding with the 25th and 97.5th percentiles in Table A.5. These are −0.675 and 1.96, respectively.

$$25\text{th percentile: } x = \mu + (z)\sigma \rightarrow x = 77 + (-0.675)10.4 \rightarrow x = 69.98$$

$$97.5\text{th percentile: } x = \mu + (z)\sigma \rightarrow x = 77 + (1.96)10.4 \rightarrow x = 97.38$$

A student in the 25th percentile would weigh 69.9 kilos. A student in the 97.5th percentile would weigh 97.4 kilos.

To reinforce this basic idea, we perform the same operations to determine the percentile for a student who is 140 centimeters tall and the percentile for a student who is 178 centimeters tall. Again, for this purpose, we know from our data for 200 sophomores at Tom, Dick, and Enrique High School that the mean height is 165 and the standard deviation is 10.51. So we merely need to convert each student's weight to a z-value and plug all these numbers into the equation.

Thus, we find:

$$140 \text{ cm student: } z = \frac{(x-\mu)}{\sigma} \rightarrow \frac{(140-165)}{10.51} = -2.38$$

$$178 \text{ cm student: } z = \frac{(x-\mu)}{\sigma} \rightarrow \frac{(178-165)}{10.51} = 1.24$$

Based on Table A.5, the percentile corresponding with a z-value of -2.38 is approximately the 1st percentile. The percentile corresponding with a z-value of 1.24 is approximately the 93rd percentile.

Now let us find the height for a student in the 25th and 97.5th percentiles based on these same data. We know from Table A.5 that the z-value for the 25th percentile is −0.675 and for the 97.5th percentile this is again, 1.96. We thus plug our numbers into the equation.

$$25\text{th percentile: } x = \mu + (z)\sigma \rightarrow x = 165 + (-0.675)10.51 \rightarrow x = 157.91$$

$$97.5\text{th percentile: } x = \mu + (z)\sigma \rightarrow x = 165 + (1.96)10.51 \rightarrow x = 185.59$$

A student in the 25th percentile would be 157.9 centimeters tall. A student in the 97.5th percentile would be 185.6 centimeters tall.

Sampling distributions, the central limit theorem, and the standard error of the mean

There is one further critical task that is made possible by the standard normal distribution. This concerns the tendency for the items in a sampling distribution to mimic the properties of the standard normal distribution. A sampling distribution is a distribution of certain values, such as the mean, for many samples drawn from the same population.

For example, rather than gathering the heights and weights of all 200 sophomores at Tom, Dick, and Enrique High School in Tweedle Dee County, we might prefer to draw 25 samples of 30 students each. We could then generate a mean height and weight for each of these 25 samples. Our sampling distribution in this case would contain the 25 mean heights and 25 mean weights for our 25 samples.

If we treat the mean of each of the 25 samples as an individual data point, we can find the mean for all 25 sample means. This will provide us with a very accurate estimate of the actual mean population height and mean population weight for all sophomores.

This technique is especially helpful when we have a small number of participants in a study and we want to estimate a population mean based on data from this study. To illustrate, let us return to our 200 high-school long-distance runners from Machel County. We want to know the mean number of daily caffeinated beverages that these long-distance runners consume.

Unfortunately, severe budget cuts have limited the athletic department to 30 photocopies or emails per month. So we cannot send out 200 surveys—only 30 at a time. We send the survey out to 30 random long-distance runners from across the county and we repeat this five times. This gives us six samples, each containing a total of 30 runners.

Note that this is an example of **sampling with replacement** because it is possible for the same person to be in more than one of these six samples. We will return to this concept shortly.

Each of our six samples produces a mean number of caffeinated beverages consumed each day for 30 runners. We then treat these six means as our sampling distribution and this allows us to find the mean of these means. See Table 9.2 for sample means.

The population mean based on these six sample means is:

$$\frac{1.5 + 1.7 + 1.8 + 1.5 + 1.6 + 1.6}{6} = 1.62$$

Given this mean, we can also calculate the population standard deviation.

$$\sigma = \sqrt{\frac{\Sigma(X-\mu)^2}{n}} \sqrt{\frac{\Sigma(X-1.62)^2}{30.0}} = 0.106$$

Note that $n = 30$ because each of the six samples has a sample size of 30.

We thus conclude that the mean number of caffeinated beverages consumed by all 200 long-distance runners in Machel County is 1.62 with a standard deviation of 0.106. One reason we have such confidence in these results is the **central limit theorem**.

Table 9.2 Six sample means for daily caffeinated beverages

Sample	1	2	3	4	5	6
Sample size	$n = 30$	$n = 30$	$n = 30$	$n = 30$	$n = 30$	$n = 30$
Mean	1.5	1.7	1.8	1.5	1.6	1.6

This theorem holds that the more random samples of 30 or more persons (with replacement) that one gathers from a population, the more that the distribution of the means from these individual samples will approximate the standard normal distribution. It is thus argued that the mean of all these sample means will approximate the actual population mean—from which we can also derive the population standard deviation.

More remarkably, so long as the size of each random sample is 30 or greater, even when the actual population distribution is *not* normal—meaning it is skewed—the distribution of the sample means will still resemble that of the standard normal distribution and reveal the population mean and standard deviation. Furthermore, if the actual population mean conforms to the standard normal distribution, the sample means will conform to the standard normal distribution, *regardless of the size of the individual samples.*

One important exception concerns dichotomous outcomes. If the outcome of interest for the population is dichotomous, then approximation of the actual population mean only holds if:

$$\min[n(p),\, n(1.0 - p)] > 5$$

Here, n is the sample size and p is the probability of "success" for the population. As previously encountered, the term "$\min[x, y]$" should be read: the smaller of either x or y. Thus, the smaller of either $n(p)$ or $n(1.0 - p)$ must be greater than 5.

The standard error of the mean—a confusion of language for a not-so-confusing notion

Let us further examine the data for Table 9.2 and our six sample means for daily caffeinated beverages in a bit more detail. We bring in the standard error for this purpose. To explore this, it helps to unravel some confusing use of language by distinguishing between the standard error of the mean (for a single sample) and the standard error of the mean (for a distribution of samples). We have encountered variations of the standard error previously and so here we add one more twist.

We begin with the standard error of the mean for a single sample. Let us reiterate the distinction between the standard error of the mean and the standard deviation in the case of a single sample. The standard deviation is an empirical statistic that makes use of basic arithmetic. It is a measure of the (actual) dispersion of scores in a single sample around the sample mean. The standard deviation thus indicates the (actual) distance between each person in a sample from the sample mean. This is a measure of variability *within a single sample.*

The standard error of the mean for a single sample is a probabilistic statistic that makes use of the central limit theorem. It estimates the (probable) distance between a sample mean and the true population mean, based on the population standard deviation and the sample size. Specifically, it estimates the variability between sample means that would result if we continued to draw more samples of the same size. The standard error of the mean for a single sample thus tells us how precise (or reliable) any particular sample mean is likely to be. This is a measure of variability *between different (hypothetical) samples from the same population.*

Mathematically, the standard error of the mean for a single sample is a function of the ratio between the population standard deviation and the size of the sample. Thus, fluctuations in the magnitude of the numerator (the population standard deviation) and the denominator (the sample size) can significantly impact the standard error.

Imagine we have a sample of 40 high-school long-distance runners and each and every one of them has a resting heart rate of 70 bpm. We happen to know that the population standard deviation is 8.3. Given this:

$$\text{standard error} \rightarrow \frac{\sigma}{\sqrt{n}} \rightarrow \frac{8.3}{\sqrt{40}} = 1.31$$

standard deviation = 0.0

In this case, a standard error of the mean of 1.31 indicates that if we were to continue drawing further samples of 40 runners from the same population, on average, the mean of these additional samples would vary from our original sample mean (70 bpm) by 1.31 bpm. Given that 1.31 is 1.87% of 70, this suggests that our sample mean very closely approximates the actual population mean.

Meanwhile, the standard deviation is 0.0 *for the sample*. This is because all persons in the sample just happen to have the same resting heart rate. Our standard deviation of 0.0 indicates nothing about how well our sample mean approximates the actual population mean. It is simply a measure of the sample data themselves.

Notice further in Table 9.3, the impact of either (a) doubling the sample size or (b) reducing the population standard deviation by one-half. The standard error of the mean falls from 1.31 to 0.93 when we double the sample size. The standard error of the mean falls even further (to 0.66) when we cut the standard deviation in half.

The principal value of the standard error of the mean for a single population is to indicate how well the mean from a single sample approximates the actual population mean, given a certain sample size. (This is critical for determining an optimal sample size.) The greater the standard error of the mean, the greater the variability between different samples (of the same size) taken from the population. In turn, this degree of variability between different sample means from the same population can directly influence the accuracy of any statistical tests.

Alternatively, the standard error of the mean for a distribution of sample means is a measure of the dispersion among the means from many samples around the true population mean. This is a measure of the variability *between different (actual) samples from the same population*. However, insofar as the six samples in our example above (Table 9.2) also represent a single sample (of six means), this is also a measure of the variability *within a single (actual) sample*—akin to a standard deviation.

The standard error here is the same as that for a single sample—the standard deviation of the population divided by the square root of the sample size.

$$\text{standard error} = \frac{\sigma}{\sqrt{n}}$$

Table 9.3 Impact of changes to sample size or standard deviation on standard error

Original standard error	Standard error after doubling sample size	Standard error after reducing population standard deviation by one-half
$SE = \frac{8.3}{\sqrt{40}} = 1.31$	$SE = \frac{8.3}{\sqrt{80}} = 0.93$	$SE = \frac{4.15}{\sqrt{40}} = 0.66$

Again, the sample size in our example is 30—the number of persons in each of the six samples that we collected! With our sample size in the denominator, it follows that the larger the sample size, the smaller the standard error. The equation for the standard error with the data from the example above is:

$$\text{standard error} = \frac{\sigma}{\sqrt{n}} \rightarrow \frac{0.106}{\sqrt{30}} = 0.019$$

Thus, the standard error of the mean provides us with a range of values that best captures the true population mean based on the standard normal distribution of our sample means. For example, given a mean of 1.62 among many sample means and a standard error of 0.019, we can surmise that the true population mean lies between 1.601 and 1.639.

$$1.62 - 0.019 = 1.601$$

$$1.62 + 0.019 = 1.639$$

Classical probability

We turn now to classical probability. The principal contribution of classical probability is the use of deductive reasoning to fill in missing pieces of a puzzle. For example, when we are presented with incomplete data regarding some situation, such as whether or not a test result might be a false positive, classical probability applies rules of formal logic to yield the missing data.

Discussions of classical probability generally introduce two challenges. **First**, there is the reliance on abstract rules. Such rules commonly take the form of law-like statements about a general relationship that we apply to specific situations. Thus, it is better to keep our focus on the specific situations rather than the abstract rules to make both more clear.

Second, there is an adamant insistence on the use of formal symbolic language. The only thing more alien and unintelligible than a general set of abstract rules, is a general set of abstract rules expressed in formal symbolic language. Algebra, by way of example, is when most of us first encounter a heavy-duty reliance on abstract, mathematical symbolic forms. For example, we learn to interpret combinations of symbols, such as: $x + y = 6$.

Once one masters the rules, a formal symbolic language provides useful shortcuts to avoid always fully writing out the rules. This makes much sense. While still mastering the rules, however, this makes almost no sense. Presenting "x + y = 6" to a 12th grader who has mastered the rules of algebra is fine. Presenting this to a 2nd grader who only learned about addition in the past year would be absurd. Both 12th and 2nd graders know how to add. The difference is their familiarity with the symbolic forms.

For the student of biostatistics, knowledge of the underlying rule may not be so onerous. However, the rule's formal symbolic language is borrowed from other subfields, mostly set theory and symbolic logic. So why should a student of introductory biostatistics be asked to learn an elaborate symbolic language that was created specifically for some other specialized subfields and which, in fact, is germane to only a very small slice of introductory biostatistics?

It is true that there are biostatistical textbooks that forgo this symbolic language with a stripped down mathematical content. The dilemma with this approach is that persons going into quantitative fields, such as health and medicine, will ultimately need elements of this symbolic language.

Let us start out with some basic rules for addition, multiplication, and subtraction. For this purpose we will draw on a specific situation (subject to amendment) to help clarify the abstract rules. We will also introduce the symbolic form of these rules, while attempting to minimize the substitution of these symbolic forms for the concrete situation.

For this, return to our 200 high-school long-distance runners in Lumumba County. As it turns out, among these runners:

- 45% compete in 5k races;
- 35% compete in 10k races; and
- 20% compete in *both* 5k and 10k races.

We will use these details—specifically, we will use the percentages—to illustrate the addition, multiplication, and subtraction rules, along with their symbolic forms.
In symbolic form, we represent these details as:

$P(A) = 0.45$
$P(B) = 0.35$
$P(A \text{ and } B) = 0.20$

P represents "probability"
A represents "competes in 5k races"
B represents "competes in 10k races"

Thus, if we randomly select one of the 200 high-school long-distance runners in Lumumba County:

"$P(A) = 0.45$" tells us that there is a 45% probability that she or he competes in 5k races.
"$P(B) = 0.35$" tells us that there is a 35% probability that she or he competes in 10k races.
"$P(A \text{ and } B) = 0.20$" tells us that there is a 20% probability that she or he competes in both 5k and 10k races.

Given this, we turn to our rules for addition, multiplication, and subtraction. Each rule has certain applications within biostatistical analysis. However, the greater importance of these rules unfolds when we combine them to develop new rules, such as **conditional probability** and the **total probability rule**. This then clears a path to **Bayes' theorem**, a specific application of conditional probability that is essential within biostatistical analysis.

The addition rule (and two situations)

The **addition rule** applies to two situations. In the first situation, we have two events that can both be true at the same time. For example, the same runner can compete in both 5k and 10k races. The purpose of the addition rule in this situation is to determine the probability of either event A or event B, *excluding* instances of A and B. For example, the probability that a runner competes in either 5k races or 10k races, includes that possibility that a runner competes in both. Our interest is the probability of event A or event B, but not both.

In the second situation, there are no runners who compete in both 5k and 10k races. If a runner competes in 5k races she or he cannot compete in 10k races. The purpose of the addition rule in this situation is again to determine the probability of event A or event B, but not both. However, the second situation stipulates that there are no runners who compete in both, whereas, the first situation stipulates that 20% of runners compete in both. (This second situation thus cannot apply to our runners in Lumumba County without some amendment.)

In symbolic form, the addition rule for the first situation is written: P(A or B) = P(A) or P(B) − P(A and B).
In symbolic form, the addition rule for the second situation is written: P(A or B) = P(A) + P(B).

To begin, we illustrate the addition rule for the first situation.
This is based on our data above.

- 45% compete in 5k races;
- 35% compete in 10k races; and
- 20% compete in *both* 5k and 10k races.

There is a 45% probability that a runner competes in 5k races and a 35% probability that a runner competes in 10k races. In addition, there is a 20% probability that a runner competes in both. But what is the probability that a runner competes in either 5k races or 10k races, but not both?

We must avoid double counting those runners (the 20%) who compete in both 5k and 10k races. For this, we first add the percentages of those competing in 5k and 10k races.

0.45 + 0.35 = 0.8

We then subtract the percentage of those competing in both races.

0.8 − 0.20 = 0.60

Thus, there is a 60% probability that a high-school long-distance runner in Lumumba County competes in either 5k or 10k races, but not both. In full symbolic form, we have:

P(A or B) = P(A) + P(B) − P(A and B) = (0.45 + 0.35) − 0.20 = 0.60

Now the second situation.
For this, we amend the details and find that:

- 45% of runners compete in 5k races, but not 10k races;
- 35% of runners compete in 10k races, but not 5k races; and
- no runners compete in both 5k and 10k races.

Thus, we have two mutually exclusive groups. If a runner belongs to the group competing in 5k races, she or he does NOT belong to the group competing in 10k races and vice versa. Now we meet the conditions for applying the addition rule to the second situation and we can insert our values into the symbolic language.

[P(A or B) = P(A) + P(B)] ➔ [P(0.45 or 0.35) = P(0.45) + P(0.35) = 0.80]

Thus, there is an 80% probability that a runner competes in either 5k or 10k races, but not both.

Notice that in both situations, 45% of high-school long-distance runners compete in 5k races and 35% compete in 10k races. However, in the first situation—in which 20% of runners compete in both races—there is a 60% probability that a runner competes in either 5k or 10k races, but not both.

In the second situation—in which no runner competes in both races—there is an 80% probability that a runner competes in either 5k or 10k races, but not both.

The multiplication rule (and two situations)

The **multiplication rule** also applies to two situations. In the first situation, we have two events that are dependent. For example, above we placed runners in three categories—(A) those who compete in 5k races, (B) those who compete in 10k races, or (A and B) those who compete in both. No runner can compete in both 5k and 10k races if one of these does not exist. Thus, for the third category of "both," event A and event B are dependent because the third category cannot exist without both.

The purpose of the multiplication rule in this situation is to determine the probability of both event A and event B. For example, the probability that a runner competes in both 5k and 10k races. The first addition rule identified those runners who competed in either the 5k or the 10k race, but *not* in both.

In the second situation, we have two events that are independent. For instance, if a coach randomly assigns runners to compete in either 5k or 10k races but never both, then a runner competing in one will not compete in the other. When two events are independent, the probability of A and B is equal to the probability of A multiplied by the probability of B. Again, this situation can only apply to our scenario after amendment. We know this requires amendment because:

$$P(A \text{ and } B) = 0.20 \text{ AND } P(A) \times P(B) = 0.45 \times 0.35 = 0.158$$

Thus, the probability of A and B is NOT equal to the probability of A multiplied by the probability of B. So we will need to amend things to demonstrate the multiplication rule in the second situation.

Let us continue with the first situation, the probability of both event A and event B. The same multiplication rule applies to both the first and second situation. In symbolic form it is written:

$$P(A \text{ and } B) = P(A) \times P(B \mid A)$$

This is read: The probability of (event A) and (event B) is equal to the probability of (event A) multiplied by the probability that if (event A) occurs, (event B) also occurs.

The symbolic form of $P(B \mid A)$ is a very common and very important construction.

An example of its application is: $P(10k \mid 5k)$. This is the probability that if a runner competes in 5k races, she or he also competes in 10k races. (Thus, the runner competes in both races.) To confirm this, we plug in our numbers, 45% compete in 5k races, 35% compete in 10k races, and 20% compete in both.

To begin, we must further untangle $P(B \mid A)$. Fortunately for us, it has been determined that:

$$P(B \mid A) = \frac{P(A \text{ and } B)}{P(A)}$$

Therefore

$$P(B \mid A) \rightarrow \frac{0.20}{0.45} = 0.444$$

Thus, there is a 44.4% probability that a runner who competes in 5k races also competes in 10k races. Now we must complete the full multiplication formula. We plug $\dfrac{P(A \text{ and } B)}{P(A)}$ into the first multiplication formula and we find:

$$P(A \text{ and } B) \rightarrow (0.45) \times \left(\frac{0.20}{0.45}\right) \rightarrow 0.45 \times (0.444) = 0.20$$

This confirms what we originally stipulated, that 20% of all runners compete in both 5k and 10k races and it further builds our toolbox for deductive reasoning when certain data are missing. However, the supreme importance of this application of the multiplication rule to the first situation—when elements are dependent—is that it provides our initial bridge to conditional probability. That is where we will turn soon.

First, we note again that this multiplication formula will work regardless of whether the elements are dependent or independent. However, if the elements are independent—as in the second situation—a far easier multiplication formula is written:

P(A and B) = P(A) × P(B)

In the first situation for the multiplication rule, event A refers to competing in a 5k race and event B refers to competing in a 10k race. We now amend this for the second situation in which event B, riding a bike to school, is independent of event A. We know that 10% of all runners ride a bike to school.

Hence, the probability that a person competes in 5k races AND rides a bike to school is:

P(A and B) = P(A) × P(B) → 0.45 × 0.10 = 0.045

Thus, 4.5% of all runners both compete in 5k races and ride a bike to school.

The subtraction rule

The **subtraction rule** is by now familiar, rather straightforward, and well ... almost simple-minded. However, its underlying principle plays an important role in more complex situations. The subtraction rule holds that the probability that A will occur is equal to 1.0 minus the probability that A will NOT occur.

This is written in symbolic form as:

P(A) = 1.0 − P(not A)

For example, continuing with our runners from Lumumba County, there is a 45% probability of randomly selecting a runner who competes in 5k races among the 200 high-school long-distance runners. Thus, the probability of selecting a runner who does NOT compete in 5k races is 1.0 − 0.45. (Remember, this is the same as 100% minus 45%.)
In symbolic form, we have:

P(0.45) = 1.0 − P(not 0.45) = 0.55

The underlying importance of the subtraction rule is that, if we know the probability that some event will occur, we can determine the probability that this event will NOT occur—and vice versa.

Remember, in classical probability, we are constantly applying deductive methods, such as this, to fill in data that we do not know based on data that we do know. For this purpose, the subtraction rule is quite helpful.

Conditional probability

The final pieces of classical probability are conditional probability, the total probability rule, and Bayes' theorem. These follow, in part, from the addition, multiplication, and subtraction rules.

The principal contribution of **conditional probability** is to provide the likely consequences if certain events occur. For example, if you fall down the stairs what is the probability you will break a leg?

We begin with a subpart of the multiplication rule that provides a core element of conditional probability. This is the formula:

$$P(B \mid A) = \frac{P(A \text{ and } B)}{P(A)}$$

Recall the details for Lumumba County:

P(A) is the probability that a runner competes in 5k races.   This is P(0.45).
P(B) is the probability that a runner competes in 10k races.   This is P(0.35).
P(A and B) is the probability that a runner competes in both races.   This is P(0.20).

Given this scenario, we determined that:

$$P(B \mid A) \rightarrow \frac{P(A \text{ and } B)}{P(A)} \rightarrow \frac{0.20}{0.45} = 0.444$$

Thus, if a runner competes in 5k races, there is a 44% probability that she or he also competes in 10k races. So we have a condition, [if a runner competes in 5k races] and we have a likely consequence [a 44% probability that she or he also competes in 10k races].

Observe how the multiplication rule allows us to generate a general probability statement based on this conditional probability.

First, we transform the multiplication rule into a subpart of the conditional probability formula.

$$[P(B \mid A) = \frac{P(A \text{ and } B)}{P(A)}] \rightarrow [P(A \text{ and } B) = P(A) \times P(B \mid A)]$$

This becomes:

$$P(A \text{ and } B) = [P(A) \times P(B \mid A)] \rightarrow 0.45 \times \left(\frac{0.20}{0.45}\right) \rightarrow [0.45 \times (0.444)] = 0.20$$

Thus, we derive a general probability statement—that there is a 20% probability that any runner competes in both 5k and 10k races—from the combination of the multiplication rule and conditional probability. This then sets in motion a great many further possibilities, including the total probability rule and Bayes' theorem.

Total probability rule

Not surprisingly, the total probability rule is an amalgam of different rules we have just reviewed. Its symbolic form is the following:

$P(B) = [P(B \mid A) \times P(A)] + [P(B \mid \text{not } A) \times P(\text{not } A)]$

We premise that:

$P(A) = 0.45$

$P(B) = 0.35$

$P(A \text{ and } B) = 0.20$

Based on this, we find that:

$P(B \mid A) = 0.444$

$P(\text{not } A) = 1.0 - P(A) = 0.55$

$P(B \text{ and not } A) = P(B) - P(A \text{ and } B) = 0.35 - 0.20 = 0.15$

Given this, and making further use of conditional probability, we first calculate:

$$P(B \mid \text{not } A) = \frac{P(B \text{ and not } A)}{P(\text{not } A)} = \frac{0.15}{0.55} = 0.273$$

To clarify, this last equation indicates that there is a 27.3% probability that a runner competes in 10k races but not 5k races. Now we have all the values we need to calculate the total probability rule.

$P(B) = [P(B \mid A) \times P(A)] + [P(B \mid \text{not } A) \times P(\text{not } A)]$

This yields:

$P(B) = [0.444 \times 0.45] + [0.273 \times 0.55] = 0.20 + 0.15 = 0.35$

Happily, the result of the total probability rule finds a 35% probability that a runner will compete in 10k races, just as we had originally premised. Now that the total probability rule has been tested and confirmed by our example, we are prepared to bring in Bayes' theorem. This theorem is built up from all those rules of classical probability that we have considered to this point.

Bayes' theorem

To begin, notice that Bayes' theorem—though comparatively sparse—combines the multiplication rule and the total probability rule. In symbolic form it is written:

$$P(A \mid B) = \frac{P\left(A \text{ and } B\right)}{P\left(B\right)}$$

As we will see, this can be rewritten in expanded form to better facilitate its application. An expanded version follows from a transformation of the shorter version via the rules of symbolic logic, the details of which need not detain us here. This is written:

$$\frac{P(A \text{ and } B)}{P(B)} = \frac{P(B|A) \times P\left(A\right)}{\left[P(B|A) \times P\left(A\right)\right] + \left[P(B|not A) \times P\left(not A\right)\right]}$$

Before proceeding, notice that there are only two actual fragments in this equation, both of which we have previously encountered.

The first fragment is **P(B | A)** × **P(A)**. This appears twice in the equation, once in the numerator and once in the denominator.

The second fragment is **P(B | *not* A)** × **P(*not* A)**. This appears once in the denominator.

To illustrate Bayes' theorem via an example of its application we retain our familiar high-school long-distance runners. However, we bring in a new scenario—health screenings.

When screening for a condition, there are five main concepts (see Table 9.4).

By way of example, recall that the symbolic form associated with sensitivity is read:

P(+T | +C): The probability that a person who has a condition (C+) will test positive for that condition (T+).

In addition, there is a tidy table to determine the sensitivity, specificity, positive predictive value, and negative predictive value of screening tests (see Tables 9.5 and 9.6).

If we combine the contents of Tables 9.4, 9.5, and 9.6, we can produce four equations to measure sensitivity, specificity, the positive predictive value, and the negative predictive value (see Table 9.7).

Table 9.4 Five concepts for health screenings

Concept	Description	Symbolic form
Prevalence	Probability any person in the population has condition	P(C)
Sensitivity	Probability person with condition has positive test	P(+T | +C)
Specificity	Probability person without condition has negative test	P(−T | −C)
Positive predictive value	Probability person with positive test has condition	P(+C | +T)
Negative predictive value	Probability person with negative test does not have condition	P(−C | −T)

Table 9.5 Grid for assessing screening tests

	Condition	No condition	Total
Screen positive	a	b	a + b
Screen negative	c	d	c + d
Total	a + c	b + d	N

Table 9.6 Interpreting cells in Table 9.4

Cells	Interpretation
a	Persons who have condition and test positive
b	Persons who do not have condition but test positive
c	Persons who have condition but test negative
d	Persons who do not have condition and test negative
a + b	All persons who test positive
c + d	All persons who test negative
a + c	All persons who have condition
b + d	All persons who do not have condition
N	Total number of persons screened

Table 9.7 Equations for health screening

Sensitivity	$\dfrac{a}{a+c}$
Specificity	$\dfrac{d}{b+d}$
Positive predictive value	$\dfrac{a}{a+b}$
Negative predictive value	$\dfrac{d}{c+d}$

Let us apply this to data for health screenings for 4,000 high-school long-distance runners across the US for hypoglycemia.

The data in Table 9.8 tell a number of stories.

There are 331 runners who are, in fact, hypoglycemic. Of these runners, 221 tested positive and 110 tested negative. Thus, the sensitivity of our test is: $\dfrac{221}{221+110} = 0.668$.

This indicates a 66.8% probability that a runner who is, in fact, hypoglycemic will receive a positive test result.

There are 3,669 runners who are not, in fact, hypoglycemic. Of these runners, 32 tested positive and 3,637 tested negative. Thus, the specificity of our test is: $\dfrac{3,637}{32+3,637} = 0.991$.

This indicates a 99.1% probability that a runner who is not, in fact, hypoglycemic will receive a negative test result.

There are 253 runners who tested positive. Of these runners, 221 were, in fact, hypoglycemic and 32 were not. Thus, our positive predictive value is: $\dfrac{221}{221+32} = 0.874$.

This indicates an 87.4% probability that a runner who tests positive is, in fact, hypoglycemic.

Table 9.8 Grid for assessing screening tests for hypoglycemia

	Hypoglycemia	No hypoglycemia	Total
Screen positive	221	32	253
Screen negative	110	3,637	3,747
Total	331	3,669	4,000

Table 9.9 Hypothetical data for Bayes' theorem example

Prevalence	$P(C) = 0.001$
Sensitivity	$P(+T \mid +C) = 0.769$
Specificity	$P(-T \mid -C) = 0.981$
Positive predictive value	$P(+C \mid +T) = ???$

There are 3,747 runners who tested negative. Of these runners, 110 were, in fact, hypoglycemic and 3,637 were not. Thus, our negative predictive value is: $\dfrac{3,637}{110+3,637} = 0.971$.

This indicates a 97.1% probability that a runner who tests negative is not, in fact, hypoglycemic.

Given the interconnectedness of these four equations, it will come as little surprise that it is often possible to derive one of these values when others are available. This, in fact, is a common ploy when applying Bayes' theorem within health and medicine. In the following example we apply Bayes' theorem to find the positive predictive value, given certain known values for prevalence, sensitivity, and specificity.

Let us now bring our high-school long-distance runners back in. The prevalence of heart arrhythmia among youth is exceptionally rare. One opportunity to screen youth for arrhythmia is during routine physicals for high-school athletes. Based on past screening campaigns, we know the test's sensitivity is 0.769 and its specificity is 0.981. In addition, past studies estimate a prevalence rate of 2.3% (or 0.023) for arrhythmia among adults.

Given this, we postulate a prevalence rate of 0.001 (or 0.10%) among all high-school athletes. (Remember, this is one-tenth of one percent, not ten percent.) This is intentionally quite low for purposes of illustration. Based on these levels of prevalence, sensitivity, and specificity, we want to know the probability that a high-school athlete who receives a positive test result does, in fact, have arrhythmia. This is the positive predictive value. See Table 9.9.

We first apply these data to Bayes' theorem to determine the probability that a high-school athlete with a positive test does, in fact, have arrhythmia. We will then repeat this for a second circumstance. All values for this second circumstance will be identical with the first, except for a higher prevalence.

Here again is Bayes' theorem.

$$P(A \mid B) = \frac{P(B|A) \times P(A)}{\left[P(B|A) \times P(A)\right] + \left[P(B|not\ A) \times P(not\ A)\right]}$$

We substitute (+C and –C) for (A and *not* A) and we substitute (+T and –T) for (B and *not* B). Again, "C" is condition. "T" is the test result.

$$P(+C\mid+T)=\frac{P(+T\mid+C)\times P(C)}{\left[P(+T\mid+C)\times P(C)\right]+\left[P(+T\mid-C)\times P(-C)\right]}$$

Given Table 9.4, we have the functional equivalent of:

$$P(+C\mid+T)=\frac{(\text{sensitivity})\times(\text{prevalence})}{\left[(\text{sensitivity})\times(\text{prevalence})\right]+\left[(1.0-\text{specificity})\times(1.0-\text{prevalence})\right]}$$

We then insert our data from Table 9.9:

$$P(+C\mid+T)=\frac{(0.769)\times(0.001)}{\left[(0.769)\times(0.001)\right]+\left[(0.019)\times(0.999)\right]}=\frac{0.0008}{0.0198}=0.040$$

Thus, given a prevalence rate of 0.001, there is a 4% probability that a high-school athlete testing positive for arrhythmia does, in fact, have arrhythmia. Notice then what happens when we then increase the prevalence rate from 0.001 to 0.01.

$$P(+C\mid+T)=\frac{(0.769)\times(0.01)}{\left[(0.769)\times(0.01)\right]+\left[(0.019)\times(0.99)\right]}=\frac{0.008}{0.0268}=0.2984$$

Suddenly, the probability that a person testing positive for arrhythmia does, in fact, have the condition leaps from 4% to 29.8%. This illustrates just how dramatically the prevalence rate can impact the positive predictive value.

Final thoughts

Finding ourselves now deep in the weeds of classical probability, we close by returning to our initial reservations about relying on certain mathematical rationale and conceptual premises that originate from highly controlled conditions and extremely constrained outcomes, such as a coin toss. To meet the conditions required for the application of such rationale and premises, the subject matter of health and medicine must be assiduously reassembled to better approximate the regularity and precision of the natural world.

At times, as with randomized controlled trials, we can get fairly close. However, adapting our research subject to fit our tools, rather than adapting our tools to fit our research subject, invariably opens one to misinterpretation and misappropriation. In this case, the need for pristine and invariant conditions, significantly distorts (and disguises) the holistic nature of our subject matter and the complex social context of its origins. Again, this is no reason to reject, or even minimize, the important contributions of biostatistical analysis. It is only to argue that we must understand, and consciously work within, the limited, tactical applications of biostatistical analysis for understanding certain facets of health and medicine.

In the main, we proceed along a holistic and contextual path, while occasionally suspending this fuller conceptual understanding of health and medicine to explore myriad quantitative aspects of our subject matter made germane at different points throughout a larger research project. Soon after, we rejoin the holistic and contextual path to carry on. This explains the need to understand the conceptual implications of probability distributions for our subject matter alongside the intricacies of its mathematical rationale.

As by now is well rehearsed, the aim of reviewing these technical steps throughout this book—at times in less-than-thrilling detail—is to explore the contentious process of preparing the complex and multi-layered social reality that comprises health and medicine for biostatistical analysis. This entails two simultaneous—and seemingly contradictory—shifts. The first is from holism to reductivism.

A complex and socially situated person becomes the (denuded) individual member of a sample. María Teresa González arrives as a full and complete human being when entering our study, via some sampling process designed to spot certain attributes or exposures. We then systematically pare down those features of her humanity that do not serve our instrumental research purposes. María Teresa—in partial form—is made the soulless fragment of a mean or standard deviation.

Then, in a twist that only a character from Chekov could have anticipated, complexity and holism return in full force. María Teresa's fragmented existence—the epitome of reductive thinking—is lifted up to join with the fragments of others, first as a discrete part within an aggregation and then as an inter-relating element within a dialectical whole.

It is these transformations that we turn to now in Chapter 10, via a conceptual distillation of descriptive statistics. Do not let this otherwise banal and unassuming chapter content throw you. In fact, it is here that the deepest mysteries of biostatistical analysis lie—in particular, those portentous moments marking the initial appropriation and conceptual reimagination of our subject matter. These developments reveal the intricacies of mathematical probability, alongside the many elaborate tools and techniques of biostatistical analysis, to be mere smoke screens that cloud our understanding of the conceptual premises that make *any* statistical analysis possible.

As alluded to above, akin to the murder weapon sitting out in the open, descriptive statistics are quite innocently—almost off-handedly—discussed in the early chapters of most all introductory biostatistics textbooks. What better way to put one off the trail of the true culprit uprooting and displacing the holistic, contextual, and contingent nature of health and medicine? Indeed, the technical minutiae of biostatistical analysis are mere pretense in this regard. By the time our first z-value appears, the crime has already been completed. We return now—via Chapter 10—to the scene of the crime.

And Finally ... We Can Now Make Sense of Descriptive Statistics

Biostatistics textbooks often warn readers about the dangers that arise when biostatistical analysis is misused—either accidentally or intentionally. Throughout this book we have warned readers, with equal alarm, about the dangers of biostatistical analysis even when—or *especially* when—it is carried out with sound methods and utmost integrity. These types of dangers begin at the beginning, with the collection, sorting, classification, and initial description of data. The purpose of this final chapter is to lay bare the nature of such dangers during the earliest stages of research and to detail their consequences for biostatistical analysis more generally.

Ironically, it is only at this point, having reached the end, that we can make sense of the beginning. For it is only after the reader has a general grasp of the various biostatistical tools and techniques—along with mathematical probability—that we apply to data that she or he can better appreciate the nature of those data. This then provides the fuller significance of the willful suspension of disbelief that is required of both novices and experienced practitioners when engaged in biostatistical analysis.

To begin, we find with uncanny consistency a basic distinction drawn between descriptive and inferential statistics across all manner of introductory biostatistics textbooks. This division follows, in part, from a separate set of rules and operations attached to each that serve contrasting purposes. For descriptive statistics there are two general purposes behind these rules and operations. First, they allow us to transform a qualitative thing into a type of thing that is appropriate for quantitative measurement. These rules and operations provide the means for recasting idiosyncratic and holistic qualities into generalizable and discrete properties. The qualitatively singular thing (the particular) is thereby erased, or at least set back into the shadows.

Second, descriptive rules and operations allow us to assure that the quantitative values that measure the general and discrete properties of one (particular) thing are commensurate with those values that measure the general and discrete properties of another (particular) thing. The rules and operations thus establish universal standards of measure for all things quantitative, such that any *distinguishing* qualitative attributes of an individual thing disappear into the unity of generalized things.

One thing with certain properties is understood *vis-à-vis* some other thing with certain properties via the application of universal units of measure. For instance, one quantitative thing can be described as longer/shorter, older/younger, heavier/lighter than another quantitative thing. Each thing thereby relates to another thing via some common third measure, as discussed in Chapter 4.

After descriptive statistics have induced the reader's participation in this exercise, aided by her or his willful suspension of disbelief, inferential statistics enter a side door and impose *their* rules and operations. These advance two further purposes. First, they allow us

DOI: 10.4324/9781003316985-10

to generalize from a sample statistic to a population parameter, such as a mean or proportion. This is obviously a pragmatic move that allows us to derive insights about populations based on a sample, saving both time and resources. The operative logic for this simple yet essential generalization resides in elements of mathematical probability discussed in Chapter 9. Configurations #1 and #6 are examples.

A second purpose behind these rules and operations of inferential statistics is to generalize from the results of a particular study to persons in the general population base on the protocols of the study. This is a specific extension of the general logic of the first purpose. It also expresses the logic behind isolating and measuring the impact of certain attributes or exposures on a given outcome (or dependent) variable. Configurations #2, #3, #4, #7, and #9 are examples of this.

Thus, descriptive and inferential statistics can be distinguished by their separate sets of rules and operations, and this is how they are understood in virtually all textbooks. Furthermore, it is assumed that the first set of rules and operations (descriptive statistics) must *logically precede* the second set (inferential statistics). Hence, even the order of methodological procedures distinguishes between the two sets.

Yet, it is also the case that we engage in the first set of rules and operations already presuming the second set—that is, in order to make the second set possible. In this sense, it is the second set (inferential statistics) that must *conceptually precede* the first set (descriptive statistics). On the one hand, each presents a unique sequence of steps. Thus, the two are separate and distinct. On the other hand, each presumes (and validates) the other. Thus, the two are conjoined and interdependent. Descriptive and inferential statistics thus seem a rather odd pair.

This pair that, at one and the same time stand in union and apart, are able to do so precisely via their intersecting, generative-conceptual roles in constituting the subject matter of health and medicine for biostatistical investigation. The principal role of descriptive statistics is to establish the predicates for the mathematical-conceptual premises distinguishing this unique subject matter. At issue here is the nature of those phenomena comprising health and medicine—and the social world more generally—that allows it to be rendered quantifiable.

The role of inferential statistics is to provide the tools and techniques for working with this quantified subject matter, based on these mathematical-conceptual premises. But these (inferential) biostatistical tools and techniques do not deviate fundamentally from those statistical tools and techniques applied more generally to other subject matter. Hence, the truly transformative work falls to descriptive statistics that allow for this radical reconstruction.

Most previous chapters have focused on inferential statistics. We have saved the "beginning" (descriptive statistics) for the end because it would otherwise be more difficult to grasp the significance and fundamental purpose of descriptive statistics. To repeat an earlier analogy, to grasp the meaning of a doorknob we must first study the house. We thus turn now to descriptive statistics—a dizzying assortment of doorknobs, windows, kitchen sinks, and more.

Our discussion has two parts. First, we turn to the discovery, collection, and classification of phenomena across the natural and social worlds as a means to bring order to a chaotic world. For this, we consider the four classifications of variables (continuous, dichotomous, ordinal, and categorical) and how these organize and guide our discovery of data.

Second, we attend the birth of data via the transformation of (subjective) descriptive observations into (objective) quantitative measures. For this, we explore sorting and measures of central tendency (the mean, median, mode) and variability (the range, variance, and standard deviation). The common theme uniting parts 1 and 2 is the role of descriptive statistics in bringing order out of chaos via the quantification of (formally) qualitative things.

Part I: Classifications of variables and our initial discovery of data

By the time of their formalization and broad adoption across health and medicine in the 1950s, quantitative methods across the natural sciences already enjoyed a significant head start. For this reason, applications of statistical analysis to the natural world provided a model for the development of biostatistical analysis and major efforts took hold to reconstitute the subject matter of health and medicine (and its analysis) within the mold of the natural world.

This "rediscovery" of health and medicine began with the development of new techniques and rationale for collecting and classifying its subject matter. Central to such efforts was a refinement of the units of measurement associated with four classifications of variables—continuous, dichotomous, ordinal, and categorical—and a reappraisal of how we discover data. We consider each of these in turn.

Classifications of variables (continuous, dichotomous, ordinal, categorical)

We saw in Chapter 3 how sampling brings order out of chaos by imposing patterns and groupings among (and relationships between) the things comprising our world. We now consider how reducing all things to the units of measure associated with four mutually exclusive classifications of variables—continuous, dichotomous, ordinal, and categorical—brings order out of chaos by further interposing a world passively populated by things with a world of things that we actively constitute.

Continuous variables do not fall from the sky and dichotomous variables are not fished from the seas. Instead, we come upon a world of random things and we appropriate these things (and thus the world they inhabit) by assigning to each thing a set of conceptual premises that make that thing what it is and allow us to distinguish one kind of thing from another kind.

After examining this world of things more closely, we "discover" that each thing possesses certain qualities and that these qualities can be further divided into properties that are either qualitative or quantitative. The quantitative properties can be represented by either continuous, dichotomous, ordinal, or categorical units of measure. In this way, each kind of thing can be investigated in a manner consistent with the nature of its properties.

Note that a categorical variable here refers to a qualitative property that is treated as a quantity that permits counting and indicates, for instance, how many or how few. For example, we can determine how many persons in a sample have the (qualitative) property of red hair.

Importantly, the language that we use to describe the process of moving between world, things, properties, and variables can be both confusing and deceiving. This follows, in part, from the incompleteness of most explanations of these four classifications of "variables" themselves and, consequently, a general failure to account for the conceptual implications attached to each.

To begin, let's think a bit more about the concept of a variable in relation to these four classifications. One of the major challenges of biostatistical analysis—especially for those less enamored with mathematics—is the use of computational symbols (such as Σ or μ) as abbreviations for complex notions that might otherwise take up several pages of exposition. However, the use of technical language (such as "dichotomous variable") can be equally mystifying and often short circuits comprehension in a similar manner. Indeed, the term dichotomous variable is a rather queer construction.

We have an adjective (dichotomous) modifying another adjective (variable). This is as nonsensical as "brave hungry." By convention, we treat "variable" as a noun. For example, we write, "A dichotomous variable is binary." Again, grammatically, this is as absurd as writing, "Brave hungry is slow." Plainly, treating "variable" as a noun is a convenient dodge to skirt some underlying confusion in the language, or in the concept. Let us look behind this dodge.

While grammar should not be the final arbiter, it can often help to more fully train our minds on what lies beneath the use of certain technical language. The present case of the missing noun is especially perplexing when there are perfectly apt alternatives to this slap-dash, double-adjective fix. Dichotomous "thing" or "phenomenon" may not roll off the tongue, but these seem closer to our true meaning than dichotomous variable. (Though we shall see that neither "thing" nor "phenomenon" are quite right either.)

In fact, the term dichotomous variable is an abbreviation. As a fully formed concept, this would read:

> The *property* of a thing (or phenomenon) that can vary in value and whose form aligns with dichotomous measurement.

It is the property of a thing that varies and not the thing itself. This property thus expresses that thing's conceptual form—such as continuous or categorical—and is what most immediately distinguishes one kind of thing from another kind of thing.

The term "dichotomous property" thus associates a specific type of measure with the (quantitative) property of a particular thing. Meanwhile, "dichotomous variable" conjures an abstraction detached from any actual thing. "Dichotomous property," in fact, retains— at least as a possibility—the qualitative and conceptual roots of a quantitative thing. (As we will see, each quantitative property was first a quality, as is the case for all quantitative properties.)

The use of "dichotomous variable" pushes us toward quantitative and mathematical modeling, while obscuring a thing's qualitative roots. Therefore, beneath these contrasting terms are opposing conceptual interpretations of the thing itself, as well as a glimpse into the implicit role of biostatistical analysis in bringing order to chaos.

The gravitational drift of biostatistical analysis toward mathematical modeling over conceptual investigation is dauntless—and in many ways laudable. It is certainly not our aim to minimize the importance of modeling. Our purpose is merely to make explicit that which is implicit—and generally unstated—within biostatistical analysis regarding its conceptual understanding (and the consequences thereof). It would otherwise be difficult to make sense of the need for our willful suspension of disbelief, as a provisional move to investigate certain aspects of health and medicine.

Thus, nurturing an appreciation for conceptual investigation at the expense of mathematical modeling would be foolhardy. However, the common default mode for biostatistical analysis—mathematical modeling at the expense of conceptual investigation—is no less myopic.

Let us start closer to the beginning. Our world is comprised of things and phenomena. Each thing (or phenomenon) possesses properties. These can be qualitative or quantitative. We appropriate things found in our world by classifying and cataloguing each of these based on its properties. For example, the properties of a rock include its color, its weight, and its shape. Though these properties belong to the rock, they may also belong to other things. These other things that share certain properties can, therefore, be grouped alongside the rock within a common classification defined by those common properties.

Given this understanding of the world, a thing is what we say it is. It existed before we *discovered* it. That is true. After discovery, however, we determine that thing's place and role in *our* world and we do so largely by identifying (and/or assigning) certain properties. Indeed, before we can even count things, we must sort things by their properties. These qualitative and quantitative properties are thus among the earliest building blocks for how we bring order to chaos.

In this mix of things and their properties, we soon land upon the notion of "variable" which seems much like a property, though not exactly. Ordinarily, a property modifies a thing. However, a variable modifies the property of a thing. Moreover, it does this by designating quantitative measures. If we say the rock is heavy, then "heavy" is a property of the rock. Heavy modifies rock. If we say the rock is nine kilos, then "nine kilos" is a property of heaviness. Nine kilos modifies heavy. Heavy thus falls away as a qualitative property—a subjective impression—and is replaced by an objective measure of the (quantitative) weight of a thing.

This progression from "heavy" to "nine kilos" follows, in part, from the fact that the rock—as an object—can be described with both qualitative and quantitative properties. However, it is initially distinguished by its *qualitative* properties. These properties differentiate it from other physical objects—trees or cars or balloons. It differs in shape from a tree. It differs in substance from a balloon. These qualitative properties are descriptive and can be expressed via language and/or visual imagery. Indeed, when we discover a new thing we first describe this in qualitative terms, either with the aid of new language (or imagery) that we create or by way of analogy to familiar things.

Of course, a rock is a physical object. It has a size, shape, and weight that can be easily measured via quantitative instruments that allow it to be neatly classified among other rocks. In this way, a rock is exemplary of how the natural sciences appropriate things in our world first via their qualitative properties before then assigning their quantitative properties—and the dimensions of those quantitative properties. This process is captured by our initial language when finding a rock. We say that it "feels" heavy or it "seems" heavy. This is soon followed by someone asking, "How heavy is it?"

Our dilemma is that the basic conceptual form of a rock, and other simple physical objects, have come to serve as prototypes for how we appropriate other things via the assignment of categorical properties and the movement from qualitative properties to quantitative properties. The universal attribution of quantitative properties to all things thus began on a large scale in the natural world before traveling to the social world, whereupon our four classifications of variables—continuous, dichotomous, ordinal, and categorical—were further refined. How we understand a rock within the natural world thus came to determine how we understand things across the social world. Let us return to the world of health and medicine to see how this works.

To begin, consider how certain areas of health and medicine in our society occupy a higher status and prioritization than others. For instance, physical health is prioritized above mental health; clinical medicine above public health; medical specializations above general practices; treating body parts (or functional systems) above holistic care; health as optimal functionality above health as quality of life; and high-tech, end-of-life interventions above low-tech, interpersonal, palliative care.

In each case, this reflects a preference for a mode of care (or a conceptual framework) with outcomes that are more in tune with quantitative (and presumptively objective) criteria rather than those outcomes requiring more qualitative, holistic, and subjective interpretation. This follows, in part, from importing how we investigate a rock into the world of health and medicine and how we investigate the health of a patient, or the health of a population.

Many factors contribute to this situation, including (quite lucrative) nonprofit healthcare systems, the insurance industry, and the nature of biomedical training. For example, one major influence is the dominance of allopathic medical doctors in shaping the broader field of health and medicine and the constrained conceptual mindset that they absorb from the medical sciences. Equally problematic is the sycophantic attitude of non-medical doctors within health and medicine toward MDs—or at least toward their heroic status within the field. For their contributions as healers this may be justified. As researchers and as conceptual thinkers, however, the training of allopathic medical doctors is, at best, parochial and incomplete.

This then is the (ordinarily missing) back story regarding the origins of the continuous, dichotomous, ordinal, and categorical classifications for variables as doctrinaire features of biostatistical analysis. On the one hand, they perpetuate a general confusion about the conceptual content of health and medicine. On the other hand, they represent the victory of a narrow band of quantitative properties for analyzing important phenomena across health and medicine, further explaining our need for the willful suspension of disbelief.

Let us then take another run at our world of things, properties, and variables. We now understand that the move from these three elements to our four classifications (continuous, dichotomous, ordinal, and categorical) results from explicit choices that commit our investigation to certain conceptual premises about the nature of health and medicine. These choices thus compel us to describe the subject matter of health and medicine in a certain way and toward a certain end.

The point here is not whether the choices are right or wrong. The only point is that the choices could have been otherwise. If they had been, we would today have a very different (or a much broader) representation of that same subject matter. In this sense, biostatistical analysis—like any singular tool of investigation—operates like a beam of light that reveals some things in stunning detail, while leaving other things hidden in the shadows.

For purposes of illustration (and persistent obsession) we will continue our focus on the resting heart rate as our property of interest. Importantly, it will be recalled that our initial research interest in Chapter 1 was cardiovascular health. More precisely, our interest was the impact of long-distance running on cardiovascular health. Yet more broadly, our original concern was simply the impact of exercise on health. The evolution from the impact of exercise on health to the impact of long-distance running on cardiovascular health to the impact of long-distance running on resting heart rates follows from the explicit choices of researchers. These choices similarly instruct our work with the four classifications of variables available to us.

All of these choices were fundamentally conceptual choices that aided in determining the nature of the thing (health) under investigation. From this, we see the increasingly narrow scope that comes to define health so as to better fit the mathematical premises of our biostatistical analysis. These were not choices based on the thing itself. There was no extensive review of the concept of health and its full galaxy of qualitative and quantitative properties. These choices were based, first, on a decidedly quantitative understanding of health and, second, on a selection of those properties most suitable for biostatistical analysis and the types of variables at hand. The qualitative origins of our subject (health) were soon extinguished.

Here then we have our familiar four classifications of variables—that is, the four "variable properties" of a resting heart rate.

We choose continuous variables when our phenomena of interest can be measured in (infinitely divisible) metric units. For example, we might wish to determine the impact of caffeine on the mean resting heart rate of high-school long-distance runners.

We choose dichotomous variables when our phenomena of interest can be measured in binary units. For example, we might wish to determine the impact of caffeine on the proportion of high-school long-distance runners with a resting heart rate above 83 bpm.

We choose ordinal variables when our phenomena of interest include nominal units with some rank order. For example, we might wish to determine the distribution of high-school long-distance runners across four rank-order levels of resting heart rates—low, moderate, elevated, and very high.

We choose categorical variables when our phenomena of interest include nominal units without rank. For example, we might wish to determine the number of high-school long-distance runners with a resting heart rate above 83 bpm based on a runner's blood type (A, B, O).

Upon further scrutiny, there is then a perplexing matter that one hates to even bring up. However faithfully we work within the grammatically challenged conceptual premises of quantitative analysis, there are troubling inconsistencies among these four classifications of "variables" that still arise. To begin, it requires little effort from the reader to realize that both dichotomous and ordinal variables operate as types (or subtypes) of categorical variables. Indeed, we have touched on this in previous chapters.

A dichotomous variable refers to the propriety of some thing (perhaps a cancer patient) that distinguishes between *categorical* binary options based on the presence or absence of some outcome (perhaps remission or non-remission). An ordinal variable refers to the variable property of some thing (perhaps caffeine consumers) that distinguishes between multiple *categories* that reflect a rank order of an outcome, such as low, moderate, and high consumption levels.

Consequently, the analysis of both dichotomous and ordinal data begins with, and is built upon, whole numbers with which we count the number of items in one category or another. With dichotomous variables, we might apply the risk ratio to assess the distribution of persons across two categories, resulting in a proportion. With ordinal variables, we might apply the chi-square goodness-of-fit test to assess the distribution of persons across three or more categories, resulting in percentages. The principle is the same. We are comparing the number of items in different (nominal) categories.

Hence, conceptually—and by the logic of biostatistical analysis itself—there are actually only two types of "variables," categorical (with two subtypes) and continuous. Given this, we soon discover that, in fact, categorical and continuous are merely synonyms for "qualitative" and "quantitative." Indeed, measures of "presence/absence" and "rank order" return us to the earliest primeval moments of investigation when our hunter-gatherer colleagues chose their cave based on "bats or no bats." Or when they carefully lined up their rocks from smallest to clobberest for hunting.

That said, it is important to keep in mind more generally that, while all categorical variables provide a form of qualitative evidence, not all qualitative evidence takes the form of categorical variables. For example, ethnographic observations or transcripts from in-depth interviews are actually more typical forms of qualitative evidence.

Thus, we all experience the world first via such qualitative properties. Indeed, our continuing efforts to bring these qualitative properties to heel within the *civilized* rules of quantitative order and decorum only result in a confusion of language and concepts that repeatedly lands us back at our beginnings. Thus, for all its mathematical complexity, an equally fundamental source of confusion for students of introductory biostatistical analysis is this underlying conceptual misunderstanding.

This may all be true. But even if so, it does not alter any of the operational rules for our nine configurations, nor does it weaken the findings that follow from our, at worst, "qualified" (no pun intended) mathematical premises. However, a further item remains. It will be recalled that alongside our four classifications of variables we had four "scales" of measurement that we also encountered some time back. But if our *four* classifications of variables are actually *two* (continuous and categorical), how is it that these can require four scales (nominal, ordinal, interval, and ratio)?

After all, even if we sort out this sordid stew of continuous, dichotomous, ordinal, and categorical variables there remains a separate, yet parallel, track on which biostatistical analysis simultaneously operates a second set of measures associated with another batch of "variables." This is bizarre, if for no other reason than basic consistency.

In Chapter 2, we illustrated applications of these scales—nominal, ordinal, interval, and ratio—based on the work of coach Dragutin Demitrijevíc, including the Demitrijevíc Self-Esteem Inventory. Our primary purpose then was to faithfully parrot how this madness was deployed in the course of biostatistical analysis. Now let us peer somewhat more closely into this intriguing use of two sets of accounting ledgers.

We just reviewed the first accounting ledger. This ledger alerts us to an ascribed conceptual form—continuous, dichotomous, ordinal, and categorical. These are held out as the four classifications of variables available to us. We have seen that a continuous or dichotomous "variable" is better understood as: The property of a thing that can vary in value and whose form permits continuous or dichotomous measurement.

We arrived here by first asking, "What kind of thing is this?" We thereby discovered that one thing can be distinguished from another thing via its properties, both qualitative and quantitative. Moreover, we have seen that these four classifications of variables can be, more precisely, reduced to two classifications, continuous and categorical, which, in fact, correspond with quantitative and qualitative properties.

Let us now bring in the second accounting ledger. This ledger claims to indicate the type of unit of measurement that is appropriate for each conceptual form. These are presented to us as four scales of measurement. The concept of a "unit of measurement" is itself very familiar to us. We know that we use meters to measure length, decibels to measure sound, kilos to measure weight, and cubic meters to measure a volume of gas. Meters, decibels, kilos, and cubic meters are all units of measurement and each pertains to a distinct type of thing. No one mistakenly provides the distance between Amman and Beirut in decibels.

But what is a "scale" of measurement? Moreover, if it is so fundamental—after all, these four scales are applied today, in one form or another, universally across biostatistical analysis—how is it that this scale did not even exist before the mid-20th century? At times, it helps to return to the original protagonist ginning up a good hullabaloo. In this case, we have one Stanley Stevens, director of the Psycho-Acoustic Laboratory at Harvard University. The year was 1946.

Fresh from animated discussions with his colleagues over the measure of "human sensation," director Stevens set off to solve this riddle. It should surprise no one that the source of contention leading to our present-day scales of measurement was how to adapt a type of thing—with arguably one foot in the social world and one foot in the natural world—for forms of measurements that originated in the natural world. Stevens' own understanding of the concept of "scales of measurement" was thus: "[M]easurement exists in a variety of forms and scales of measurement fit within certain classes. These classes are determined both by the empirical operations invoked in the process of 'measuring' and by the formal (mathematical) properties of the scales" (Stevens, 1946:677).[1]

This does not initially advance matters beyond replacing "scales" with "classes." However, reference to the "formal (mathematical) properties of the scales" moves the needle a bit. On the one hand, we can view these four scales as applications of formal mathematical rules. On the other hand, these rules apply to specific conceptual forms. This better explains the need for two ledgers.

The first ledger (four classifications of variables) is the transformation of a general thing into a type of thing with certain quantitative properties. The second ledger (four scales) takes over *only after* the first transformation and merely formalizes and universalizes the operational rules that we apply to such classifications of things, based on formal mathematical rules. Thus, by the 1950s, the four scales of measurement served both to reify (and carry forward) the conceptual premises wrapped in the four classifications of variables and to legitimize this new consensus via the respected rigor of mathematics.

A scale, however, was not actually a property of the thing itself. So hold on to your hat now. Technically, a scale of measurement (such as interval or ratio) is a property of the property of a property of a thing. For example, a ratio scale is a property of nine kilos. Nine kilos is a property of heaviness. Heaviness is a property of a thing (a rock). Hence, the propensity for confusion.

Furthermore, this "property" (the ratio scale) is nothing more than a set of mathematical rules. Thus, it is the actual instrument possessing universal units of measure (such as a yard stick) that does not itself alter when measuring different rocks. However, nine kilos is a specific quantity. A specific quantity—such as a measure of heaviness—is, of course, likely to alter with each rock that one measures. In this sense, the scale (or instrument) itself is not a *variable* property. It acts as a universal and unchanging measuring rod by which other properties—lengths, sounds, speeds—vary. This is why scales of measurement are associated with abstract mathematical rules, not empirical things, that is, the properties of the properties of the properties of a thing.

The scales of measurement that we associate with categorical, dichotomous, and ordinal properties—and that vary by quantity—are, respectively, the nominal, nominal, and ordinal scales. This makes even more clear that dichotomous and ordinal variables (or properties) are actually subtypes of categorical variables (or properties)! The ratio scale of measurement then pertains to continuous variables (or properties) that vary by quantity. This leaves us that most mysterious creature of all, the interval scale of measurement.

There is no direct correlate with this scale among our four classifications of variables. The interval scale has two features. The intervals along the scale are all of equal distance and there is no zero point. Thus, we can compare the difference between two absolute values. For example, the distance between 36 and 46 is equal to the distance between 110 and 120. But we cannot determine the ratio between two values. For instance, on a ratio scale, a 20-kg rock is 5 kg more than a 15-kg rock *and* a 20-kg rock weighs 33% more than a 15-kg rock.

Likewise, on an interval scale, we can determine that one room that is 20 degrees Celsius is 10 degrees more than a second room that is 10 degrees Celsius. However, we cannot determine the ratio between these two rooms, and thus we cannot claim that the first room is 50% warmer than the second room.

We can only calculate the ratio between two values on a scale that has a true zero point. The Celsius scale arbitrarily sets zero to the freezing point of water. The Kelvin scale is a true ratio scale because zero is set to the absolute absence of thermal energy. The interval scale is, therefore, reserved for those measures that, but for having no zero point, would utilize a continuous scale. For all intents and purposes it is a subtype of the continuous scale. But don't take my word for it. Here is the original source. "With the interval scale we come to a form that is 'quantitative' in the ordinary sense of the word. Almost all the usual statistical measures are applicable here, unless they are the kinds that imply a knowledge of a 'true' zero point" (Stevens, 1946:679).[2]

It is most telling that phenomena requiring the interval scale are almost exclusively human creations. It is difficult to find phenomena in the natural world, whose measurement lacks a true zero point. Even the popular example of temperature is merely a matter of convenience for human beings for whom the extremes of the Kelvin scale prove impractical. Zero on the Kelvin scale, for instance, leaves us at a nippy −459.67 Fahrenheit.

Hence, interval scales nearly always result from a continuing effort on the part of social and behavioral scientists to contrive quantitative measures for what are arguably qualitative phenomena, such as measures of intelligence, depression, physical pain, autism, not to mention a gymnast's floor routine or two people's romantic compatibility. Thus, in addition to their intended applications, these interval scales are also apt measures of our relentless search for objective and quantifiable measures of all aspects of the human condition.

Therefore, to engage with biostatistical analysis we must resolve ourselves to work with four classifications of variable properties—those susceptible to either continuous, dichotomous, ordinal, or categorical units of measure. This does not originate from the nature of things in the world of health and medicine. It is merely that this is the most widely agreed-upon lens available to us for such purposes. Indeed, with this lens we have made world-changing medical discoveries. When relied upon in isolation, however, this lens offers only a partial understanding of the broader subject matter across health and medicine.

Hence, the same tool that brings order out of chaos for some aspects of our world, buries other aspects in obscurity. All this explains the ubiquitous transformation of the (initially) qualitative properties of phenomena across health and medicine into things principally identified by quantitative properties outfitted as continuous, dichotomous, ordinal, and categorical variables.

These then are the necessary conceptual premises that precede (and permit) the application of biostatistical analysis. Indeed, it is telling that the natural sciences provide no language for turning quantitative things into qualitative things. We can quantify things or make things quantifiable. But we are reduced to gibberish when trying to "qualitatify" things or make things "qualitatable."

Part 2: Sorting, central tendency, and variability—the origins of data and our transformation of qualitative things

Our four classifications of variables and how these guide our discovery of data thus help bring a degree of order to our chaotic world of things. The next step in this process is a most remarkable reconstruction of data across three sets of operations. These are sorting-by-frequency, measures of central tendency, and measures of variability. Biostatistical analysis would be all but unthinkable without these. The mathematical rules for these operations are elementary. However, as we shall see, this simplicity belies a number of other-worldly consequences.

For instance, after a sample enters these operations, a remarkable transformation takes hold and each member of the original sample suddenly finds its individual self-expression only in unison with the other members, *through* its integration with the whole. In this sense, a sample takes on the form of a collective, insofar as each individual's identity is folded into an oddly contrived communal totality. Individual self-expression thus finds itself supplanted by collective expression via various quantitative measures, such as a mean or proportion.

But we must not get ahead of the story. Let us begin with a basic rendition of these three operations. To illustrate each, we will work from a single data set of resting heart rates gathered by coach Yukio Mishima for 40 long-distance runners at League of the Divine

Table 10.1 Unsorted resting heart rates for a random sample of long-distance runners at League of the Divine Wind High School in Jimmu County, n = 40

76	95	73	78	41	71	67	70
80	105	75	77	74	66	74	67
80	72	78	78	71	71	66	67
88	75	74	101	61	41	69	69
76	88	76	78	75	69	75	70

Table 10.2 Resting heart rates for a random sample of long-distance runners at League of the Divine Wind High School in Jimmu County, sorted by size, n = 40

41	67	69	71	74	76	78	88
41	67	70	72	75	76	78	88
61	67	70	73	75	76	78	95
66	69	71	74	75	77	80	101
66	69	71	74	75	78	80	105

Wind High School in Jimmu County. Coach Mishima began by thanking all 40 runners for their supreme sacrifice, the spirit of which he promised would live on forever. He then gathered the data we find in Table 10.1.

Sorting-by-frequency

Sorting-by-frequency is uncomplicated. The task is to combine same with same. The goal is to organize our (unsorted) sample into numerous groups that are simple aggregations of similar things. We have already rehearsed, in Chapter 3, the conceptual complexity behind the sampling that precedes sorting-by-frequency and that determines the properties by which we identify sameness and difference. Here we begin by first ordering the unsorted data collected by coach Mishima from slowest to fastest resting heart rate. See Table 10.2.

This first sort-by-frequency for heart rates is both crucial and cataclysmic. In the original unsorted data set (Table 10.1), the value in a given cell represents a specific individual who entered the sample with her or his full identify and by her or his own agency. All that ends after our first sort. It is true that, if needed, we could probably trace the value in the third cell of the first column (61) back to a specific individual in the sample. This is true for any non-repeating value at this stage. However, after this first sort, the chief property that we assign to any value in any cell is its ordinal position—its relation (slower or faster) to values in other cells.

This signals the first submergence of the individuality attached to each value—that is, the memory of the person to whom this property (a resting heart rate) was originally attached. That said, there are limitations for working with Table 10.2, insofar as we still have 40 individual cells with data to analyze. Our next step, therefore, is to aggregate our cells.

This step in sorting-by-frequency requires a simple count, after combining same with same. This is illustrated in Table 10.3. The left column contains the rank order for each resting heart rate that coach Mishima recorded. The middle column provides the actual value of the resting heart rates. The right column indicates the number of persons (cases) with a resting heart rate at each value. For example, four persons have a resting heart rate of 75 bpm and two persons have a resting heart rate of 88 bpm.

We have 19 unique values between 41 and 105 in Table 10.3. Seven of these 19 values fit only one person in the sample, while 12 fit two to four persons. Thus, 33 of the 40 persons

Table 10.3 Aggregation of cases, n = 40

Rank order	Resting heart rate	Number of cases
1	41	✿✿
2	61	✿
3	66	✿✿
4	67	✿✿✿
5	69	✿✿✿
6	70	✿✿
7	71	✿✿✿
8	72	✿
9	73	✿
10	74	✿✿✿
11	75	✿✿✿✿
12	76	✿✿✿
13	77	✿
14	78	✿✿✿✿
15	80	✿✿
16	88	✿✿
17	95	✿
18	101	✿
19	105	✿

Table 10.4 Cases aggregated by group intervals, n = 40

Interval group	Number of cases
≤ 65	✿✿✿ (3)
66–70	✿✿✿✿✿✿✿✿✿✿ (10)
71–75	✿✿✿✿✿✿✿✿✿✿✿✿ (12)
76–80	✿✿✿✿✿✿✿✿✿✿ (10)
≥ 81	✿✿✿✿✿ (5)

in the sample have been absorbed into a group of at least two values. There are some values at the extremes, but otherwise the values in Table 10.3 are mostly clustered between 67 and 78. To better represent this, our next sort forms groups comprising five-unit intervals.

With Table 10.4, we have removed any final remnants of individuality. Each value that was originally attached to a particular person in our sample (Table 10.1) is now lost within one of five interval groups, as simple aggregations. Indeed, because individual values are no longer available, even one's membership in a particular group cannot be cleanly discerned.

For example, if a person is in the second interval group, her or his value may be 66, 67, 68, 69, or 70. However, with regard to the 10 cases in the second column for this second interval group (66–70), it is impossible to know which case represents which value. They may all be 67. None may be 67. We have form but no substance. The particular disappears.

Our 40 individuals have thus been reconstituted as five interval groups with a certain number of cases. All we know about these groups is (1) the number of (disembodied) cases that each contains, (2) the range of the values for the cases in each group, and (3) the relation of each group to the other groups by size (more, fewer, or the same number of cases) and by speed of resting heart rates (slower or faster).

This suggests two salient points. First, the steps taken thus far for sorting-by-frequency are indifferent to either the source of the data or the purpose for which it has been collected. This is not the case for sampling or for classifying the properties of a thing so that it can be quantified. It is the purpose behind the creation of a sample that determines the criteria for inclusion or exclusion and, thus, its membership. It is the role of a thing within a study that determines which quantitative properties of that thing we wish to measure and, thereby, which classification—continuous, dichotomous, ordinal, or categorical—we choose.

When reaching the stage of sorting-by-frequency, however, neither the source of our data nor its purpose continue to play any role. Our only mandate is to relentlessly combine same with same.

With regard to sorting-by-frequency the data collected by coach Mishima, the criterion for sameness is pure quantitative value, shorn of any individualizing properties. This results in the "universalization" of the individual "self-sacrifices" by those who enter aggregations via the erasure of their personal identities. For instance, the attachment of any of the 40 persons in the sample to her or his resting heart rate is now removed. In this sense, their individual identity has been *sacrificed*. Each individual resting heart rate is replaced by a set of group resting heart rates that is determined by the range of interval values.

Thus, this range of interval values for resting heart rates is the same—it is "universal"— for all members of an interval group. This is regardless of an individual member's actual resting heart rate. This then allows each individual to fall within a five-unit interval.

A second point is that the stage of sorting-by-frequency, overall, adds nothing new. It merely rearranges our data. The five interval groups in Table 10.4 are simple aggregations that combine the values from different cells as individual things. These groups are formed by basic counting. There is no interaction among the things being counted (or summed) in each group and their combination does not lead to any new type of thing—just a new arrangement of our original 40 things into five aggregations.

Thus, sorting-by-frequency thus introduces no new findings or insights. Its only purpose is to prepare our data for the next operation, or stage of transformation. First, we universalize our data by stripping them of any individual identity and, second, we prepare these data for the next stage.

In this sense, sorting-by-frequency has much in common with the work of a slaughter-house. First, the butchers reduce each hog to its various (discrete) parts. Then, these parts are mixed and matched so that the identity of any original hog is lost in the mounds of aggregated ribs, hoofs, entrails, etc. However, the work of the slaughterhouse is merely to prepare these hogs (much like the members of our sample) for the next stage.

For the hog, this next stage is the rendering plant. For the members of our sample, the next stage is collectivization. This entails subjecting our sample to two further sets of operations—measures of central tendency and measures of variability. Let us see then how an aggregation becomes a collective.

Central tendency (mean, median, and mode)

A principal outcome of sorting-by-frequency is the initial vanishing of the individual. Measures of central tendency—the mean, median, and mode—then build on this igno-minious start. Central tendency refers to the degree to which the values in a data set con-gregate around a single value, the mean. As seen in Chapter 9, one feature of the standard normal distribution is that data form a symmetrical, bell-shaped curve and the values of the mean, median, and mode closely align.

Thus, a good gauge of central tendency is the degree of similarity between the mean, median, and mode. Importantly, no single statistic allows for comparison of central tendency across multiple data sets. For example, if one sample has a mean of 4.25 and another sample has a mean of 4 million this alone tells us nothing about how the central tendencies of the two samples compare.

We begin with the median and the mode. In fact, each of these is functionally just a further application of sorting-by-frequency. Both rely on a frequency distribution from the smallest to largest value that stops short of aggregation, as in Table 10.2. The median is the midpoint value in a frequency distribution. For the data collected by coach Mishima, the median value for resting heart rates is 74. The sample contains an even number of 40 values.' We, therefore, pull the 20th and 21st values and find the average of these for our midpoint value. In this case, the value of each is 74, so this is the median. One half of all values lie below 74 and one half above.

Hence, the median occupies an ordinal position *vis-à-vis* all other values. It is derived not from the actual values in the cells ("75" or "66") but from the ordinal position of each *vis-à-vis* the others, first to fortieth. Two "groups" form out of this. The first group contains those values that occupy the 1st through 20th ordinal positions. The second group contains those values occupying the 21st through 40th positions. With regard to the median, the members of each of these groups form an undifferentiated aggregation via a count (or summation) of the members. This is similar to the manner by which the members within a five-unit interval are aggregated in our example above for sorting-by-frequency in Table 10.4.

The mode is the single most common value among the 40 cells in our sample. In our data, the values of 75 and 78 both occur four times, which is more often than any other value. Given that two values account for the highest number of occurrences, this frequency distribution has two modes. It is "bimodal." This indicates that the central tendency is likely to not be as strong as the frequency distribution of another data set with a single mode. Given that both of these modes (75, 78) fall to the right of the median (74), we know that our data are skewed toward larger values.

This notion of "skewed" data refers to the degree of alignment between the mean, median, and mode. The greater the misalignment, the greater the skew. When the mean sits to the right of the median, we say that it is skewed right. When the mean sits to the left of the median, it is skewed left. In addition, when data are skewed, this indicates that one side of a frequency distribution curve will have a longer "tail" than the other. We have a "positive" skew if the longer tail is to the right and a "negative" skew if the tail is to the left. See Figures 10.1 and 10.2.

The mean is a simple calculation of the arithmetic mean. For our data, the mean resting heart rate for all 40 runners is 73.93. Hence, our mean (73.93) and our median (74) are closed aligned. Our bimodal values suggest some degree of spread. The central tendency is otherwise fairly strong (or symmetrical). See Figure 10.3.

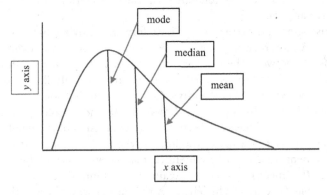

Figure 10.1 Right-skewed or (positive-skewed) distribution curve

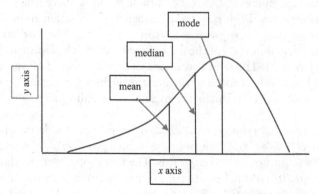

Figure 10.2 Left-skewed or (negative-skewed) distribution curve

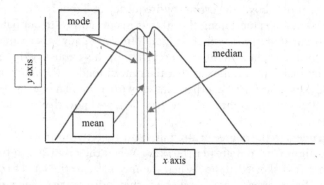

Figure 10.3 Bimodal distribution curve for coach Mishima's date, n = 40

Let us now more closely examine this notion of the mean, as an aspect of central tendency. We saw how sorting-by-frequency converts data (values) derived from the members of a sample—thus initially linked to specific individuals—into groups organized by interval ranges. For example, the group in row two of Table 10.4 contains 10 anonymous cases and each of these has a value between 66 and 70. We do not know who these 10 cases are or the actual value of any one of these. This individual-level information is replaced by a single, general descriptor—the values between 66 and 70—that pertains to everyone in this interval group. These aggregations thus convey generality via the elimination of any individual bearing her or his particular data.

The mean takes over at this point and carries the process forward, moving us from an aggregation to a formal whole. An aggregation is a simple summation of parts. A formal whole is formed from relationships between the parts and the whole. To produce a mean we return to the original unsorted data. With this step, all individuality suddenly floods back in. Each of the 40 values is re-attached to a specific individual in the sample, along with (at least potentially) her or his full identity. In this way, all members of the sample are *active contributors* to (or parts of) our end result—the sample mean as an expression of the whole.

Soon we learn, however, that it is this measure of the formal whole (the mean) that is all that matters in this new arrangement. In the same moment that an individual contributes to the creation of the formal whole (the mean), that person again vanishes into that whole. The mean is a value representing a *singular* entity. This entity is the formal whole to which all individuals have contributed. This is thus a formal whole—whose expression is the mean—for which each member of the sample has sacrificed her or his individual identity.

This formal whole, expressed as a mean, is now the sole voice speaking on behalf of each individual. The mean, a fundamental measure within biostatistical analysis, saves the individual from extinction within an aggregation, only to prepare that same individual for life as a hollow and mute instrument of our formal whole.

We participate in the creation of a formal whole each time we calculate a mean. Imagine we have the resting heart rates from a sample of 10 runners. We first display our data.

$$77, 81, 66, 65, 55, 73, 75, 66, 88, 82$$

This first step provides an array of data that retains a strong sense of individuality. The members of our sample stand out—quite visibly—from their aggregation within this array. At this point, each value represents a person from our random sample, with a certain height, weight, age, etc. Thus, if we wished to do so, we could associate each value with the fuller details of each individual.

Next, we sum these values.

$$77 + 81 + 66 + 65 + 55 + 73 + 75 + 66 + 88 + 82 = 728$$

This second step results in a simple aggregation that submerges individuality. No individual person remains. The value of 728 itself is an empty abstraction. It is the summation of all resting heart rates for persons in the sample. It is the mathematical equivalent of a mound of hog's hoofs in the slaughterhouse and thus holds no particular meaning.

We now divide this aggregation by the number of persons in the sample. From this, our mean appears.

$$\frac{728}{10} = 72.8$$

In this third step our individuals return briefly in oblique form, as part of a number count (10) in the denominator. Each individual's expression and purpose are, thereafter, supplied by (and through) the formal whole. The mean (72.8) is everything. The individual—our only empirical link to the original data—and her or his value is nothing, outside its contribution to the mean ... to the formal whole.

Thus, the hog-rendering plant now comes more fully into view. The plant's operation is analogous to the formal whole that takes in the members of a sample and churns out statistical measures, such as the mean. The plant's goal is to take in as many hogs as possible, at the fastest possible clip, and to turn out a great bevy of delectable treats. Each treat contains parts from perhaps hundreds of hogs, though each part is untraceable to any particular hog.

The byproducts of biostatistical analysis are, likewise, only possible through the contributions of everyone. But each individual's contribution is absorbed within the anonymity of the formal whole. Unnerving as this may be, more is yet to come as we turn now to measures of variability.

Measures of variability (full range, interquartile range, variance, and standard deviation)

To frame our discussion of measures of variability, we are guided by two considerations. First, there is the peculiar construction of the variance and standard deviation—and the mean as well. After first introducing each of these via their elementary mathematical operations, we discover upon closer inspection that the conceptual grounding for these supposedly empirical measures feels eerily metaphysical.

A second consideration is the nature of the thing whose mean or standard deviation we calculate. Continuing with our resting heart rate, we now know that this "thing" is a fragment of a person that originates from the steps taken prior to determining a mean, variance, or standard deviation. Without sampling, sorting, and the classification of variables there is no thing for which a mean, variance, or standard deviation can be calculated. Hence, these are as much *measures* of these prior steps, and their reductive rationale, as they are measures of the fragmented products of these steps and rationale.

Given these origins, it can be very easy to confuse a mean or a standard deviation for a measure of the world as we find it, rather than a measure of the world as we construct it. Indeed, the facility of the calculations for a mean or standard deviation and the robustness of their statistical consequences only further obscure the crucial (and consequential) role of these prior steps. Thus, the conceptual integrity of the mean or standard deviation follows not from the logic of the mathematical operations behind these two measures, but from the intentional construction (and quantification) of the thing under study.

All this signals two familiar themes guiding our entire introduction to biostatistics. These are an ongoing effort to bring order out of chaos via the tools and techniques of biostatistical analysis and, relatedly, the grave conceptual distortions that result when treating qualitative things as quantitative things. Let us then continue.

There are two forms of variability. The first form is absolute variability. This includes the full range and the interquartile range. These are absolute measures because each represents the actual difference (via subtraction) between two values based on their original units of measure.

The second form is relative variability. This includes the variance and the standard deviation. These are relative measures because they take the form of ratios. The variance is a ratio whose numerator is the sum of the squared differences between individual values and the sample mean. The denominator is the sample size. The standard deviation is the square root of the variance. We begin with absolute variability.

Like the median and mode, the full range and the interquartile range are values pertaining to a frequency distribution that precedes aggregation. The full range is a measure of the distance between the smallest and largest values in a data set. In our sample collected by coach Mishima the range is: $105 - 41 = 64$. As a measure of variability this can be tricky to interpret. Consider two data sets, each with 10 values.

Data set 1: (2, 2, 2, 2, 2, 2, 2, 2, 2, 20)

Data set 2: (2, 4, 6, 8, 10, 12, 14, 16, 18, 20)

The full range of each data set is 18. (For both, this is: $20 - 2 = 18$.) But the values in data set 1—with one exception—have literally zero variation, while no two values in data set 2 are the same. Notice further that for determining the full range, two values (the lowest and highest) are all that matter. Each of these relates to the other, but to no other values in the data set. We simply sort our data from lowest to highest, leaving us the two values of interest at either end. Consequently, the full range itself—18 for both data set 1 and data set 2—is meaningless *vis-à-vis* any individual value in either of these data sets.

Lastly, unlike the variance or the standard deviation, the full range itself plays no significant role in deriving any other statistic. We have managed, for instance, to traverse the entirety of this book—including consideration of our 10 configurations—without once needing to calculate a full range.

Thus, the ordinary role of the full range is to flag outliers and to compare two like things. For example, in two high schools that are reasonably alike it might be informative to know that the full range for resting heart rates among long-distance runners is 35 in the first school and 11 in the second school. This could indicate greater variability within the data at the first school, or the presence of outliers.

The interquartile range is slightly more informative than the full range. For this range, we again sort our data from lowest to highest. We then identify the point below which 25% of all items lie. This is Q1, or the first quartile. The point below which 50% of all items lie is Q2 and the point below which 75% of all items lie is Q3. The distance between Q1 and Q3 is the interquartile range. This contains 50% of the data, excluding the top 25% and the bottom 25%.

Thus, the interquartile range removes outliers and provides a more targeted view of variation in the mid-range, where half of the data reside. In our example, the interquartile range for data set 1 is: $2 - 2 = 0$. For data set 2, this is: $16 - 6 = 10$. Therefore, the interquartile range provides a more accurate sense of the variation in these two data sets than the full range, which is 18 for each.

The second form of variability, relative variability, centers on the degree to which the distance between the individual data values in a sample and the mean of that sample differ across all the values in a data set. We notice immediately that it is each *individual* data value *vis-à-vis* the formal whole (the mean) that matters most for relative variability.

For the mean, what most matters is the ratio between an aggregation of values (such as the sum of Mishima's 40 resting heart rates) and an aggregation of cases (such as the sum of 40 persons in Mishima's sample). As we will see, this return of individual data values to calculate relative variability is what lies behind the resurrection of the 40 original individuals *vis-à-vis* a most disturbing relation of (living) self to (entombed) self.

We proceed then. Again, we have two measures of relative variability, the variance and the standard deviation. We calculated the variance in Chapter 7, when introducing correlation coefficients. We have made use of the standard deviation throughout many chapters. But we have had little to say about the conceptual premises of either until now.

The principal distinction between the variance and the standard deviation is that the latter returns the values of a given measure to the original scale of the units in which the data were reported. For example, from the data in Table 9.5 in Chapter 9, we found that the standard deviation for student weights was 10.4, with a mean student weight of 77 kg. The variance for these student weights was 108.2. The standard deviation (10.4) thus provides a more intuitive interpretation of the relative variability of these student weights than the variance (108.2).

Because the standard deviation is only one step removed from the variance, we will focus here on the standard deviation with a bonus reveal of the variance along the way. (Again, the standard deviation is simply the square root of the variance. Hence, the one extra step.) As detailed below, both the mean and the standard deviation result from procedures that methodically snuff out the individual. However, each does so through slightly different maneuvers.

Let us demonstrate the mean and standard deviation for the same two data sets from above. Notice in working through this demonstration how few complications the technical steps present and, by contrast, how convoluted the conceptual implications of these technical steps can seem at times. This underscores the reasoning behind our insistence to present the technical and conceptual aspects of biostatistical analysis side-by-side throughout this text. Often the simplest procedures harbor considerable complexity.

Data set 1: (2, 2, 2, 2, 2, 2, 2, 2, 2, 20)

Data set 2: (2, 4, 6, 8, 10, 12, 14, 16, 18, 20)

First, we find the mean for each data set.

Data set 1: $\dfrac{2+2+2+2+2+2+2+2+2+20}{10} = 3.8$

Data set 2: $\dfrac{2+4+6+8+10+12+14+16+18+20}{10} = 11.0$

For each data set, the individual values again vanish within the formal whole. It is true that the values expressed by each formal whole differ, a mean of 3.8 versus a mean of 11.0. Therefore, given that each data set has 10 persons, we can surmise that at least one of the individual values concealed within each mean must also differ. However, any number of combinations of values could account for each mean. In this way, individual values are concealed within each mean. After this first step, we thus again have our formal whole, which results from the self-sacrifice of individuality.

For our second step, we subtract the mean from each individual value and square the result.

$$\text{Data set 1:} (2-3.8)^2 + (2-3.8)^2 + (2-3.8)^2 + (2-3.8)^2 + (2-3.8)^2 + (2-3.8)^2$$
$$+ (2-3.8)^2 + (2-3.8)^2 + (2-3.8)^2 + (20-3.8)^2$$

$$\text{Data set 2:} (2-11)^2 + (4-11)^2 + (6-11)^2 + (8-11)^2 + (10-11)^2 + (12-11)^2$$
$$+ (14-11)^2 + (16-11)^2 + (18-11)^2 + (20-11)^2$$

This second step proves most chilling, indeed. After burying each body within the formal whole in the first step, each individual now rejoins the living, again expressing her or his individual value. This presents a macabre scene, wherein each person is placed in relation to the disembodied remnant of her- or himself as a fragment—such as a resting heart rate—within the formal whole.

Let us examine things from the standpoint of the person who contributed one of the values of "2" in data set 1 and the person contributing the value of "4" in data set 2. Each appears in the second step as either $(2-3.8)^2$ for data set 1 or $(4-11)^2$ for data set 2.

Note that "2" stands in relation to the mean of "3.8." But "3.8" is itself an expression of the whole (the mean) into which the lifeless body of "2" has been consigned. In this manner, we have a relation of living self and former self. The resurrected individual ("2") confronts its remnant (as a fragment of "3.8") to create a new zombie form ("3.24"). We derive 3.24 from: $(2-3.8)^2 = 3.24$. This zombie form then joins with the other zombies from data set 1 to form a new type of whole in the third step below. In similar harrowing fashion, "4" is placed in relation to "11" in data set 2. Surely now the sights and smells of the hog-rendering plant grow in strength.

The products of the second step are the 10 new values (or zombies) in each data set that now appear in the third step. These 10 values result from the relation of each (resurrected) individual to the formal whole (the mean). This is thus a relation of parts to whole in which the individual is both a part—as "2" in data set 1 or "4" in data set 2—while also being an integral fragment within the formal whole.

Both this part and this formal whole are then re-absorbed into a new type of whole in the third step, a collective whole. As seen below, a collective whole is formed via the reciprocally conditioning relationships between part and part and between part and whole.

In this third step we find the mean for these (zombie) values.

$$\text{Data set 1: } \frac{3.24 + 3.24 + 3.24 + 3.24 + 3.24 + 3.24 + 3.24 + 3.24 + 3.24 + 262.44}{10 - 1} = 32.4$$

$$\text{Data set 2: } \frac{81 + 49 + 25 + 9 + 1 + 1 + 9 + 25 + 49 + 81}{10 - 1} = 36.7$$

This third step returns each individual to the shadows via the formation of a new collective whole. This is also known as the variance. (Note that we prefer $n - 1$ for calculating the variance of a small data set.) Certainly, "2" and "4," whoever they were, are no more. This collective whole is no longer comprised of the discrete values of the 10 individuals from each of the original data sets. Rather, this collective whole is now comprised of 10 values (such as "3.24" in data set 1) that are expressions of the relationships between the original values of those 10 individuals and the formal whole (the mean)—which had at least still contained the husks for the original values.

Now preserved within our collective whole (or variance) we have, at best, a composite measure of the relationships between each original value and the formal whole. Remarkably, insofar as that formal whole contained the original value of each person in the sample, we can say that this collective whole is built up from relations that reflect the self back into itself. In this manner, astonishingly, we preserve the individual by erasing the individual.

In fact, we find that it is this relationship of the individual to her or his fragment within the formal whole that provides the foundational grounds for relative variability within *ANY* data set! Furthermore, this serves as a fundamental source of variability across biostatistical analysis. The individual returns to obscurity. After first erasing her or his identity (including her or his quantitative value) within the formal whole (the mean), our collective whole (the variance) now redefines the individual within a transformed relation of part to whole—a part that *is* the individual and a whole that *itself contains the individual*.

This relationship of part to whole is quantified as the distance of each part (that is, a fragment of each member of the sample) from the mean. Again, a mean that is an expression of all members absorbed into the formal whole. These distances, in combination, become a measure of the unity of the whole. The individual thus returns as the basis for a perverse relation between part (an individual) and whole (a fragment of that same individual), to form a collective whole.

Crucially, all this follows *only* from an empirical description of what happens (conceptually) when we apply the elementary mathematical operations for creating a mean, variance, and standard deviation to a sample comprised of human subjects. No *external* metaphysical conjecture is required.

The work of the rendering plant is thus complete. It is now only a matter of shipping the hogs' final products to market to be packaged, labeled, and sold. For us, the equivalent final step is to find the square root of the collective whole, or variance. This yields the standard deviation.

$$\text{Data set 1: } \sqrt{32.4} = 5.69$$

$$\text{Data set 2: } \sqrt{36.7} = 6.06$$

This step restores our units of measure to their original scale after we had squared each of the values in the second step above to remove any negative values. These values (5.69 and 6.06) are the products "shipped out" to become elements of biostatistical analysis.

Notice incidentally the proximity of the standard deviations for these two data sets—5.69 and 6.06. We find this, notwithstanding the nearly complete homogeneity of data set 1 and the significant variability in data set 2. This demonstrates the influence of a single outlier, the value of "20" in data set 1. If we remove the value of "20" from each data set, the standard deviation for data set 1 becomes 0.0 and for data set 2 it becomes 5.48.

Concluding thoughts

In this chapter we have described how the tools and techniques of descriptive statistics help us to transform qualitative things into quantitative things in a bid to bring order out of chaos. This introduces considerable distortions of the content of health and medicine after examining their conceptual premises, leaving now even the empirical nature of biostatistical analysis uncertain.

Notice, for instance, that the empirical world we first encounter is concrete, disordered, and qualitative, while the collective whole that results from the interaction of statistical analysis with that world is abstract, orderly, and quantitative. Ultimately, what we create via descriptive statistics appears to conform more closely to what we envision than what we see.

The peculiar conceptual consequences for the mean, variance, and standard deviation made visible here reflect, in part, the efforts of biostatistical analysis to reconstitute the qualitative subject matter of health and medicine as quantitative (and pseudo-concrete) things ready for investigation. In the ordinary course of introducing biostatistics, instructors review the elementary operations of the mean, the variance, and the standard deviation without pausing to consider the conceptual premises of these operations that allow for such radical reconstitution of the subject matter.

Yet, given their fundamental roles at the earliest stages of biostatistical investigation, these conceptual premises that result in aggregates, formal wholes, and collective wholes necessarily have consequences that carry forward throughout all of biostatistical analysis regarding how we construct the subject matter that we study. This, of course, is no less true for the conceptual premises of our four classifications of variables—continuous, dichotomous, ordinal, and categorical—and for sorting.

This is why we purposely end our introduction to biostatistical analysis back at the beginning, with descriptive statistics. These are the principal tools and techniques underwriting all of biostatistical analysis and, thereby, granting authority to all of their claims. It stands to reason that the troubling conceptual integrity (and dubious empirical methods) that they introduce should be matters of considerable apprehension for those conceiving of biostatistical analysis as a finished product, or an end-in-itself.

However, for those who view biostatistical analysis as a temporary and willful suspension of disbelief before returning to a more complete and holistic understanding of health and medicine, such "misrepresentations" of its content serve a vital though limited purpose. This is the viewpoint that we have tried to maintain and validate throughout the book.

It is true that the assorted tools and techniques of biostatistical analysis that we have reviewed throughout this book are designed to drive out idiosyncrasy, to decontextualize phenomena, and to undo holistic thinking and that this undermines our understanding of a subject matter that originates with human beings and historical societies and cultures. Nonetheless, properly understood and treated as a strategic and temporary departure from a fuller reality, this submission to the tendentious workings of biostatistical analysis is reasonably benign.

We began this book with the observation that most introductory biostatistics textbooks emphasize technical steps over conceptual understanding. For this reason, biostatistical tools and techniques receive great attention, while the underlying subject matter tends to be marginal and is included primarily to illustrate various technical steps. We thus argued, early on, that students tend to learn much more about the tools and techniques of biostatistical analysis than about the content of health and medicine from these textbooks.

Consequently, the bar we set for ourselves from the beginning was ambitious and clearcut. By the book's end, our goal was that a reader would learn as much about the conceptual nature of health and medicine as she or he would learn about the tools and techniques of biostatistical analysis. How well we did in this regard is for each student to determine.

Ultimately, our insistence upon grounding our conceptual understanding of health and medicine within a broader, holistic perspective makes it no less essential to learn from the reductionist perspective of biostatistical analysis and to then fold this back into a larger holistic framework. Biostatistical analysis is *not adjunctive* to a holistic perspective. Indeed, it is as integral to a whole and complete understanding of health and medicine as global capitalism, religion, or poetry. To wit,

> As when a Cancer in the Body feeds,
> And gradual Death from Limb to Limb proceeds;
> So does the Chilness to each vital Part
> Spread by degrees, and creeps into her Heart;
> 'Till hard'ning ev'ry where, and speechless grown,
> She sits unmov'd, and freezes to a Stone.
> But still her envious Hue and sullen Mien
> Are in the Sedentary Figure seen.
>
> (*Ovid's Metamorphoses in Fifteen Books.*
> Translated by the Most Eminent
> Hands, 1717)

Notes

1 Stanley Smith Stevens (1946) "On the Theory of Scales of Measurement." *Science.* 103(2684): 677–680.
2 Ibid.

Appendix

Table A.1 Standard normal distribution and probabilities of z-values

z-Score	Proportion in body (larger part)	Proportion in tail (smaller part)	Proportion between mean and z
0.00	.5000	.5000	.0000
0.01	.5040	.4960	.0040
0.02	.5080	.4920	.0080
0.03	.5120	.4880	.0120
0.04	.5160	.4840	.0160
0.05	.5199	.4801	.0199
0.06	.5239	.4761	.0239
0.07	.5279	.4721	.0279
0.08	.5319	.4681	.0319
0.09	.5359	.4641	.0359
0.10	.5398	.4602	.0398
0.11	.5438	.4562	.0438
0.12	.5478	.4522	.0478
0.13	.5517	.4483	.0517
0.14	.5557	.4443	.0557
0.15	.5596	.4404	.0596
0.16	.5636	.4364	.0636
0.17	.5675	.4325	.0675
0.18	.5714	.4286	.0714
0.19	.5753	.4247	.0753
0.20	.5793	.4207	.0793
0.21	.5832	.4168	.0832
0.22	.5871	.4129	.0871
0.23	.5910	.4090	.0910
0.24	.5948	.4052	.0948
0.25	.5987	.4013	.0987
0.26	.6026	.3974	.1026
0.27	.6064	.3936	.1064
0.28	.6103	.3897	.1103
0.29	.6141	.3859	.1141
0.30	.6179	.3821	.1179
0.31	.6217	.3783	.1217
0.32	.6255	.3745	.1255
0.33	.6293	.3707	.1293
0.34	.6331	.3669	.1331
0.35	.6368	.3632	.1368
0.36	.6406	.3594	.1406
0.37	.6443	.3557	.1443
0.38	.6480	.3520	.1480
0.39	.6517	.3483	.1517
0.40	.6554	.3446	.1554

Table A.1 Cont.

z-Score	Proportion in body (larger part)	Proportion in tail (smaller part)	Proportion between mean and z
0.41	.6591	.3409	.1591
0.42	.6628	.3372	.1628
0.43	.6664	.3336	.1664
0.44	.6700	.3300	.1700
0.45	.6736	.3264	.1736
0.46	.6772	.3228	.1772
0.47	.6808	.3192	.1808
0.48	.6844	.3156	.1844
0.49	.6879	.3121	.1879
0.50	.6915	.3085	.1915
0.51	.6950	.3050	.1950
0.52	.6985	.3015	.1985
0.53	.7019	.2981	.2019
0.54	.7054	.2946	.2054
0.55	.7088	.2912	.2088
0.56	.7123	.2877	.2123
0.57	.7157	.2843	.2157
0.58	.7190	.2810	.2190
0.59	.7224	.2776	.2224
0.60	.7257	.2743	.2257
0.61	.7291	.2709	.2291
0.62	.7324	.2676	.2324
0.63	.7357	.2643	.2357
0.64	.7389	.2611	.2389
0.65	.7422	.2578	.2422
0.66	.7454	.2546	.2454
0.67	.7486	.2514	.2486
0.68	.7517	.2483	.2517
0.69	.7549	.2451	.2549
0.70	.7580	.2420	.2580
0.71	.7611	.2389	.2611
0.72	.7642	.2358	.2642
0.73	.7673	.2327	.2673
0.74	.7704	.2296	.2704
0.75	.7734	.2266	.2734
0.76	.7764	.2236	.2764
0.77	.7794	.2206	.2794
0.78	.7823	.2177	.2823
0.79	.7852	.2148	.2852
0.80	.7881	.2119	.2881
0.81	.7910	.2090	.2910
0.82	.7939	.2061	.2939
0.83	.7967	.2033	.2967
0.84	.7995	.2005	.2995
0.85	.8023	.1977	.3023
0.86	.8051	.1949	.3051
0.87	.8078	.1922	.3078
0.88	.8106	.1894	.3106
0.89	.8133	.1867	.3133
0.90	.8159	.1841	.3159
0.91	.8186	.1814	.3186
0.92	.8212	.1788	.3212
0.93	.8238	.1762	.3238
0.94	.8264	.1736	.3264

(continued)

Table A.1 Cont.

z-Score	Proportion in body (larger part)	Proportion in tail (smaller part)	Proportion between mean and z
0.95	.8289	.1711	.3289
0.96	.8315	.1685	.3315
0.97	.8340	.1660	.3340
0.98	.8365	.1635	.3365
0.99	.8389	.1611	.3389
1.00	.8413	.1587	.3413
1.01	.8438	.1562	.3438
1.02	.8461	.1539	.3461
1.03	.8485	.1515	.3485
1.04	.8508	.1492	.3508
1.05	.8531	.1469	.3531
1.06	.8554	.1446	.3554
1.07	.8577	.1423	.3577
1.08	.8599	.1401	.3599
1.09	.8621	.1379	.3621
1.10	.8643	.1357	.3643
1.11	.8665	.1335	.3665
1.12	.8686	.1314	.3686
1.13	.8708	.1292	.3708
1.14	.8729	.1271	.3729
1.15	.8749	.1251	.3749
1.16	.8770	.1230	.3770
1.17	.8790	.1210	.3790
1.18	.8810	.1190	.3810
1.19	.8830	.1170	.3830
1.20	.8849	.1151	.3849
1.21	.8869	.1131	.3869
1.22	.8888	.1112	.3888
1.23	.8907	.1093	.3907
1.24	.8925	.1075	.3925
1.25	.8944	.1056	.3944
1.26	.8962	.1038	.3962
1.27	.8980	.1020	.3980
1.28	.8997	.1003	.3997
1.29	.9015	.0985	.4015
1.30	.9032	.0968	.4032
1.31	.9049	.0951	.4049
1.32	.9066	.0934	.4066
1.33	.9082	.0918	.4082
1.34	.9099	.0901	.4099
1.35	.9115	.0885	.4115
1.36	.9131	.0869	.4131
1.37	.9147	.0853	.4147
1.38	.9162	.0838	.4162
1.39	.9177	.0823	.4177
1.40	.9192	.0808	.4192
1.41	.9207	.0793	.4207
1.42	.9222	.0778	.4222
1.43	.9236	.0764	.4236
1.44	.9251	.0749	.4251
1.45	.9265	.0735	.4265
1.46	.9279	.0721	.4279
1.47	.9292	.0708	.4292
1.48	.9306	.0694	.4306
1.49	.9319	.0681	.4319

Table A.1 Cont.

z-Score	Proportion in body (larger part)	Proportion in tail (smaller part)	Proportion between mean and z
1.50	.9332	.0668	.4332
1.51	.9345	.0655	.4345
1.52	.9357	.0643	.4357
1.53	.9370	.0630	.4370
1.54	.9382	.0618	.4382
1.55	.9394	.0606	.4394
1.56	.9406	.0594	.4406
1.57	.9418	.0582	.4418
1.58	.9429	.0571	.4429
1.59	.9441	.0559	.4441
1.60	.9452	.0548	.4452
1.61	.9463	.0537	.4463
1.62	.9474	.0526	.4474
1.63	.9484	.0516	.4484
1.64	.9495	.0505	.4495
1.65	.9505	.0495	.4505
1.66	.9515	.0485	.4515
1.67	.9525	.0475	.4525
1.68	.9535	.0465	.4535
1.69	.9545	.0455	.4545
1.70	.9554	.0446	.4554
1.71	.9564	.0436	.4564
1.72	.9573	.0427	.4573
1.73	.9582	.0418	.4582
1.74	.9591	.0409	.4591
1.75	.9599	.0401	.4599
1.76	.9608	.0392	.4608
1.77	.9616	.0384	.4616
1.78	.9625	.0375	.4625
1.79	.9633	.0367	.4633
1.80	.9641	.0359	.4641
1.81	.9649	.0351	.4649
1.82	.9656	.0344	.4656
1.83	.9664	.0336	.4664
1.84	.9671	.0329	.4671
1.85	.9678	.0322	.4678
1.86	.9686	.0314	.4686
1.87	.9693	.0307	.4693
1.88	.9699	.0301	.4699
1.89	.9706	.0294	.4706
1.90	.9713	.0287	.4713
1.91	.9719	.0281	.4719
1.92	.9726	.0274	.4726
1.93	.9732	.0268	.4732
1.94	.9738	.0262	.4738
1.95	.9744	.0256	.4744
1.96	.9750	.0250	.4750
1.97	.9756	.0244	.4756
1.98	.9761	.0239	.4761
1.99	.9767	.0233	.4767
2.00	.9772	.0228	.4772
2.01	.9778	.0222	.4778
2.02	.9783	.0217	.4783
2.03	.9788	.0212	.4788

(continued)

Table A.1 Cont.

z-Score	Proportion in body (larger part)	Proportion in tail (smaller part)	Proportion between mean and z
2.04	.9793	.0207	.4793
2.05	.9798	.0202	.4798
2.06	.9803	.0197	.4803
2.07	.9808	.0192	.4808
2.08	.9812	.0188	.4812
2.09	.9817	.0183	.4817
2.10	.9821	.0179	.4821
2.11	.9826	.0174	.4826
2.12	.9830	.0170	.4830
2.13	.9834	.0166	.4834
2.14	.9838	.0162	.4838
2.15	.9842	.0158	.4842
2.16	.9846	.0154	.4846
2.17	.9850	.0150	.4850
2.18	.9854	.0146	.4854
2.19	.9857	.0143	.4857
2.20	.9861	.0139	.4861
2.21	.9864	.0136	.4864
2.22	.9868	.0132	.4868
2.23	.9871	.0129	.4871
2.24	.9875	.0125	.4875
2.25	.9878	.0122	.4878
2.26	.9881	.0119	.4881
2.27	.9884	.0116	.4884
2.28	.9887	.0113	.4887
2.29	.9890	.0110	.4890
2.30	.9893	.0107	.4893
2.31	.9896	.0104	.4896
2.32	.9898	.0102	.4898
2.33	.9901	.0099	.4901
2.34	.9904	.0096	.4904
2.35	.9906	.0094	.4906
2.36	.9909	.0091	.4909
2.37	.9911	.0089	.4911
2.38	.9913	.0087	.4913
2.39	.9916	.0084	.4916
2.40	.9918	.0082	.4918
2.41	.9920	.0080	.4920
2.42	.9922	.0078	.4922
2.43	.9925	.0075	.4925
2.44	.9927	.0073	.4927
2.45	.9929	.0071	.4929
2.46	.9931	.0069	.4931
2.47	.9932	.0068	.4932
2.48	.9934	.0066	.4934
2.49	.9936	.0064	.4936
2.50	.9938	.0062	.4938
2.51	.9940	.0060	.4940
2.52	.9941	.0059	.4941
2.53	.9943	.0057	.4943
2.54	.9945	.0055	.4945
2.55	.9946	.0054	.4946
2.56	.9948	.0052	.4948
2.57	.9949	.0051	.4949
2.58	.9951	.0049	.4951

Table A.1 Cont.

z-Score	Proportion in body (larger part)	Proportion in tail (smaller part)	Proportion between mean and z
2.59	.9952	.0048	.4952
2.60	.9953	.0047	.4953
2.61	.9955	.0045	.4955
2.62	.9956	.0044	.4956
2.63	.9957	.0043	.4957
2.64	.9959	.0041	.4959
2.65	.9960	.0040	.4960
2.66	.9961	.0039	.4961
2.67	.9962	.0038	.4962
2.68	.9963	.0037	.4963
2.69	.9964	.0036	.4964
2.70	.9965	.0035	.4965
2.71	.9966	.0034	.4966
2.72	.9967	.0033	.4967
2.73	.9968	.0032	.4968
2.74	.9969	.0031	.4969
2.75	.9970	.0030	.4970
2.76	.9971	.0029	.4971
2.77	.9972	.0028	.4972
2.78	.9973	.0027	.4973
2.79	.9974	.0026	.4974
2.80	.9974	.0026	.4974
2.81	.9975	.0025	.4975
2.82	.9976	.0024	.4976
2.83	.9977	.0023	.4977
2.84	.9977	.0023	.4977
2.85	.9978	.0022	.4978
2.86	.9979	.0021	.4979
2.87	.9979	.0021	.4979
2.88	.9980	.0020	.4980
2.89	.9981	.0019	.4981
2.90	.9981	.0019	.4981
2.91	.9982	.0018	.4982
2.92	.9982	.0018	.4982
2.93	.9983	.0017	.4983
2.94	.9984	.0016	.4984
2.95	.9984	.0016	.4984
2.96	.9985	.0015	.4985
2.97	.9985	.0015	.4985
2.98	.9986	.0014	.4986
2.99	.9986	.0014	.4986
3.00	.9987	.0013	.4987
3.01	.9987	.0013	.4987
3.02	.9987	.0013	.4987
3.03	.9988	.0012	.4988
3.04	.9988	.0012	.4988
3.05	.9989	.0011	.4989
3.06	.9989	.0011	.4989
3.07	.9989	.0011	.4989
3.08	.9990	.0010	.4990
3.09	.9990	.0010	.4990
3.10	.9990	.0010	.4990
3.11	.9991	.0009	.4991

Table A.2 t Distribution and critical values of *t*

Level of significance for one-tailed test

	0.10	0.05	0.025	0.01	0.005	0.0005

Level of significance for two-tailed test

df	0.20	0.10	0.05	0.02	0.01	0.001
1	3.08	6.31	12.71	31.82	63.66	636.62
2	1.89	2.92	4.30	6.97	9.93	31.60
3	1.64	2.35	3.18	4.54	5.84	12.94
4	1.53	2.13	2.78	3.75	4.60	8.61
5	1.48	2.02	2.57	3.37	4.03	6.86
6	1.44	1.94	2.45	3.14	3.71	5.96
7	1.42	1.90	2.37	3.00	3.50	5.41
8	1.40	1.86	2.31	2.90	3.36	5.04
9	1.38	1.83	2.26	2.82	3.25	4.78
10	1.37	1.81	2.23	2.76	3.17	4.59
11	1.36	1.80	2.20	2.72	3.11	4.44
12	1.36	1.78	2.18	2.68	3.06	4.32
13	1.35	1.77	2.16	2.65	3.01	4.22
14	1.35	1.76	2.15	2.62	2.98	4.14
15	1.34	1.75	2.13	2.60	2.95	4.07
16	1.34	1.75	2.12	2.58	2.92	4.02
17	1.33	1.74	2.11	2.57	2.90	3.97
18	1.33	1.73	2.10	2.55	2.88	3.92
19	1.33	1.73	2.09	2.54	2.86	3.88
20	1.33	1.73	2.09	2.53	2.85	3.85
21	1.32	1.72	2.08	2.52	2.83	3.82
22	1.32	1.72	2.07	2.51	2.82	3.79
23	1.32	1.71	2.07	2.50	2.81	3.77
24	1.32	1.71	2.06	2.49	2.80	3.75
25	1.32	1.71	2.06	2.49	2.79	3.73
26	1.32	1.71	2.06	2.48	2.78	3.71
27	1.31	1.70	2.05	2.47	2.77	3.69
28	1.31	1.70	2.05	2.47	2.76	3.67
29	1.31	1.70	2.05	2.46	2.76	3.66
30	1.31	1.70	2.04	2.46	2.75	3.65
40	1.30	1.68	2.02	2.42	2.70	3.55
60	1.30	1.67	2.00	2.39	2.66	3.46
120	1.29	1.66	1.98	2.36	2.62	3.37
∞	1.28	1.65	1.96	2.33	2.58	3.29

Table A.2 Cont.

Level of significance for one-tailed test

	.10	.05	.025	.01	.005	.0005

Level of significance for two-tailed test

df	.20	.10	.05	.02	.01	.001
1	3.078	6.314	12.706	31.821	63.657	636.619
2	1.886	2.920	4.303	6.965	9.925	31.598
3	1.638	2.353	3.182	4.541	5.841	12.941
4	1.533	2.132	2.776	3.747	4.604	8.610
5	1.476	2.015	2.571	3.365	4.032	6.859
6	1.440	1.943	2.447	3.143	3.707	5.959
7	1.415	1.895	2.365	2.998	3.499	5.405
8	1.397	1.860	2.306	2.896	3.355	5.041
9	1.383	1.833	2.262	2.821	3.250	4.781
10	1.372	1.812	2.228	2.764	3.169	4.587
11	1.363	1.796	2.201	2.718	3.106	4.437
12	1.356	1.782	2.179	2.681	3.055	4.318
13	1.350	1.771	2.160	2.650	3.012	4.221
14	1.345	1.761	2.145	2.624	2.977	4.140
15	1.341	1.753	2.131	2.602	2.947	4.073
16	1.337	1.746	2.120	2.583	2.921	4.015
17	1.333	1.740	2.110	2.567	2.898	3.965
18	1.330	1.734	2.101	2.552	2.878	3.922
19	1.328	1.729	2.093	2.539	2.861	3.883
20	1.325	1.725	2.086	2.528	2.845	3.850
21	1.323	1.721	2.080	2.518	2.831	3.819
22	1.321	1.717	2.074	2.508	2.819	3.792
23	1.319	1.714	2.069	2.500	2.807	3.767
24	1.318	1.711	2.064	2.492	2.797	3.745
25	1.316	1.708	2.060	2.485	2.787	3.725
26	1.315	1.706	2.056	2.479	2.779	3.707
27	1.314	1.703	2.052	2.473	2.771	3.690
28	1.313	1.701	2.048	2.467	2.763	3.674
29	1.311	1.699	2.045	2.462	2.756	3.659
30	1.310	1.697	2.042	2.457	2.750	3.646
40	1.303	1.684	2.021	2.423	2.704	3.551
60	1.296	1.671	2.000	2.390	2.660	3.460
120	1.289	1.658	1.980	2.358	2.617	3.373
∞	1.282	1.645	1.960	2.326	2.576	3.291

Source: R. A. Fisher and F. Yates (1974) Statistical Tables for Biological, Agricultural, and Medical Research (6th ed.). London: Longman Group. Reprinted with permission of Addison-Wesley Longman.

Table A.3 Chi-square distributions and critical values of chi-square

df	0.20	0.10	0.05	0.02	0.01	0.001
1	1.64	2.71	3.84	5.41	6.64	10.83
2	3.22	4.61	5.99	7.82	9.21	13.82
3	4.64	6.25	7.82	9.84	11.34	16.27
4	5.99	7.78	9.49	11.67	13.28	18.47
5	7.29	9.24	11.07	13.39	15.09	20.52
6	8.56	10.65	12.59	15.03	16.81	22.46
7	9.80	12.02	14.07	16.62	18.48	24.32
8	11.03	13.36	15.51	18.17	20.09	26.13
9	12.24	14.68	16.92	19.68	21.67	27.88
10	13.44	15.99	18.31	21.16	23.21	29.59
11	14.63	17.28	19.68	22.62	24.73	31.26
12	15.81	18.55	21.03	24.05	26.22	32.91
13	16.99	19.81	22.36	25.47	27.69	34.53
14	18.15	21.06	23.69	26.87	29.14	36.12
15	19.31	22.31	25.00	28.26	30.58	37.70
16	20.47	23.54	26.30	29.63	32.00	39.25
17	21.62	24.77	27.59	31.00	33.41	40.79
18	22.76	25.99	28.87	32.35	34.81	42.31
19	23.90	27.20	30.14	33.69	36.19	43.82
20	25.04	28.41	31.41	35.02	37.57	45.32
21	26.17	29.62	32.67	36.34	38.93	46.80
22	27.30	30.81	33.92	37.66	40.29	48.27
23	28.43	32.01	35.17	38.97	41.64	49.73
24	29.55	33.20	36.42	40.27	42.98	51.18
25	30.68	34.38	37.65	41.57	44.31	52.62
26	31.80	35.56	38.89	42.86	45.64	54.05
27	32.91	36.74	40.11	44.14	46.96	55.48
28	34.03	37.92	41.34	45.42	48.28	56.89
29	35.14	39.09	42.56	46.69	49.59	58.30
30	36.25	40.26	43.77	47.96	50.89	59.70

Table A.4 F distribution and critical values of F

$p = 0.05$

df2 ↓ / df1 →	1	2	3	4	5	6	8	12	24	∞
1	161.4	199.5	215.7	224.6	230.2	234.0	238.9	243.9	249.0	254.3
2	18.51	19.00	19.16	19.25	19.30	19.33	19.37	19.41	19.45	19.50
3	10.13	9.55	9.28	9.12	9.01	8.94	8.84	8.74	8.64	8.53
4	7.71	6.94	6.59	6.39	6.26	6.16	6.04	5.91	5.77	5.63
5	6.61	5.79	5.41	5.19	5.05	4.95	4.82	4.68	4.53	4.36
6	5.99	5.14	4.76	4.53	4.39	4.28	4.15	4.00	3.84	3.67
7	5.59	4.74	4.35	4.12	3.97	3.87	3.73	3.57	3.41	3.23
8	5.32	4.46	4.07	3.84	3.69	3.58	3.44	3.28	3.12	2.93
9	5.12	4.26	3.86	3.63	3.48	3.37	3.23	3.07	2.90	2.71
10	4.96	4.10	3.71	3.48	3.33	3.22	3.07	2.91	2.74	2.54
11	4.84	3.98	3.59	3.36	3.20	3.09	2.95	2.79	2.61	2.40

Table A.4 Cont.

p = 0.05

df1 →	1	2	3	4	5	6	8	12	24	∞
df2 ↓										
12	4.75	3.88	3.49	3.26	3.11	3.00	2.85	2.69	2.50	2.30
13	4.67	3.80	3.41	3.18	3.02	2.92	2.77	2.60	2.42	2.21
14	4.60	3.74	3.34	3.11	2.96	2.85	2.70	2.53	2.35	2.13
15	4.54	3.68	3.29	3.06	2.90	2.79	2.64	2.48	2.29	2.07
16	4.49	3.63	3.24	3.01	2.85	2.74	2.59	2.42	2.24	2.01
17	4.45	3.59	3.20	2.96	2.81	2.70	2.55	2.38	2.19	1.96
18	4.41	3.55	3.16	2.93	2.77	2.66	2.51	2.34	2.15	1.92
19	4.38	3.52	3.13	2.90	2.74	2.63	2.48	2.31	2.11	1.88
20	4.35	3.49	3.10	2.87	2.71	2.60	2.45	2.28	2.08	1.84
21	4.32	3.47	3.07	2.84	2.68	2.57	2.42	2.25	2.05	1.81
22	4.30	3.44	3.05	2.82	2.66	2.55	2.40	2.23	2.03	1.78
23	4.28	3.42	3.03	2.80	2.64	2.53	2.38	2.20	2.00	1.76
24	4.26	3.40	3.01	2.78	2.62	2.51	2.36	2.18	1.98	1.73
25	4.24	3.38	2.99	2.76	2.60	2.49	2.34	2.16	1.96	1.71
26	4.22	3.37	2.98	2.74	2.59	2.47	2.32	2.15	1.95	1.69
27	4.21	3.35	2.96	2.73	2.57	2.46	2.30	2.13	1.93	1.67
28	4.20	3.34	2.95	2.71	2.56	2.44	2.29	2.12	1.91	1.65
29	4.18	3.33	2.93	2.70	2.54	2.43	2.28	2.10	1.90	1.64
30	4.17	3.32	2.92	2.69	2.53	2.42	2.27	2.09	1.89	1.62
40	4.08	3.23	2.84	2.61	2.45	2.34	2.18	2.00	1.79	1.51
60	4.00	3.15	2.76	2.52	2.37	2.25	2.10	1.92	1.70	1.39
120	3.92	3.07	2.68	2.45	2.29	2.17	2.02	1.83	1.61	1.25

p = 0.01

df1 →	1	2	3	4	5	6	8	12	24	∞
df2 ↓										
1	4052	4999	5403	5625	5764	5859	5981	6106	6234	6366
2	98.49	99.01	99.17	99.25	99.30	99.33	99.36	99.42	99.46	99.50
3	34.12	30.81	29.46	28.71	28.24	27.91	27.49	27.05	26.60	26.12
4	21.20	18.00	16.69	15.98	15.52	15.21	14.80	14.37	13.93	13.46
5	16.26	13.27	12.06	11.39	10.97	10.67	10.27	9.89	9.47	9.02
6	13.74	10.92	9.78	9.15	8.75	8.47	8.10	7.72	7.31	6.88
7	12.25	9.55	8.45	7.85	7.46	7.19	6.84	6.47	6.07	5.65
8	11.26	8.65	7.59	7.01	6.63	6.37	6.03	5.67	5.28	4.86
9	10.56	8.02	6.99	6.42	6.06	5.80	5.47	5.11	4.73	4.31
10	10.04	7.56	6.55	5.99	5.64	5.39	5.06	4.71	4.33	3.91
11	9.65	7.20	6.22	5.67	5.32	5.07	4.74	4.40	4.02	3.60
12	9.33	6.93	5.95	5.41	5.06	4.82	4.50	4.16	3.78	3.36
13	9.07	6.70	5.74	5.20	4.86	4.62	4.30	3.96	3.59	3.16
14	8.86	6.51	5.56	5.03	4.69	4.46	4.14	3.80	3.43	3.00
15	8.68	3.36	5.42	4.89	4.56	4.32	4.00	3.67	3.29	2.87
16	8.53	6.23	5.29	4.77	4.44	4.20	3.89	3.55	3.18	2.75
17	8.40	6.11	5.18	4.67	4.34	4.10	3.79	3.45	3.08	2.65
18	8.28	6.01	5.09	4.58	4.25	4.01	3.71	3.37	3.00	2.57
19	8.18	5.93	5.01	4.50	4.17	3.94	3.63	3.30	2.92	2.49

(continued)

Table A.4 Cont.

p = 0.01

df 1 →	1	2	3	4	5	6	8	12	24	∞
df2 ↓										
20	8.10	5.85	4.94	4.43	4.10	3.87	3.56	3.23	2.86	2.42
21	8.02	5.78	4.87	4.37	4.04	3.81	3.51	3.17	2.80	2.36
22	7.94	5.72	4.82	4.31	3.99	3.76	3.45	3.12	2.75	2.31
23	7.88	5.66	4.76	4.23	3.94	3.71	3.41	3.07	2.70	2.26
24	7.82	5.61	4.72	4.22	3.90	3.67	3.36	3.03	2.66	2.21
25	7.77	5.57	4.68	4.18	3.86	3.63	3.32	2.99	2.62	2.17
26	7.72	5.53	4.64	4.14	3.82	3.59	3.29	2.96	2.58	2.13
27	7.68	5.49	4.60	4.11	3.78	3.56	3.26	2.93	2.55	2.10
28	7.64	5.45	4.57	4.07	3.75	3.53	3.23	2.90	2.52	2.06
29	7.60	5.42	4.54	4.04	3.73	3.50	3.20	2.87	2.49	2.03
30	7.56	5.39	4.51	4.02	3.70	3,47	3.17	2.84	2.47	2.01
40	7.31	5.18	4.31	3.83	3.51	3.29	2.99	2.66	2.29	1.80
60	7.08	4.98	4.13	3.65	3.34	3.12	2.82	2.50	2.12	1.60
120	6.85	4.79	3.95	3.48	3.17	2.96	2.66	2.34	1.95	1.38
∞	6.64	4.60	3.78	3.32	3.02	2.80	2.51	2.18	1.79	1.00

Table A.5 Standard normal distribution and z-values for percentiles

Percentile	z-Value
1st	−2.326
2.5th	−1.960
5th	−1.645
10th	−1.282
25th	−0.675
50th	0.0
75th	0.675
90th	1.282
95th	1.645
97.5th	1.960
99th	2.326

Table A.6 Standard normal distribution and z-values for confidence intervals

Confidence interval	z-Value
99.9%	3.291
99%	2.576
95%	1.960
90%	1.645
80%	1.282
75%	1.150
50%	0.674

Index

Printed in the United States
by Baker & Taylor Publisher Services